T0342453

Pediatric Audiologic Rehabilitation
From Infancy to Adolescence

Pediatric Audiologic Rehabilitation
From Infancy to Adolescence

Elizabeth M. Fitzpatrick, PhD, LSLS Cert. AVT
Associate Professor
Audiology and Speech-Language Program
Faculty of Health Sciences
University of Ottawa
Ottawa, Ontario, Canada

Suzanne P. Doucet, MEd, DipEd Deaf, LSLS Cert. AVT
Specialized Teacher and Coordinator for Continuing Education
Services for Students with Hearing Loss
Department of Education and Development of Early Childhood—New Brunswick
Moncton, New Brunswick, Canada

Thieme
New York · Stuttgart

Thieme Medical Publishers, Inc.
333 Seventh Ave.
New York, NY 10001

Acquisition Editor: Emily Ekle
Editorial Assistant: Elizabeth D'Ambrosio
Senior Vice President, Editorial, and E-Product Development: Cornelia Schulze
Production Editor: Kenneth L. Chumbley
International Production Director: Andreas Schabert
Vice President, Finance and Accounts: Sarah Vanderbilt
President: Brian D. Scanlan
Compositor: Prairie Papers Inc.
Printer: Sheridan Books

Library of Congress Cataloging-in-Publication Data
Fitzpatrick, Elizabeth M.
  Pediatric audiologic rehabilitation : from infancy to adolesence / Elizabeth M. Fitzpatrick, Suzanne P. Doucet.
    p. ; cm.
  Includes bibliographical references.
  ISBN 978-1-60406-695-1 (alk. paper)–ISBN 978-1-60406-696-8 (eISBN)
  I. Doucet, Suzanne P. II. Title.
  [DNLM: 1. Rehabilitation of Hearing Impaired. 2. Adolescent. 3. Child. 4. Infant. WV 271]
  617.80083–dc23

                                                                            2012036221

Important note: Medical knowledge is ever-changing. As new research and clinical experience broaden our knowledge, changes in treatment and drug therapy may be required. The authors and editors of the material herein have consulted sources believed to be reliable in their efforts to provide information that is complete and in accord with the standards accepted at the time of publication. However, in view of the possibility of human error by the authors, editors, or publisher of the work herein or changes in medical knowledge, neither the authors, editors, nor publisher, nor any other party who has been involved in the preparation of this work, warrants that the information contained herein is in every respect accurate or complete, and they are not responsible for any errors or omissions or for the results obtained from use of such information. Readers are encouraged to confirm the information contained herein with other sources. For example, readers are advised to check the product information sheet included in the package of each drug they plan to administer to be certain that the information contained in this publication is accurate and that changes have not been made in the recommended dose or in the contraindications for administration. This recommendation is of particular importance in connection with new or infrequently used drugs.

Some of the product names, patents, and registered designs referred to in this book are in fact registered trademarks or proprietary names even though specific reference to this fact is not always made in the text. Therefore, the appearance of a name without designation as proprietary is not to be construed as a representation by the publisher that it is in the public domain.

Printed in the United States of America

5 4 3 2 1

ISBN 978-1-60406-695-1
eISBN 978-1-60406-696-8

Contents

Preface

■ Authors' Perspectives

The "overwhelming" majority of children with hearing loss have the potential to develop listening and spoken language. Although we recognize that no single audiologic rehabilitation approach is appropriate for all children, new developments in technology and interventions permit the majority of children *access* to spoken language. This book focuses on rehabilitation for children with hearing loss whose parents have opted for a spoken language approach and inclusion with their family and peers with normal hearing.

A book provides an opportunity to take a topic like pediatric hearing loss and package the science and practical applications. Different authors absorb and present the array of information in their own personalized style. This book attempts to build on previous contributions to child hearing loss by taking a contemporary perspective on auditory rehabilitation from birth to adolescence (identification through the school years). In light of the rapid progress in hearing technology, the shift to identification of hearing loss in the first few months of life, and the interest and growth in research on spoken language outcomes, a new overview of the current world of pediatric audiologic rehabilitation is timely. Although practiced by many types of practitioners, and borrowing extensively from child language or speech-language pathology fields, as the title implies, we view auditory rehabilitation as "grounded" in audiology because hearing and hearing technology are essential to spoken language development.

This book is not intended as a comprehensive guide to rehabilitation and education of all children with hearing loss as our emphasis is on listening and spoken language, and therefore the book does not address alternative methods of developing communication. Lively debates about educational philosophies for children with hearing loss, best practices, and even appropriate terminology have reigned in our field for hundreds of years. It is our premise that the potential for age-appropriate spoken language has increased for all children, particularly those with severe to profound hearing loss. Where there is evidence, we do our utmost to present it, but we are cognizant that some of what we describe and propose related to intervention is lacking solid scientific evaluation. Where there is limited evidence, we draw on our clinical and educational experience to present our understanding of the best available information.

Expectations for developmental outcomes for children with hearing loss have greatly evolved in recent years given that most children in developed countries are early-identified and have access to hearing technology. As technology changes, the expected outcomes for children's listening and spoken language development have become a "moving target" (Geers, 2006). Numerous reviews in the last decade summarize evidence supporting the view that spoken language acquisition is achievable when optimal technology and learning conditions are in place (Dornan, Hickson, Murdoch, & Houston, 2008; Eriks-Brophy, 2004; Rhoades, 2006; Spencer & Marschark, 2010; Thoutenhoofd et al, 2005). However, it is well accepted that technology alone is not generally sufficient for most children with permanent hearing loss to develop competent spoken language. Rather, it is the combination of technology and the application of evidence-based intervention from multiple disciplines, including audiology, education, speech-language pathology, medicine and psychology, that is expected to generate the most promising results.

Audiologic rehabilitation is fundamental to successful participation in a typical classroom where the majority of today's children will be educated. As regular classrooms are natural listening and spoken language settings, it is important to develop listening skills from the earliest possible age. It is well recognized that the complexity of deafness and its impact on the child and family makes specialized guidance and support necessary. In this book, we underscore the importance of partnerships with parents and other professionals in facilitating listening and spoken language development from infancy through the learning years.

▨ Objectives of the Book

The objectives of *Pediatric Audiologic Rehabilitation* are simple—to present evidence-based information on hearing accessibility and on the clinical and educational management of children with hearing loss who are learning spoken language from infancy through adolescence. Much is known in pediatric hearing, much remains to be known. In this book, our goal was to bring together the best available evidence and to apply what we currently know and understand to practice. In this sense, this book provides not only theoretical knowledge but also a collection of practical strategies that practitioners can use to guide parents in developing their child's spoken language. This book was written to assemble in a single resource, up-to-date information for graduate students and practitioners in audiology, speech-language pathology, and education of the deaf and hard of hearing that covers the spectrum of auditory and spoken language development throughout childhood.

▨ Terminology

A plethora of terminology exists to describe individuals with hearing loss—deaf and hard of hearing, hearing-impaired, children with hearing loss, children with hearing disorders. We have adopted the term children with hearing loss. Similarly, the field of rehabilitation has evolved to include various professionals, each with expertise in common and different areas related to hearing loss, who in general complement each other in servicing children and their families. Professionals are known in different countries and regions under different titles (some regulated by their respective professional bodies) as audiologists, speech-language pathologists, teachers of the deaf and hard-of hearing, or the more generic forms of therapists, interventionists, and specialists. Given that practitioners work in clinical, community, and educational settings, we have opted to use the generic term clinician/teacher to refer to specialists in rehabilitation. Multiple terms are also used to describe intervention approaches for developing spoken language in children with hearing loss, some of the more common being auditory-oral, auditory-verbal, aural, oral, and cued speech approaches. Rather than focus on a specific philosophy or intervention method, we have chosen to place the emphasis in this book on creating/providing optimal learning environments through technology and parent-guided interventions to achieve the desired outcomes in auditory and spoken language development.

▨ General Approach to the Book

Drawing on our numerous years as clinician and educator, we have taken an approach that follows the child through his/her development from infancy to early adulthood, presenting ages and stages of development in multiple domains. We are indebted to the contributions from our colleagues, Drs. Giguère, Ching, Madell, and Flexer, who, in chapters 2, 3, and 8, shared their expertise to enhance our understanding of the importance of hearing and technology in helping children access the best possible acoustic information. We are also grateful to our many colleagues, who either directly through their writing or through our discussions with them, contributed their insights to this book.

The text has been organized into two main sections. The first section (chapters 1–4) provides important foundations about typical auditory development and the impact of childhood hearing loss on spoken language acquisition. These chapters also describe how to optimize the child's listening potential through acoustic and implantable hearing technologies; in other words, how to provide the fundamental access to hearing that the child requires to develop spoken language. The subsequent section (chapters 5–11) presents a description of how to maximize daily learning environments to facilitate auditory and spoken language development, not only in the critical early years but throughout the child's school years. This section is broadly organized along developmental lines from early intervention in infancy through to adolescence. Finally, in chapter 12, professionals from around the world share their perspectives on spoken language development.

No one textbook can provide comprehensive coverage of all areas of pediatric audiologic rehabilitation, and we too had to make choices. In reviewing the useful material already published, special focus is given in this book to clinical management of children with hearing loss and continued development of spoken language and literacy during the school years. Throughout the text, we have provided case examples to illustrate the topic areas from a very practical clinical and/or educational perspective. We are indebted to the many clinicians who provided us with meaningful cases to elucidate key concepts. These examples were selected to present the reader with an overview of how intervention is applied in real-world settings.

It is our hope that this text can provide useful foundations for many different individuals who have an interest in pediatric auditory rehabilitation: students in audiology, speech-language pathology and education, practicing clinicians and teachers, and parents, as well as other professionals who desire to learn about children with hearing loss.

Acknowledgments

Throughout this project, we benefitted from the guidance, professionalism, and especially an incredibly efficient approach from the entire editorial group at Thieme. In addition to the direct contributions from our chapter authors and clinician-authors throughout the text, we are grateful to many other individuals who contributed directly or indirectly to the realization of this project. The many discussions, as well as studies conducted with our research colleagues in Ottawa, undoubtedly shaped the content of this book. JoAnne Whittingham at the Child Hearing Laboratory in Ottawa and several students from the University of Ottawa who worked or trained in Elizabeth Fitzpatrick's lab also assisted with tables, figures, and review of references. Glenn Collins, Jessica Fitzpatrick, Tim Johnstone, and Hilaire Chiasson were immensely helpful in reviewing and clarifying sections of the text. We thank Daniel Dostie, graphic artist, for transposing our ideas into illustrations to capture core themes. We are grateful to the many children and families who taught us so much and who have shaped our understanding and perspectives throughout our careers. Finally, we thank our partners, Glenn and Hilaire, for their encouragement and enthusiasm for our work with children.

Elizabeth M. Fitzpatrick
Suzanne P. Doucet

References

Dornan, D., Hickson, L., Murdoch, B., & Houston, T. (2008). Speech and language outcomes for children with hearing loss educated in auditory-verbal therapy programs: A review of the evidence. *Communicative Disorders Review, 2* (3-4), 157–172.

Eriks-Brophy, A. (2004). Outcomes of auditory-verbal therapy: A review of the evidence and a call for action. *The Volta Review, 104*(1), 21–35.

Geers, A. E. (2006). Spoken language in children with cochlear implants. In P. E. Spencer & M. Marschark (Eds.), *Advances in the spoken language development of deaf and hard-of-hearing children*. New York: Oxford University Press.

Rhoades, E. A. (2006). Research outcomes of auditory-verbal intervention: Is the approach justified? *Deafness & Education International, 8*(3), 125–143. 10.1002/dei.197.

Spencer, P. E., & Marschark, M. (2010). *Evidence-based practice in educating deaf and hard-of-hearing students*. New York: Oxford University Press.

Thoutenhoofd, E. D., Archbold, S. M., Gregory, S., Lutman, M. E., Nikolopoulos, T. P., & Sach, T. H. (2005). *Paediatric cochlear implantation: Evaluating outcomes*. London: Whurr Publishers Ltd.

About the Authors

Elizabeth M. Fitzpatrick, PhD, LSLS Cert. AVT, is an associate professor in the School of Rehabilitation Sciences at the University of Ottawa, where she teaches courses in audiology and listening and spoken language development. She has been working in the area of pediatric hearing loss since 1982. Prior to joining the university, she practiced as a clinical audiologist and listening and spoken language specialist for over 20 years in a variety of clinical settings. Dr. Fitzpatrick's research is focused on early intervention practices in audiology and rehabilitation, services for families, and outcomes in both children and adults with hearing loss.

Suzanne P. Doucet, MEd, DipEd Deaf, LSLS Cert. AVT, has worked as an itinerant teacher for preschool and school age students with hearing loss for over 30 years in New Brunswick, Canada. She is responsible for continuing education services for teachers of the deaf and hard of hearing and has developed numerous educational resources in the field of audition, speech, and language intervention. In 2000, she established a postgraduate program at the Université de Moncton, specializing in the education of children with hearing loss based on auditory-verbal practice. She has been a member of the Alexander Graham Bell Academy for Listening and Spoken Language committees on certification and mentorship.

Contributors

Cindy Bell
Parent
Kuala Lumpur, Malaysia

Anita Bernstein, MSc, LSLS Cert. AVT
Director of Therapy and Training Programs
VOICE for Hearing Impaired Children
Hamilton, Canada

Teresa Y. C. Ching, PhD
Senior Research Scientist
Head, Rehabilitation Procedures Section
National Acoustic Laboratories
Sydney, Australia

Cheryl L. Dickson, PhD, LSLS Cert. AVT
Director
Auditory-Verbal Independent Consultant
Sydney, Australia

Dimity Dornan, AM, A/Prof, PhD, HonDUniv, BSpThy, FSPAA, CpSp, LSLS Cert. AVT
Executive Director and Founder
Hear and Say
Toowong, Australia

Suzanne P. Doucet, MEd, DipEd Deaf, LSLS Cert. AVT
Specialized Teacher and Coordinator for
 Continuing Education
Services for Students with Hearing Loss
Department of Education and Development
 of Early Childhood–New Brunswick
Moncton, New Brunswick, Canada

Jill Duncan, PhD, LSLS Cert. AVT
Head of Graduate Studies and Conjoint Senior
 Lecturer
Royal Institute for Deaf and Blind Children
RIDBC Renwick Centre
University of Newcastle
Sydney, Australia

Warren Estabrooks, MEd, DipEdDeaf Cert., LSLS Cert. AVT
President and CEO
WE Listen International, Inc.
Toronto, Canada

Elizabeth M. Fitzpatrick, PhD, LSLS Cert. AVT
Associate Professor
Audiology and Speech-Language Program
Faculty of Health Sciences
University of Ottawa
Ottawa, Ontario, Canada

Carol Flexer, PhD, CCC-A, LSLS Cert. AVT
Distinguished Professor Emeritus
Department of Audiology
University of Akron
Akron, Ohio

Jasmine Gallant, BÉd, MÉd, LSLS Cert. AVT
Agente pédagogique pour les élèves ayant un
 handicap sensoriel
Ministère de l'Education et du
 Développement de la petite enfance du
 Nouveau-Brunswick
Fredericton, Canada

Christian Giguère, PhD
Professor
Faculty of Health Sciences
University of Ottawa
Ottawa, Canada

Erin Gilbert
Parent
Kemptville, Canada

Donald M. Goldberg, PhD, LSLS Cert. AVT
Professor
College of Wooster
Wooster, Ohio
Consultant
Professional Staff
Cleveland Clinic
Cleveland, Ohio

Bruno and Sonia Leprette
Parents
Poissy, France

Stephanie Y. C. Lim, EdD, LSLS Cert. AVT
Chief Listening and Spoken Language
    Specialist
NOVENA Hearing Health and Cochlear
    Implant Unit
NOVENA ENT-Head and Neck Surgery
    Specialist Centre
Singapore

Jane R. Madell, PhD, CCC-A/SLP, LSLS Cert. AVT
Director
Pediatric Audiology Consulting
New York, New York

Mary McGinnis, PhDc, LSLS Cert. AVT
Director
John Tracy Clinic Graduate and Professional
    Programs
John Tracy Clinic
Los Angeles, California

**Erin McSweeney, MClSc, S-LP (C), LSLS Cert.
    AVT**
Speech-Language Pathologist
Auditory-Verbal Therapist
Audiology Department
Children's Hospital of Eastern Ontario
Ottawa, Canada

Jean Sachar Moog, MS, CED, LSLS Cert. AVEd
Founding Director
The Moog Center for Deaf Education
St. Louis, Missouri

Deirdre Neuss, PhD, LSLS Cert. AVT
Auditory-Verbal Therapist
Audiology Department
Children's Hosptial of Eastern Ontario
Ottawa, Canada

Jan North, CertTeach, BSpecEd, MEd, MACE
Director, Children's Services
Royal Institute for Deaf and Blind Children
Sydney, Australia

Kelly Rabjohn, MEd, LSLS Cert. AVT
Auditory-Verbal Therapist
Audiology Department
Children's Hospital of Eastern Ontario
Ottawa, Canada

Ellen A. Rhoades, EdS, LSLS Cert. AVT
Auditory-Verbal Independent Consultant
Lecturing, Mentoring International
Auditory Verbal Training
Ft. Lauderdale, Florida

Rosemary Somerville, BA, BE, LSLS Cert. AVT
Credential Auditory Verbal Therapist
Audiology Department
Children's Hospital of Eastern Ontario
Ottawa, Canada

Pamela Steacie, MSc, LSLS Cert. AVT
Auditory-Verbal Therapist
Audiology Department
Children's Hospital of Eastern Ontario
Ottawa, Canada

**Jacqueline Stokes, BEd, Dip TEFL, MSc, LSLS
    Cert. AVT**
Director and Therapist
Auditory Verbal UK
Chesterton, England

1 Audition as the Basis for Spoken Communication

The acquisition of spoken language is a naturally occurring phenomenon in all cultures. Audition is the foundation of spoken language development (Saffran, Werker, & Werner, 2006), and children exposed to spoken language models, regardless of the native language, typically become proficient speakers. Sometimes the process of language acquisition is interrupted before, during, or after birth, such as when hearing loss occurs. Before we discuss the impact of hearing loss on typical language and communication, it is important to understand the basic notions underlying audition, speech, and language development.

In this chapter we present an overview of how audition, speech, and language are usually acquired, as well as neurobiological evidence for auditory development. A rudimentary knowledge of typical language development is essential to understanding the consequences of hearing loss. Our goal in this chapter is to present a cursory description of typical speech and language development, providing the reader with a foundation for undertaking rehabilitation involving children with hearing deficits.

▣ Audition as the Foundation for Spoken Language Development

Typical Development in Audition, Speech, and Language

Permanent childhood hearing loss negatively affects several areas of typical child development, most notably spoken language (Kennedy et al, 2006; Sininger, Grimes, & Christensen, 2010; Yoshinaga-Itano, Sedey, Coulter, & Mehl, 1998). A brief overview of typical development in audition, speech, and language is presented here to provide a basic frame of reference for expectations and information considered important prior to a discussion of the effects of hearing loss on the child and family. For more in-depth study of typical language development, refer to textbooks such as Paul and Norbury (2012) and Owens (2012).

Stages of Auditory Development

Audition plays a critical role in the development of oral communication in children with normal hearing. Studies have shown that by the 26th week of gestation, the fetus not only has the capacity to detect sounds (Hepper & Shahidullah, 1994), but also shows reaction to sounds and seems to have the capacity to store auditory information. DeCasper and Fifer (1980) have demonstrated that right after birth, babies are more likely to respond to familiar sounds, such as rhymes repeated by their mothers, than to novel stimuli to which they have not been exposed.

In practical terms, babies are ready to hear and learn at birth and can perceive the melody and rhythm of language. Soon after birth, an infant shows a preference for the mother's voice and can even distinguish between the voice of the mother and that of another female (DeCasper & Fifer, 1980; DeCasper & Spence, 1986). However, research also suggests there is sensory immaturity in the infant's auditory system, resulting in a lack of auditory fine tuning in the early months of life (Leibold, Yarnell Bonino, & Fleenor, 2007). From birth to 6 months, there is rapid maturation of the auditory system (middle ear and auditory pathways of the brainstem) in its capacity to track and differentiate sounds (Werner, 2002, 2007). In the first 6 months, the infant's neural networks are organized to discriminate speech and other sounds (Vouloumanos & Werker, 2007). During these early months, babies learn to distinguish phonetic features in both their native language and non-native languages. However, they soon learn to differentiate their native language from others, first on the basis of rhythmic structure (Nazzi, Bertoncini, & Mehler, 1998; Werker & Tees, 2005; Werker & Yeung, 2005), and later they appear to become more sensitive to phonetic characteristics in the language. In the first year of life, babies can be observed to perform several distinct auditory behaviors. Examples from everyday home settings detailed in **Table 1.1** describe early observed auditory events.

In the first year of life, children discriminate a variety of speech sounds, including the sounds of foreign languages, but at around 12 months of age there is a neural reorganization in the brain that may be viewed as a refinement or pruning, enabling the child to focus mainly on speech sounds from his or her own language (Werker & Tees, 2005). Effectively, children become more skillful in discriminating speech sounds from their own language and gradually lose the ability to discriminate sounds to which they are not exposed on a daily basis. Throughout this developmental period, which continues until around age 5, there is a maturation of the ability to focus on specific characteristics of speech sounds such that the auditory system becomes increasingly more efficient (Werner, 2007).

Research has also shown that infants and young children have a strong interest in auditory stimuli over visual stimuli (Sloutsky & Napolitano, 2003). For example, in experiments conducted by Sloutsky and Napolitano, children presented with auditory versus visual stimuli choices showed a preference for auditory stimuli, suggesting that in the early stages of language acquisition, auditory information is of greater interest. Preference for sound stimuli continues into the preschool years but tends to decrease with maturity, and the researchers suggested that this reduction could be due to the fact that once language is acquired, it is no longer important for the child to favor the auditory modality. During the early developmental years, the child becomes more selective and flexible in the ability to process auditory information. As auditory skills mature, the child is able to process speech with less acoustic information available, such as in difficult listening conditions (Werner, 2007).

The usual stages of auditory development can be interrupted or delayed by hearing impairment in early childhood. Usually, the longer the hearing loss is present—that is, the longer the child is deprived of adequate access to sound (e.g., through amplification or cochlear implants, discussed in Chapters 3 and 4)—the greater the impact on the child's development (Yoshinaga-Itano, 2003).

Stages of Speech Development

As noted above, children are born with an overall preference for speech sounds and, in spite of the complexity of speech perception and production, are programmed for spoken language acquisition (Vouloumanos, Hauser, Werker, & Martin, 2010; Vouloumanos & Werker, 2007).

Starting with words and moving on to phrases, children must progressively master speech sounds and the suprasegmental aspects of speech to achieve speech intelligibility. At first, infant speech is mainly characterized by suprasegmentals, namely intensity, duration, and

Table 1.1 Examples of auditory behaviors in the first year

Auditory behavior	Approximate age	Example from home environment
Baby quiets to sound	1 month	Baby is fussing, apparently wanting to be fed. Mother uses an animated voice, saying, "Oh, you are hungry," and baby quiets briefly.
Baby turns head to sound	3 to 6 months	Four-year-old sister enters the kitchen loudly singing a nursery rhyme, and baby turns his head and tries to locate sound.
Baby localizes sounds	6 to 9 months	Baby is lying on a blanket on the floor and mother is preparing lunch in the kitchen about 6 feet away; baby turns head slightly toward mother when she calls his name.
Baby turns to locate a sound from behind	9 to 12 months	Baby is crawling on the floor and is moving toward the heater. Mother, who is several feet behind him, calls, "Don't touch." Baby turns around and grins at her.

pitch variations (De Boysson-Bardies, 1996), sounds that are often described as gurgles, cries, and intonation patterns. These vocalizations are used not only to express emotions, such as discomfort and delight, but also enable the infant to practice using motor skills associated with speech patterns. As covered in Chapter 2, speech sounds are produced through complex articulatory movements. This developmental stage is believed to be a precursor to phonetic development (preceding sound production) and is an important period as the child practices using the articulatory system (lungs, trachea, larynx, vocal folds, etc.) (Oller, 2000).

Around the age of 6 months, phonemes appear gradually in the child's speech, and in spite of individual variations, the order of emergence is fairly constant (Oller, 2000; Oller, Eilers, Neal, & Schwartz, 1999). At first these phonemes consist of full vowels and "raspberries," and soon the child produces a greater variety and improved quality of vocalizations, moving into what has been labeled the canonical stage, when the child produces well-formed syllables and reduplicated sequences, for example, [ba-ba, ga-ga]. Maturation of the central auditory system as discussed above is required for the development of the ability to perceive differences among speech sounds (e.g., intensity, duration, and pitch), which in turn enables the child to produce a variety of sounds (Werker & Tees, 2005). Chapter 2 provides further details on specific acoustic characteristics of speech.

Of importance in this introductory section is the notion that a child must hear and react instantly to auditory cues that define the production of words to process acoustic information in speech sounds. There is considerable variability in the acquisition of phonemes, and children take several years to acquire the complete repertoire of speech sounds in their language. For English, it can take children up to 6 to 7 years to master all of the phonemes (Sander, 1972). Vowels are generally easily acquired by typically developing children by age 3 (Donegan, 2002; Oller, 2000), while consonant production is physiologically more complex. Consonant acquisition tends to follow a general sequence of development with a range in the age of emergence of new sounds among children. Typical sequences of consonant development in English are described in several resources (e.g., Sander, 1972; Oller, 2000). One simple classification is provided by Shriberg (1993), where the 24 English consonants are categorized developmentally into three groups according to order of acquisition. Early developing consonants include phonemes such as /m/ and /p/, followed by middle developing phonemes such as /t/ and /d/, and finally by later phonemes such as /s/ and /z/. For the majority of children with normal hearing and typical development, acquisition of speech sounds occurs effortlessly. By 24 months of age, typically developing children achieve around 70% accuracy in their production of consonants in target words compared with adults (Stoel-Gammon, 1987, 1991). The presence of hearing loss, which restricts access to important acoustic features of speech sounds, is one of the reasons that some children require intervention to facilitate speech sound acquisition.

Stages of Language Development

Preverbal Stage

Children with normal hearing usually develop competent oral communication skills, allowing them to express themselves in complete sentences and be understood, by about 3 or 4 years of age (Owens, 2012). Various aspects of language, such as complexity of grammar, vocabulary growth, and overall communicative competence, are mastered well into adolescence and beyond (Nippold, 2007; Paul & Norbury, 2012). In fact, during the preverbal stage in the first year or so, that is, before the emergence of first words, children seem to be preparing for communication more generally and developing numerous prerequisites to spoken language.

Several researchers have identified key communicative interactions, such as joint reference, turn taking, and signaling intention, that occur well before the end of the first year and that are considered fundamental to typical language acquisition (Owens, 2012; Paul & Norbury, 2012). Joint reference to an object or activity is an interaction where the child and caregiver show a common interest in an event or object—for example, when the caregiver and baby are both looking at (and listening to) a mobile above the baby's crib. With this joint attention, the mother and baby share an interest and the mother has the opportunity to teach the baby new information, such as the specific name of the object and its qualities and function. In early infancy, joint referencing is established largely through gazing and pointing, and later on through spoken language alone as the child learns to associate speech meaningfully with objects and events in his or her environment. Specific research on infants and caregivers shows that turn taking, such as when the mother engages in a "babble" conversation with the infant, also promotes later verbal interaction. During this period, children appear to be laying important groundwork for spoken communication.

Although in the first months of life, an infant's movements and vocalizations are considered to be primarily reflexive and without specific communicative intent, the infant soon learns to use gestures and eventually vocalizations to signal intention, that is, to communicate about something. Effectively, during this period the child is learning that conversation is a social event and that certain rules govern interaction, whether the communication is verbal or nonverbal. For example, a 10-month-old child, sitting in her high chair, who throws a spoon on the floor and looks expectantly at her mother, has learned to signal an intention to communicate. Gradually, these communicative acts become more elaborate and sophisticated and the child becomes a more effective communicator even before the first "real" words are evident. **Table 1.2** describes interactions between a 10-month-old child and a caregiver, highlighting how these communication exchanges occur naturally and effortlessly in typical home or playgroup activities.

First Words and Beyond

Most children acquire their first words around 1 year of age, although, as with other developmental aspects, there is considerable variation among children. Research provides us with general guidelines about vocabulary development, suggesting that most children use about 10 words by 12 to 15 months of age, and 50 words at 15 to 20 months of age, continuing to progress rapidly from there. By the time the child reaches 24 months, he is likely to have 200 to 300 words, with vocabulary increasing to over 2,000 words by age 5 (Fenson et al, 1994; Owens, 2012).

Most children start combining words at 18 to 24 months. Between ages 3 and 5, it is well documented that there is a rapid explosion in the child's spoken language, not only in sentence length but also in complexity (Owens, 2012) as more syntactical forms and morphological markers are added. In children who experience no language difficulties, all of these aspects of typical language development occur without specific attention paid to the various developmental stages. **Table 1.3** provides excerpts from parent–child exchanges to illustrate language abilities during interactive play sessions at different stages of development. As illustrated, children's language skills as well as their parents' vocabulary and language structures become increasingly sophisticated. Our examples are intended

Table 1.2 Examples of communicative interaction between mother and 10-month-old child

Mother:	Catch the ball.
Jenny:	Ba ba
Mother:	Yes! It's the ball.
Mother:	Roll, roll, roll the ball! Get the ball! Oops, it's going under the table.
Jenny:	Bah bah
Mother:	Yeah! You rolled the ball! I caught it. Your turn. Oh, it's rolling fast.
Mother:	Here comes the ball again! Oh, it's a bouncy ball.
Jenny:	Oh

Table 1.3 Interactions during play activities between caregiver and 12-, 24-, and 36-month-old children with normal hearing

Child	Conversation
Female, age 12 months	M: Doesn't go? Does the doggy go? [Child puts the doggy in.] M: Oh, the doggy goes in! Where does the girl go? C: [Unintelligible words] Do! M: Doggy! C: Do-do-do do-do-do M: Is he like Scooby-Doo? C: Yeah! M: Don't eat the doggy! C: [Shakes head no] M: No, that's right. C: Do do doggy M: No. C: That—do no M: Yeah, that's the dog. Does he have a nose? C: Huh?

Female, age 24 months	M: Oh she's gonna go in the dog house? Uh oh, or the crate. I dunno,
	    is—is she too big or too small?
	C: Too small.
	M: Too small? Well, she's too big; the crate's too small.
	    [Child tries to ride the toy tricycle.]
	C: Yeh, ni ni way
	M: You're gonna ride the bike?
	C: [Nods]
	M: Are you too big? You're too big for that.
	C: Woo
	M: Paige, it's too small for you. Is it OK for me?
	C: You're—you're too big.
	M: I'm too big, you're right. I'm way too big.

Male, age 36 months	M: And where do you go down the slide? In the . . . C: Park. M: That's right. C: Just leave it there [puts the slide near the house]. M: OK. It's just gonna be outside the girl's house, isn't it? C: Yeah. I love this. M: You love it, that's nice. I think somebody should make a play on the slide. C: Someone. M: Yeah who's gonna play on it? Who would you like to play on the slide? C: I can't 'cause somebody's bum s-sat on it. M: Somebody's bum to slide on it? C: Yeah. M: OK, who—the doggie or the little girl? Which one? Which one? C: I don't know.

Abbreviations: M, mother; C, child.

to provide only a very introductory description of typical language development. We encourage the reader to consult the numerous helpful resources for a more in-depth understanding of typical language acquisition (for example, see Owens, 2012; Paul & Norbury, 2012).

One of the most important factors underlying typical language development is a rich learning environment. In a now well-known longitudinal study of 42 children and parents, Hart and Risley (1995) demonstrated that children's exposure to language models and vocabulary acquisition differed immensely as a function of their early learning environment. By age 3, children in higher-educated families were much more advanced in language skills compared with children in families of lower socioeconomic level (referred to as welfare families in the study). Children in families with low-income were exposed to 600 words per hour compared with 2,100 words per hour for children in families with at least one professional parent. Subsequent research with a subset of 29 children showed that early experience strongly predicted vocabulary and language abilities at age 9 to 10 years. Similarly, when hearing loss occurs early in childhood, auditory access to rich language models is more difficult to achieve and linguistic development is affected in a large percentage of children.

■ Neurobiological Evidence for Audition

Critical Period for Auditory Development

The definition of early intervention has changed substantially in the current context of universal newborn hearing screening where children can be identified with hearing loss in the first months of life. However, the notion of early auditory stimulation was a prevailing theme in early rehabilitation literature (Ling & Ling, 1978; Ross, 1982). Historically, researchers and clinicians have been convinced that audition plays a critical role in the development of spoken language (Beebe, 1953; Ling & Ling, 1978; Pollack, Goldberg, & Caleffe-Schenck, 1997). Early clinical work suggested that children whose hearing loss was identified earlier were more likely to develop better spoken language skills (Ling & Ling, 1978), and early research reported on the concept of a sensitive period for language development (Lennenberg, 1967). In addition, a substantial body of clinical work indicated that children who had little residual hearing, and therefore limited auditory experience, had more difficulty developing spoken language (Ling & Ling, 1978; Pollack et al, 1997).

There has been a plethora of research supporting the notion of audition as the foundation of oral language as well as other, related skills, including literacy (Dehaene, 2009; Perfetti & Sandak, 2000). Investigators have suggested that audition not only permits typical language acquisition but also shapes one's conception of the environment. The field of neurobiology has developed and broadened considerably in recent years, and evoked potential measures and brain imaging techniques have led to improved methods to study auditory functioning. In particular, animal studies have increased support for the concept of a critical period in which there is optimal formation of areas of the brain that are highly tuned for sensory processing, including auditory processing (Harrison, 2011; Harrison, Nagasawa, Smith, Stanton, & Mount, 1991; Hashisaki & Rubel, 1989). In contrast, sensory deprivation, such as lack of auditory experience, prevents the brain from forming the neural connections required during the developmental or "plastic" period to ensure optimal development of these areas. Furthermore, there is evidence that cross-modal plasticity occurs when a region of the brain is unused for its typical tasks; that is, reorganization occurs to the point that an area of the brain typically associated with processing one type of sensory information becomes reassigned to processing another type of sensory input. For example, in individuals with congenital blindness, the visual cortex can become used for somatosensory processing (Sadato et al, 1996), and visual processing has been shown to occur in auditory areas of the brain in individuals who are deaf (Neville, Schmidt, & Kutas, 1983).

In addition, cochlear implantation for individuals with profound deafness has provided an unparalleled opportunity to study neural functioning in children who were born deaf and later gained access to hearing through cochlear implantation. Using cortical evoked potential measures, studies with children following cochlear implantation point to the first 3 to 4 years as a critical period of plasticity with respect to auditory development (Sharma & Dorman, 2005, 2006; Sharma, Dorman, & Spahr, 2002). Further cochlear implant studies that used auditory brainstem measures to examine the ability of the auditory system to establish binaural processes also provide evidence for the advantage of early auditory stimulation (Gordon & Papsin, 2009; Gordon, Valero, van Hoesel, & Papsin, 2008). These findings support the concept that developmental aspects occur in a synchronous fashion. In other words, there appears to be a clearly defined period when the human brain is at its optimal capacity for auditory development, and when appropriate and sufficient external auditory stimulation occurs, there is developmental synchrony with respect to auditory-based language acquisition. For example, a 2-year-old child with normal hearing abilities growing up in a rich-language stimulation environment seemingly develops spoken language effortlessly. In this situation, proper formation of the brain regions specifically primed for this type of sensory activity occurs. At this young age, the brain has often been described as a "sponge" ready to absorb whatever auditory and other information is available in the environment.

Even when the perceived input is less than perfect relative to the normal hearing system, such as that provided through hearing aids and cochlear implants, the brain is adept enough to extract a sufficient amount of useful information to enable auditory development. Furthermore, although research points to optimal periods of development for certain activities, there is evidence, particularly from animal studies, for the notion of some degree of plasticity of the brain, that is, for the ability of the brain to reorganize itself at all ages (Jones & Pons, 1998; Recanzone, Schreiner, & Merzenich, 1993; Schwaber, Garraghty, & Kaas, 1993). Essentially, these studies suggest that with training, new pathways can be created to permit learning of new experiences even in older children and adults (Wright & Zhang, 2006). However, current understanding suggests that plasticity in the auditory pathways is greatly reduced with increasing age (Harrison, 2011).

Epidemiology of Childhood Hearing Loss

Prevalence of Permanent Childhood Hearing Loss

Hearing loss of any degree of severity can act as a barrier to spoken language development. Prevalence estimates for permanent childhood hearing loss vary widely depending on the definition of hearing disorder used. Historically, bilateral hearing loss of moderate degree or greater, which affects approximately 1 in 1,000 live births (Fortnum, Summerfield, Marshall, Davis, & Bamford, 2001; Russ et al, 2003; Watkin & Baldwin, 2011), has been of greatest concern and the subject of considerable newborn hearing screening research because of the documented negative effects on spoken language (Kennedy et al, 2006; Wake, Poulakis, Hughes, Carey-Sargeant, & Rickards, 2005). Compelling evidence for the impact of specific degrees of hearing loss has led some countries to implement newborn screening programs that target hearing loss of moderate degree or greater. Other screening programs have aimed at the early identification of milder degrees of hearing loss and include the management of unilateral hearing loss on the basis that hearing loss of any degree potentially affects the child's development (Hyde, 2005; Prieve & Stevens, 2000). When mild and unilateral hearing loss are taken into account, the prevalence of childhood hearing loss is 3 to 4 per 1,000 live births (Prieve & Stevens, 2000; Watkin & Baldwin, 2011), making it one of the most common congenital disorders in children (Erenberg et al, 1999).

A report from follow-up of a newborn hearing screening cohort in the United Kingdom (UK) suggests that in screening programs that target hearing loss of moderate degree or greater, about half of all childhood hearing loss can be expected to be identified in the newborn period (Watkin & Baldwin, 2011). Based on a newborn screening cohort of 35,668 children, these investigators reported a prevalence of 3.64 children with permanent hearing loss per 1,000 by the end of the first year of school. Population-based data from one Canadian region specifically examining mild bilateral and unilateral hearing loss characteristics found that of

75 children who underwent newborn screening, 20 (26.7%) who passed screening or had normal hearing at first assessment presented with delayed onset by age 2 years (Fitzpatrick, 2011). Over all, these data suggest that a substantial number of children with hearing loss are identified after the first 6 months of life regardless of whether newborn hearing screening is in place, and that a substantial amount of permanent hearing loss may be of later onset.

Etiology of Childhood Hearing Loss

The Joint Committee on Infant Hearing (JCIH) (2007) has identified 11 risk factors that are associated with congenital or delayed-onset hearing loss. These risk factors serve as a guide for increased vigilance or targeted screening in areas where universal newborn screening is not available, and for surveillance of children who pass newborn screening but who are at increased risk for later onset of hearing loss or for the presence of mild hearing loss. The etiology of childhood hearing loss remains unknown in 25% or more of affected children. Genetic mutations contribute to over half of hearing loss cases, with the *GJB2* gene identified as contributing from an estimated 21% (Morton & Nance, 2006) to as much as 50% of nonsyndromic genetic hearing loss in some populations (Hood & Keats, 2011). In 70% of genetic cases, sensorineural hearing loss is nonsyndromic, that is, not accompanied by other clinical abnormalities, while 30% of known genetic hearing loss is associated with syndromic features with or without other disabilities (Morton & Nance, 2006). With increased interest in genome sequencing and better integration of genomics into audiology programs, progress can be expected to continue toward understanding the relationship between certain genetic hearing losses and the audiologic profiles and other clinical characteristics of affected individuals.

The remaining approximately 25% of permanent hearing loss cases appear to be due to environmental causes. The most common known cause of nongenetic hearing loss is cytomegalovirus (CMV), an infection that reportedly affects 1 to 2% of newborns and accounts for up to 20% of congenital sensorineural hearing loss (Nance, Lim, & Dodson, 2006). CMV has also been reported to be one of the major causes of delayed-onset deafness (Nance et al, 2006). Other congenital diseases known to affect hearing include toxoplasmosis and congenital syphilis (Almond & Brown, 2009). The use of ototoxic drugs during pregnancy also place a child at risk for hearing loss.

Radiologic abnormalities of the inner ear occur in roughly 20% of individuals affected with congenital hearing loss (Coticchia, Gokhale, Waltonen, & Sumer, 2006; Jackler, Luxford, & House, 1987). These inner ear conditions have frequently been categorized under the broad term *Mondini dysplasia*, but involve a constellation of conditions that include complete absence of all inner ear structures, cochlear anomalies (e.g., complete absence of the cochlea, an underdeveloped cochlea), malformation of the semicircular canals, malformations of the cochlear and vestibular aqueducts (e.g., enlarged vestibular aqueduct), and abnormalities of the neural structures. This information can be of importance in determining the clinical profile and course of the hearing loss. For example, enlarged vestibular aqueduct syndrome has been associated with deterioration of hearing loss to profound levels in 40% or more of affected individuals (Govaerts et al, 1999). Nance et al (2006) reported that causes of enlarged vestibular aqueduct are major factors in the development of delayed-onset prelingual deafness. Information about inner ear structures is also of utmost importance in determining radiologic status for cochlear implantation (see Chapter 4).

Impact of Hearing Loss on Auditory Development

Hearing Loss as a Barrier to Acoustic Information

Types of Hearing Loss

Childhood hearing loss acts as a barrier to spoken language development and can interfere with the trajectory of language acquisition. Hearing loss can affect one ear only (unilateral) or both ears (bilateral), and can be temporary or permanent. Permanent hearing loss is not amenable to medical intervention and is generally associated with sensorineural hearing loss (cochlea or auditory nerve is affected). Temporary hearing loss is usually referred to as a conductive impairment. The most common cause in children is otitis media, with effusion affecting 70 to 90% of children during the first 2 years of life (Canadian Working Group on Childhood Hearing, 2005). Conductive hearing loss occurs due to difficulty with the transmission of sounds to the inner ear, and in some children may persist for a period of time. Usually these conditions are responsive to medical treatment or resolve on their own (Buchman, Adunka, Zdanski, & Pillsbury, 2011). Persistent cases of otitis media may be managed through myringotomy and surgical insertion of tympanostomy tubes (Canadian

Working Group on Childhood Hearing, 2005; Paradise & Bluestone, 2005; Rosenfeld & Bluestone, 1999).

This book is concerned with permanent childhood hearing loss because of its potential negative effects on spoken language development and communication. Some permanent hearing loss is conductive, in which case it is not associated with transient middle ear pathology but is associated with structural deficits, such as atresia of the external auditory canals. It is important to emphasize that children with sensorineural hearing loss are not immune to temporary or long-term conductive involvement associated with middle ear dysfunction, and that when such a condition results in a mixed hearing loss, it can create an additional barrier for the child who is developing language.

Severity of Hearing Loss

In audiometric terms, hearing loss is classified according to severity, ranging from mild to profound. More specific information on the measurement of hearing loss and the effects of various levels of hearing impairment is presented in Chapter 2. In the Watkin and Baldwin (2011) study of 130 children identified with permanent hearing loss, 12 (9.2%) had profound, 12 (9.2%) severe, and 30 (23.1%) moderate degrees of hearing loss based on average audiometric thresholds in the better-hearing ear. The remaining 76 (58.5%) children had mild bilateral (36.2%) or unilateral (22.3%) hearing loss. **Fig. 1.1** shows the distribution of hearing loss based on research from a population study of 709 children identified with hearing loss who were born from 1980 to 2003 in one Canadian region of approximately

1 million people. Considerable clinical attention is directed toward severe and profound hearing loss because of its immediate and serious effects on auditory and spoken language development. However, severe and profound hearing loss accounts for about 20 to 30% of permanent hearing loss in children, moderate and moderately severe hearing loss accounts for an additional 20 to 30%, and mild and unilateral hearing loss makes up 40 to 50% of hearing loss cases (Durieux-Smith, Fitzpatrick, & Whittingham, 2008; Fitzpatrick, 2011; Fitzpatrick, Durieux-Smith, & Whittingham, 2010). As discussed in a subsequent section, degree of hearing loss seems to be one determinant of spoken language development (Ching, 2012; Fitzpatrick, Durieux-Smith, Eriks-Brophy, Olds, & Gaines, 2007; Sininger et al, 2010).

■ Consequences of Hearing Loss for Auditory Learning and Spoken Language Acquisition

As discussed in Chapters 3 and 4, modern technology in the form of hearing aids and cochlear implants now provides children with hearing loss access to speech sounds more efficiently than at any other time in our history. Children with hearing loss tend to follow the same pathways of auditory and language development at the same rate or with the same ease as in children with normal hearing. However, it is important to understand that even when the

child is fitted with the best available technology, hearing function is not restored to normal, and the impairment may prevent some of the typical auditory behaviors from occurring at the rate or with the ease they do in their peers with normal hearing. Hearing loss reduces access to sounds, which translates into difficulties with such auditory and related behaviors as localization, distance hearing, overhearing, and incidental learning, all of which can inter-

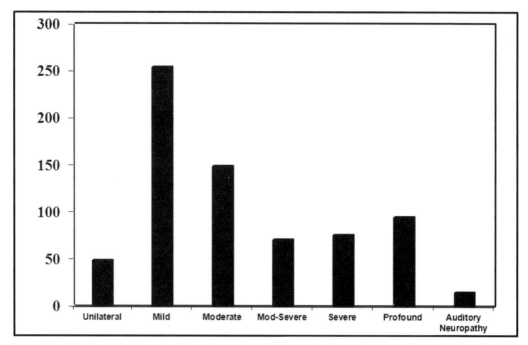

Fig. 1.1   Distribution of number of children with various degrees of permanent hearing loss in a clinical population of 709 children. (Data from a study published as Durieux-Smith, A., Fitzpatrick, E., & Whittingham, J. (2008). Universal newborn hearing screening: A question of evidence. *International Journal of Audiology, 47*(1), 1–10.)

fere with the ease of language learning (**Fig. 1.2**). While hearing technology can offer the child considerable access to the speech spectrum, it does not "cure" hearing loss; that is, the child armed with the best possible technology will not hear in all situations as well as a child whose hearing is within normal limits. Early-onset hearing loss has often been described as an acoustic filter that distorts and limits or eliminates incoming sounds (Flexer, 1999).

The specific consequences of childhood hearing loss for any individual child vary according to factors, such as the severity of loss, the environment, and family circumstances, as discussed in a subsequent section. Therefore, the actual impact or the extent to which hearing loss interferes with participation in society varies from child to child. However, in general, we can summarize some of the practical audition-related consequences for children with hearing loss.

Localization, Distance, Overhearing, and Incidental Learning

Even babies equipped with optimal hearing technology will have difficulty with acoustic access because of the reduced ability to hear sounds from a distance and to localize the source of sounds (see stages in **Table 1.1**). Children with hearing loss are particularly at a disadvantage when listening in unfavorable acoustic environments. The quality of the speech signal received and the limited earshot (distance over which the signal can be detected and processed) affect the usual process of learning for children, increase lis-

tening effort, and reduce the ability to overhear sounds and to benefit from natural or incidental learning. One has only to think of the situation where a young child spills her glass of milk and exclaims, "D—," to which her mother responds, "I didn't teach her that!" to understand that young children continuously learn new vocabulary and expressions from overhearing others in their environment. In playgroups, children constantly learn new vocabulary and social language through incidental learning simply by being exposed to

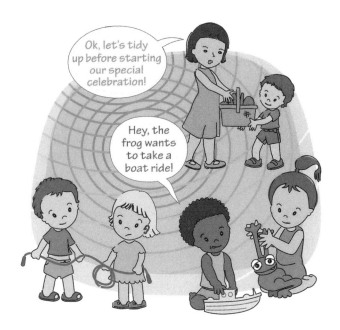

Fig. 1.2 Relative to children with normal hearing, children who wear hearing technology will have more difficulty accessing all of the acoustic information in natural play and learning environments. They are particularly at risk of missing out on incidental learning and distance hearing.

different models of language. Children with hearing loss have fewer opportunities for expanding their vocabulary and expressions through natural, everyday learning. As we will see in subsequent chapters, audiologic intervention is aimed at providing embellished language-rich environments to compensate for the barriers to learning.

Quality of Speech Signal

Not only does permanent hearing loss reduce the intensity of the acoustic signal, making access to sound more difficult, but sensorineural hearing loss (that is, cochlear hearing loss) also affects the quality of the speech signal. In practical terms, a child with a sensorineural hearing loss may understand the sentence "Go get your coat" as "Go get your goat," or "This is a pain" as "This is a cane." A practical example from a school lesson is a child whose teacher says, "Turn to page 15" and the child then looks for the assigned exercise on page 16. Because of reduced sound quality and distance limitations, individuals with hearing loss require a more favorable signal-to-noise ratio (SNR); that is, relative to individuals with normal hearing, speech must be louder compared with background noise. This concept is further elaborated in Chapter 8.

As discussed in the next chapter, the severity and configuration of hearing loss can have an important impact on the child's ability to access speech sounds. Specific examples of how different degrees of hearing loss affect accessibility to speech sounds are presented in Chapter 2, along with an overview of acoustic phonetics of speech.

Impact of Hearing Loss on Parent–Child Interaction

The overwhelming majority of children with hearing loss (up to 95%) are born to parents with normal hearing (Mitchell & Karchmer, 2004), and therefore are expected to grow up in typical hearing and speaking environments. It is not surprising that, for parents, the effect of learning about their child's hearing loss is very different from the impact of such news on the minority of parents who themselves have hearing loss. Parents often describe the emotional aspect of finding out about their child's hearing loss as a shock, using words like *devastating* and *overwhelming* to describe this impact on the family (Fitzpatrick, Angus,

Durieux-Smith, Graham, & Coyle, 2008; Fitzpatrick, Graham, Durieux-Smith, Angus, & Coyle, 2007; Luterman, 2006; Young & Tattersall, 2007). With time and support, which are discussed in later chapters, most parents are able to move forward and take action to provide the recommended early auditory stimulation. From an auditory development perspective, one of the greatest concerns is that mother–child bonding and, ultimately, the natural learning environment for the child, will be affected. Parents generally support screening but speak of the difficulty of learning about hearing loss in their child shortly after birth. One mother said, "I think I didn't enjoy my new baby like others do 100%; I think I didn't enjoy her as much as other mothers." A mother whose son was born before the availability of screening said, "To be completely honest, I had a happy year at home with him, in that quiet land of happy baby, so ignorance is bliss" (Fitzpatrick, 2007).

In addition to the emotional impact of hearing loss on the family, parent–child interaction patterns can be disrupted (Cole, 1992). For example, parents may provide less auditory stimulation and speak less to their children,

presumably because of the reduced feedback from the child and their expectations that the child will not hear them. Relative to parents of children with normal hearing, parents of children with hearing loss have been reported to employ directive speech patterns rather than the typical infant-directed talk (also referred to as motherese) observed in typical parent–child interactions, which involves repetition, enhanced acoustic patterns, and greater use of suprasegmental and melodic speech (Cooper & Aslin, 1989; Werker & McLeod, 1989). Characteristics of adult speech to children with hearing loss are summarized in Cole and Flexer (2007) and include less time spent talking with the child, fewer language expansions, more self-repetition, more rejections of the child's communicative attempts, and use of speech that is less fluent and audible. In other words, by virtue of their child's hearing loss, adults are at risk for developing communication behaviors that are misaligned with typical interactions that enhance auditory and language growth. These findings point to the need for specialized intervention to guide parents in developing their child's audition-based communication.

Factors Affecting Auditory Development

Hearing loss reduces access to speech sounds, and therefore creates barriers to the usual trajectory of auditory and communication development. There is major consensus that one of the most obvious effects of hearing loss is on the acquisition of spoken language (Ching et al, 2010; Fitzpatrick, Durieux-Smith, et al, 2007; Kennedy et al, 2006; Sininger et al, 2010; Wake, Hughes, Poulakis, Collins, & Rickards, 2004), which has consequences for social development as well as literacy and later academic learning (Geers, Strube, Tobey, Pisoni, & Moog, 2011; Karchmer & Mitchell, 2003; Marschark, Rhoten, & Fabich, 2007). Throughout this book, we will discuss the development of listening and spoken language for children of various ages. As we will see, the consequences of hearing loss on development and learning will vary according to the child's particular circumstances. This is because outcomes are related to a myriad of factors, some of which affect the child's development more generally, independent of the hearing disorder.

The notion of multiple outcomes and multiple influencing factors associated with childhood hearing is captured in a framework (**Fig. 1.3**) adapted from the International Classification of Disability and Functioning (World Health Organization, 2001). The framework (Fitzpatrick, 2010) provides a reference for the approach to audiologic rehabilitation elaborated in this book. Research findings reinforce the importance of focusing on rehabilitation outcomes beyond typical child communication measures, and suggest that consideration should be accorded to clinical processes as well as to family-perceived benefits (Fitzpatrick, Graham, et al, 2007; Nelson, Bougatsos, & Nygren, 2008; Tattersall & Young, 2006; Young & Tattersall, 2007). For example, research conducted with parents shows that while quality therapy and audiology services are of primary importance to all families, other valued characteristics of service provision include a service model that is well coordinated and that facilitates access to ongoing medical, technical,

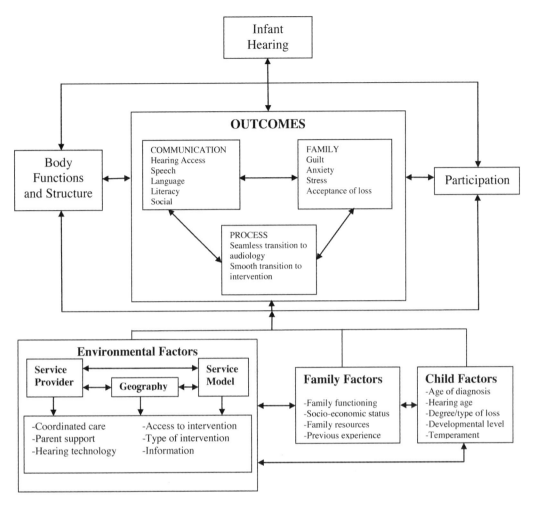

Fig. 1.3 A framework for the factors affecting childhood hearing and development. (Adapted and reprinted with permission from Fitzpatrick, E. (2010). A framework for research and practice in infant hearing. *Canadian Journal of Speech-Language Pathology and Audiology, 34*(1), 25–32.)

prognostic, and resource information. In addition, access to support from other parents of children with hearing loss has been identified as having benefits for the family (Fitzpatrick, Graham, et al, 2007).

In this framework, outcomes are conceptualized as three interrelated products: communication outcomes, process outcomes, and family impact outcomes. Each outcome category has been defined to incorporate research findings. The outcomes have been arranged to emphasize that they are not discrete and separate phenomena, but rather have the potential to have interaction with one another. For example, in one

study, families who perceived that their children had access to hearing (communication outcome) described the positive impact of early identification of hearing loss on the family, whereas other families who were concerned about their child's poor communication skills attributed it to late diagnosis and referred to increased guilt and anxiety at the family level. Families who experienced difficulty with the referral process to audiology (process outcome) also associated this experience with increased stress, frustration, and anxiety for the family and with reduced opportunities for the child to learn through hearing (Fitzpatrick, Graham, et al, 2007).

Influencing and interrelated factors affecting infant hearing development are categorized in the framework as follows:

Environmental factors: hearing technology, geographic location, type of intervention, access to intervention and other services, and service delivery models

Child factors: age of identification, severity of hearing loss, developmental level, and temperament

Family factors: family functioning, socioeconomic status, family resources, and previous experience

Environmental factors appear to closely interact with family characteristics to facilitate or hinder progress toward meeting families' needs. For example, families who mentioned financial hardship, which in turn interfered with timely access to hearing technology, described a barrier that is directly influenced by family circumstances (Fitzpatrick et al, 2008). This has the potential to impact the child's access to hearing, and influences eventual outcomes in multiple domains. In this framework, service providers, geography, and service models are seen as dynamic and interrelated factors that can determine the availability of other components, such as access to hearing technology and audiologic rehabilitation.

▨ Summary

Given the evidence presented here for developmental synchrony and the progress made in the early identification of hearing loss, opportunities for auditory and spoken language development through typical and embellished developmental models are available to many children. The premise of this book is that audition forms the basis of spoken language communication. Optimal development of audition in children with hearing loss requires an understanding of typical auditory and language development as well as an awareness of the many environmental, child, and family factors that interact to impact an individual child's development. Chapter 2 provides more detailed information on the acoustic aspects of speech and how hearing loss interferes with acquisition.

▨ References

Almond, M., & Brown, D. J. (2009). The pathology and etiology of sensorineural hearing loss and implications for cochlear implantation. In J. K. Niparko (Ed.), *Cochlear implants: Principles and practices* (2nd ed., pp. 43–87). Philadelphia, PA: Lippincott Williams & Wilkins.

Beebe, H. (1953). *A guide to help the severely hard of hearing child.* New York: Karger.

Buchman, C. A., Adunka, O. F., Zdanski, C. J., & Pillsbury, H. C. (2011). Medical considerations for infants and children with hearing loss: The otologists' perspective. In R. Seewald & A.-M. Tharpe (Eds.), *Comprehensive handbook of pediatric audiology.* San Diego, CA: Plural Publishing, Inc.

Canadian Working Group on Childhood Hearing. (2005). Early hearing and communication development: Canadian Working Group on Childhood Hearing (CWGCH) resource document. Ottawa.

Ching, T. Y. C. (2012). Predicting developmental outcomes of early- and late-identified children with hearing impairment, including those with special needs: Findings from a population study. Paper presented at the Newborn Hearing Screening 2012, Cernobbio, Italy.

Ching, T. Y. C., Crowe, K., Martin, V., Day, J., Mahler, N., Youn, S., . . . Orsini, J. (2010). Language development and everyday functioning of children with hearing loss assessed at 3 years of age. *International Journal of Speech-Language Pathology, 12*(2), 124–131 10.3109/17549500903577022.

Cole, E. B. (1992). *Listening and talking: A guide to promoting spoken language in young hearing-impaired children.* Washington, DC: Alexander Graham Bell Association for the Deaf.

Cole, E. B., & Flexer, C. (2007). *Children with hearing loss: Developing listening and talking, birth to six.* San Diego, CA: Plural Publishing, Inc.

Cooper, R. P., & Aslin, R. N. (1989). The language environment of the young infant: Implications for early perceptual development. *Canadian Journal of Psychology, 43*(2), 247–265.

Coticchia, J. M., Gokhale, A., Waltonen, J., & Sumer, B. (2006). Characteristics of sensorineural hearing loss in children with inner ear anomalies. *American Journal of Otolaryngology, 27*(1), 33–38.

De Boysson-Bardies, B. (1996). *Comment la parole vient aux enfants.* Paris: Editions Odile Jacob.

DeCasper, A. J., & Fifer, W. P. (1980). Of human bonding: Humans prefer their mother's voices. *Science, 6*(208), 1174–1176.

DeCasper, A. J., & Spence, M. J. (1986). Prenatal maternal speech influences newborns' perception of speech sounds. *Infant Behavior and Development, 9*(2), 133–150.

Dehaene, S. (2009). *Reading in the brain: The new science of how we read.* New York: Penguin Books.

Donegan, P. (2002). Normal vowel development. In M. J. Ball & F. E. Gibbon (Eds.), *Vowel disorders* (pp. 1–35). Woburn, MA: Butterworth-Heinemann.

Durieux-Smith, A., Fitzpatrick, E., & Whittingham, J. (2008). Universal newborn hearing screening: A question of evidence. *International Journal of Audiology, 47*(1), 1–10.

Erenberg, A., Lemons, J., Sia, C., Trunkel, D., & Ziring, P.; American Academy of Pediatrics. (1999). Newborn and infant hearing loss: Detection and intervention. American Academy of Pediatrics. Task Force on Newborn and Infant Hearing, 1998–1999. *Pediatrics, 103*(2), 527–530.

Fenson, L., Dale, P. S., Reznick, J. S., Bates, E., Thal, D. J., & Pethick, S. J. (1994). Variability in early communicative development. *Monographs of the Society for Research in Child Development, 59*(5), 1–173, discussion 174–185.

Fitzpatrick, E. (2007). Population infant hearing screening to intervention: Determinants of outcome from the parents' perspective. Doctoral thesis, University of Ottawa, Ottawa.

Fitzpatrick, E. (2010). A framework for research and practice in infant hearing. *Canadian Journal of Speech-Language Pathology and Audiology, 34*(1), 25–32.

Fitzpatrick, E., Angus, D., Durieux-Smith, A., Graham, I. D., & Coyle, D. (2008). Parents' needs following identification of childhood hearing loss. *American Journal of Audiology, 17*(1), 38–49.

Fitzpatrick, E., Durieux-Smith, A., Eriks-Brophy, A., Olds, J., & Gaines, R. (2007). The impact of newborn hearing screening on communication development. *Journal of Medical Screening, 14*(3), 123–131.

Fitzpatrick, E., Graham, I. D., Durieux-Smith, A., Angus, D., & Coyle, D. (2007). Parents' perspectives on the impact of the early diagnosis of childhood hearing loss. *International Journal of Audiology, 46*(2), 97–106.

Fitzpatrick, E. M. (2011). Newborn hearing screening: Making it work. Paper presented at the Canadian Association of Speech-Language Pathology and Audiology Conference 2011, Montreal, Canada.

Fitzpatrick, E. M., Durieux-Smith, A., & Whittingham, J. (2010). Clinical practice for children with mild bilateral and unilateral hearing loss. *Ear and Hearing, 31*(3), 392–400.

Flexer, C. (1999). *Facilitating hearing and listening in young children.* San Diego, CA: Singular.

Fortnum, H. M., Summerfield, A. Q., Marshall, D. H., Davis, A. C., & Bamford, J. M. (2001). Prevalence of permanent childhood hearing impairment in the United Kingdom and implications for universal neonatal hearing screening: Questionnaire based ascertainment study. *BMJ (Clinical Research Ed.), 323*(7312), 536–540.

Geers, A. E., Strube, M. J., Tobey, E. A., Pisoni, D. B., & Moog, J. S. (2011). Epilogue: Factors contributing to long-term outcomes of cochlear implantation in early childhood. *Ear and Hearing, 32*(1, Suppl.), 84S–92S.

Gordon, K. A., & Papsin, B. C. (2009). Benefits of short interimplant delays in children receiving bilateral cochlear implants. *Otology & Neurotology, 30*(3), 319–331.

Gordon, K. A., Valero, J., van Hoesel, R., & Papsin, B. C. (2008). Abnormal timing delays in auditory brainstem responses evoked by bilateral cochlear implant use in children. *Otology & Neurotology, 29*(2), 193–198.

Govaerts, P. J., Casselman, J., Daemers, K., De Ceulaer, G., Somers, T., & Offeciers, F. E. (1999). Audiological findings in large vestibular aqueduct syndrome. *International Journal of Pediatric Otorhinolaryngology, 51*(3), 157–164.

Harrison, R. V. (2011). Development of the auditory system from periphery to cortex. In R. Seewald & A.-M. Tharpe (Eds.), *Comprehensive handbook of pediatric audiology.* San Diego, CA: Plural Publishing, Inc.

Harrison, R. V., Nagasawa, A., Smith, D. W., Stanton, S., & Mount, R. J. (1991). Reorganization of auditory cortex after neonatal high frequency cochlear hearing loss. *Hearing Research, 54*(1), 11–19.

Hart, B., & Risley, T. R. (1995). *Meaningful differences in the everyday experience of young American children.* Baltimore, MD: Paul H. Brookes Publishing Co.

Hashisaki, G. T., & Rubel, E. W. (1989). Effects of unilateral cochlea removal on anteroventral cochlear nucleus neurons in developing gerbils. *Journal of Comparative Neurology, 283*(4), 5–73.

Hepper, P. G., & Shahidullah, B. S. (1994). Development of fetal hearing. *Archives of Disease in Childhood, 71*(2), F81–F87.

Hood, L. J., & Keats, B. J. B. (2011). Genetics of childhood hearing loss. In R. Seewald & A.-M. Tharpe (Eds.), *Comprehensive handbook of pediatric audiology.* San Diego, CA: Plural Publishing, Inc.

Hyde, M. L. (2005). Newborn hearing screening programs: Overview. *Journal of Otolaryngology, 34*(Suppl. 2), S70–S78.

Jackler, R. K., Luxford, W. M., & House, W. F. (1987). Congenital malformations of the inner ear: A classification based on embryogenesis. *Laryngoscope, 97*(3 Pt. 2, Suppl. 40), 2–14.

Joint Committee on Infant Hearing, American Academy of Pediatrics. (2007). Year 2007 position statement: Principles and guidelines for early hearing detection and intervention programs. *Pediatrics, 120*(4), 898–921.

Jones, E. G., & Pons, T. P. (1998). Thalamic and brainstem contributions to large-scale plasticity of primate somatosensory cortex. *Science, 282*(5391), 1121–1125.

Karchmer, M. A., & Mitchell, R. E. (2003). Demographic and achievement characteristics of deaf and hard-of-hearing students. In M. Marschark & P. Spencer (Eds.), *Oxford handbook of deaf studies, language and education* (pp. 21–37). New York: Oxford University Press.

Kennedy, C. R., McCann, D. C., Campbell, M. J., Law, C. M., Mullee, M. A., Petrou, S., . . . Stevenson, J. (2006). Language ability after early detection of permanent childhood hearing impairment. *New England Journal of Medicine, 354*(20), 2131–2141.

Leibold, L. J., Yarnell Bonino, A., & Fleenor, L. (2007). The importance of establishing a time course for typical auditory development. In R. Seewald (Ed.), *Phonak Conference* (pp. 35–42). Chicago: Phonak.

Lennenberg, E. H. (1967). *Biological foundations of language*. New York: John Wiley & Sons.

Ling, D., & Ling, A. H. (1978). *Aural habilitation: The foundations of verbal learning in hearing-impaired children*. Washington, DC: Alexander Graham Bell Association of the Deaf, Inc.

Luterman, D. (2006). The emotional impact of hearing loss. In D. Luterman (Ed.), *Children with hearing loss: A family guide* (pp. 9–35). Sedona, AZ: Auricle Ink Publishers.

Marschark, M., Rhoten, C., & Fabich, M. (2007). Effects of cochlear implants on children's reading and academic achievement. *Journal of Deaf Studies and Deaf Education, 12*(3), 269–282 10.1093/deafed/enm013.

Mitchell, R., & Karchmer, M. (2004). Chasing the mythical ten percent: Parental hearing status of deaf and hard of hearing students in the United States. *Sign Language Studies, 4*, 138–163.

Morton, C. C., & Nance, W. E. (2006). Newborn hearing screening—a silent revolution. *New England Journal of Medicine, 354*(20), 2151–2164.

Nance, W. E., Lim, B. G., & Dodson, K. M. (2006). Importance of congenital cytomegalovirus infections as a cause for pre-lingual hearing loss. *Journal of Clinical Virology, 35*(2), 221–225.

Nazzi, T., Bertoncini, J., & Mehler, J. (1998). Language discrimination by English-learning 5-month-olds: Effects of rhythm and familiarity. *Journal of Memory and Language, 43*, 1–19.

Nelson, H. D., Bougatsos, C., & Nygren, P.; 2001 US Preventive Services Task Force. (2008). Universal newborn hearing screening: Systematic review to update the 2001 US Preventive Services Task Force Recommendation. *Pediatrics, 122*(1), e266–e276 10.1542/peds.2007-1422.

Neville, H. J., Schmidt, A., & Kutas, M. (1983). Altered visual-evoked potentials in congenitally deaf adults. *Brain Research, 266*(1), 127–132.

Nippold, M. (2007). *Later language development: School-age children, adolescents, and young adults* (3rd ed.). Austin, TX: Pro-Ed.

Oller, D. K. (2000). *The emergence of the speech capacity*. Mahwah, NJ: Lawrence Erlbaum Associates Inc.

Oller, D. K., Eilers, R. E., Neal, A. R., & Schwartz, H. K. (1999). Precursors to speech in infancy: The prediction of speech and language disorders. *Journal of Communication Disorders, 32*(4), 223–245.

Owens, R. E., Jr. (2012). *Language development: An introduction* (8th ed.). Upper Saddle River, NJ: Pearson.

Paradise, J. L., & Bluestone, C. D. (2005). Consultation with the specialist: Tympanostomy tubes: A contemporary guide to judicious use. *Pediatrics Review, 26*(2), 61–66.

Paul, R., & Norbury, C. F. (2012). *Language disorders from infancy through adolescence: Listening, speaking, reading, writing, and communicating* (4th ed.). St. Louis, MO: Elsevier, Inc.

Perfetti, C. A., & Sandak, R. (2000). Reading optimally builds on spoken language: Implications for deaf readers. *Journal of Deaf Studies and Deaf Education, 5*(1), 32–50.

Pollack, D., Goldberg, D., & Caleffe-Schenck, N. (1997). *Educational audiology for the limited-hearing infant and preschooler: An auditory-verbal program* (3rd ed.). Springfield, IL: Charles C Thomas.

Prieve, B. A., & Stevens, F. (2000). The New York State universal newborn hearing screening demonstration project: Introduction and overview. *Ear and Hearing, 21*(2), 85–91.

Recanzone, G. H., Schreiner, C. E., & Merzenich, M. M. (1993). Plasticity in the frequency representation of primary auditory cortex following discrimination training in adult owl monkeys. *Journal of Neuroscience, 13*(1), 87–103.

Rosenfeld, R. M., & Bluestone, C. D. (Eds.) (1999). *Evidence-based otitis media*. Hamilton, BC: Decker, Inc.

Ross, M. (1982). *Hard of hearing children in regular schools*. Englewood Cliffs, NJ: Prentice-Hall, Inc.

Russ, S. A., Poulakis, Z., Barker, M., Wake, M., Rickards, F., Saunders, K., & Oberklaid, F. (2003). Epidemiology of congenital hearing loss in Victoria, Australia. *International Journal of Audiology, 42*(7), 385–390.

Sadato, N., Pascual-Leone, A., Grafman, J., Ibañez, V., Deiber, M. P., Dold, G., & Hallett, M. (1996). Activation of the primary visual cortex by Braille reading in blind subjects. *Nature, 380*(6574), 526–528.

Saffran, J. R., Werker, J. F., & Werner, L. A. (2006). The infant's auditory world: Hearing, speech and the beginnings of language. In R. Siegler & D. Kuhn (Eds.), *Handbook of child development* (Vol. 6, pp. 58–108). New York: Wiley.

Sander, E. K. (1972). When are speech sounds learned? *Journal of Speech and Hearing Disorders, 37*(1), 55–63.

Schwaber, M. K., Garraghty, P. E., & Kaas, J. H. (1993). Neuroplasticity of the adult primate auditory cortex following cochlear hearing loss. *American Journal of Otology, 14*(3), 252–258.

Sharma, A., & Dorman, M. (2005). The clinical use of P1 latency as a biomarker for assessment of central auditory development in children with hearing impairment. *Audiology Today, 17*(3), 18–19.

Sharma, A., & Dorman, M. F. (2006). Central auditory development in children with cochlear implants: Clinical implications. *Advances in Oto-Rhino-Laryngology, 64,* 66–88.

Sharma, A., Dorman, M. F., & Spahr, A. J. (2002). A sensitive period for the development of the central auditory system in children with cochlear implants: Implications for age of implantation. *Ear and Hearing, 23*(6), 532–539.

Shriberg, L. D. (1993). Four new speech and prosody-voice measures for genetics research and other studies in developmental phonological disorders. *Journal of Speech and Hearing Research, 36*(1), 105–140.

Sininger, Y. S., Grimes, A., & Christensen, E. (2010). Auditory development in early amplified children: Factors influencing auditory-based communication outcomes in children with hearing loss. *Ear and Hearing, 31*(2), 166–185.

Sloutsky, V. M., & Napolitano, A. C. (2003). Is a picture worth a thousand words? Preference for auditory modality in young children. *Child Development, 74*(3), 822–833.

Stoel-Gammon, C. (1987). Phonological skills of two year olds. *Language, Speech, and Hearing Services in Schools, 18,* 323–329.

Stoel-Gammon, C. (1991). Normal and disordered phonology in two year olds. *Topics in Language Disorders, 11*(4), 21–32.

Tattersall, H., & Young, A. (2006). Deaf children identified through newborn hearing screening: Parents' experiences of the diagnostic process. *Child: Care, Health and Development, 32*(1), 33–45.

Vouloumanos, A., Hauser, M. D., Werker, J. F., & Martin, A. (2010). The tuning of human neonates' preference for speech. *Child Development, 81*(2), 517–527.

Vouloumanos, A., & Werker, J. F. (2007). Listening to language at birth: Evidence for a bias for speech in neonates. *Developmental Science, 10*(2), 159–164.

Wake, M., Hughes, E. K., Poulakis, Z., Collins, C., & Rickards, F. W. (2004). Outcomes of children with mild-profound congenital hearing loss at 7 to 8 years: A population study. *Ear and Hearing, 25*(1), 1–8.

Wake, M., Poulakis, Z., Hughes, E. K., Carey-Sargeant, C., & Rickards, F. W. (2005). Hearing impairment: A population study of age at diagnosis, severity, and language outcomes at 7-8 years. *Archives of Disease in Childhood, 90*(3), 238–244.

Watkin, P. M., & Baldwin, M. (2011). Identifying deafness in early childhood: Requirements after the newborn hearing screen. *Archives of Disease in Childhood, 96*(1), 62–66.

Werker, J. F., & McLeod, P. J. (1989). Infant preference for both male and female infant-directed talk: A developmental study of attentional and affective responsiveness. *Canadian Journal of Psychology, 43*(2), 230–246.

Werker, J. F., & Tees, R. C. (2005). Speech perception as a window for understanding plasticity and commitment in language systems of the brain. *Developmental Psychobiology, 46*(3), 233–251.

Werker, J. F., & Yeung, H. H. (2005). Speech perception bootstraps word learning in infancy. *Trends in Cognitive Sciences, 9*(11), 519–527.

Werner, L. A. (2002). Infant auditory capabilities. *Current Opinion in Otolaryngology & Head & Neck Surgery, 10*(5), 398–402.

Werner, L. A. (2007). What do children hear? How auditory maturation affects speech perception. *ASHA Leader, 12*(6–7), 32–33.

World Health Organization. (2001). *International classification of functioning, disability and health: ICF.* Geneva: WHO.

Wright, B. A., & Zhang, Y. (2006). A review of learning with normal and altered sound-localization cues in human adults. *International Journal of Audiology, 45*(Suppl. 1), S92–S98.

Yoshinaga-Itano, C. (2003). From screening to early identification and intervention: Discovering predictors to successful outcomes for children with significant hearing loss. *Journal of Deaf Studies and Deaf Education, 8*(1), 11–30.

Yoshinaga-Itano, C., Sedey, A. L., Coulter, D. K., & Mehl, A. L. (1998). Language of early- and later-identified children with hearing loss. *Pediatrics, 102*(5), 1161–1171.

Young, A., & Tattersall, H. (2007). Universal newborn hearing screening and early identification of deafness: Parents' responses to knowing early and their expectations of child communication development. *Journal of Deaf Studies and Deaf Education, 12*(2), 209–220.

2 Understanding Hearing Loss: Implications for Speech Perception

Christian Giguère

▦ Basic Concepts in Childhood Hearing Loss

Spoken language enables social contact and interactions between individuals. While not the only means of human communication, speech offers distinct advantages in conveying simple messages and complex thoughts efficiently and comprehensively over a wide range of situations in daily life (Borden, Harris, & Raphael, 2003; Kent, 1997). The acquisition of spoken language in infants and young children is made possible through the normal process of speech communication itself. Thus, childhood hearing loss may not only be an obstacle to daily communication needs, but it can negatively impact the development of the auditory skills necessary for the processing of speech sounds and the acquisition of language (Northern & Downs, 2002; also see Chapter 1). It is therefore crucially important to detect the presence of hearing loss as early as possible in children and put in place effective rehabilitative strategies to alleviate the impact of hearing loss.

A range of behavioral and physiologic techniques are available to assist the audiologist in assessing hearing in infants and young children for screening and clinical purposes (Madell & Flexer, 2008; Northern & Downs, 2002). Behavioral testing procedures include behavioral observation audiometry (BOA) for infants up to 6 months, visual reinforcement audiometry (VRA) for children 5 to 36 months, and conditioned play audiometry (CPA) for children 30 months to 5 years. Traditional air and bone conduction audiometric techniques may generally be used for older children. Cognitive age, instead of chronological age, is used to select the most appropriate behavioral test, since these tests actively involve the infant or child. Physiologic procedures, such as acoustic immittance, auditory brainstem response (ABR) audiometry, and otoacoustic emission (OAE) testing, provide objective results for all age groups and are often used in conjunction with behavioral procedures to ensure reliable pediatric assessments.

Hearing loss is typically categorized by the type or origin of the dysfunction and the degree of severity. The three basic types are conductive, sensorineural, and mixed hearing losses. A conductive hearing loss affects sound transmission at the level of the external ear or middle ear before it reaches the sensory organ of hearing. Conductive loss may occur due to congenital malformation or absence of the ear canal, a perforated eardrum, reduced mobility of the ossicular chain in the presence of middle ear fluid, or simply excessive accumulation of cerumen, among other causes. In a sensorineural hearing loss, the origin of the damage is located in the sensory organ of hearing (cochlea), typically at the level of the hair cells, or in the auditory nerve up to the first relay stations in the brainstem. A mixed hearing loss includes a conductive and a sensorineural component.

The degree of hearing loss specifies the severity of the dysfunction using broad categories of decrement in hearing sensitivity based on absolute hearing threshold measurements. One of the most common classifications (ASHA, 2011) uses seven categories for the degree of hearing loss (where dB HL represents "decibels hearing level"): normal (thresholds ≤ 15 dB HL), slight (16 to 25 dB HL), mild (26 to 40 dB HL), moderate (41 to 55 dB HL), moderately severe (56 to 70 dB HL), severe (71 to 90 dB HL), and profound (≥ 91 dB HL). It is important to note, however, that hearing thresholds are frequency dependent, and when a single designation is needed, the degree of hearing loss is based on the frequency range thought to be most important for speech understanding—for example, from 500 to 3,000 Hz. Hearing loss is described as unilateral if it affects only one ear, or bilateral if both ears are affected. Bilateral hearing loss may be further designated as symmetrical or asymmetrical depending on whether the degree of hearing loss (or configuration of hearing thresholds) differs across the two ears.

Sample audiograms for two children with bilateral sensorineural hearing losses are illustrated in **Fig. 2.1**. Child A has hearing thresh-

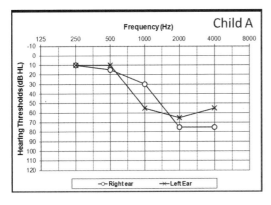 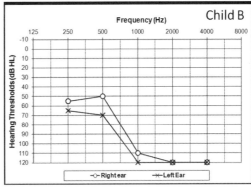

Fig. 2.1   Sample audiograms for two children.

olds just within normal limits in both ears up to 500 Hz, but a moderately severe hearing loss in the left ear and a mild to severe hearing loss in the right ear above 500 Hz. Child B has a moderately severe hearing loss in the left ear and a moderate hearing loss in the right ear up to 500 Hz, while a profound hearing loss is present in both ears above 500 Hz. Child A would normally be prescribed hearing aids, while Child B may be a candidate for cochlear implants. (See Chapters 3 and 4 for discussions of hearing technology.)

Hearing loss is multifaceted and not characterized only by elevated hearing thresholds. Suprathreshold deficits are also common in sensorineural and mixed hearing losses, such as a reduced dynamic range for hearing due to an abnormal growth of loudness with increasing sound level above threshold. A reduced frequency resolution or ability to separate out audible sounds according to frequency content is also a common condition, as is reduced temporal resolution or ability to extract useful signal information during brief gaps or pauses in masking noises. These effects can strongly impact speech understanding in quiet or noisy environments in real life, but they are not well predicted by hearing thresholds. Consequently, there is not an exact relationship between the degree of hearing loss and its impact on speech communication. Furthermore, a variety of disorders collectively referred to as auditory

processing disorders (APDs) affect the transmission and processing of auditory information in some children and adults, mainly in the central auditory system, despite the apparent loss of hearing sensitivity. A wide range of audiologic and other factors (e.g., age, cognitive skills, listening environments, child and family needs) must be considered before establishing a treatment plan and selecting the most appropriate rehabilitation interventions necessary to optimize speech understanding and communication for each individual child (see Chapters 3 to 7).

Over all, the goal of rehabilitation is to consider all aspects of a child's hearing loss and its impact on speech communication and the development of spoken language skills. A primary focus of intervention is invariably to maximize audibility of all speech cues in the diverse listening environments encountered by the child. This may be realized in whole or in part by proper use of rehabilitative technologies (e.g., hearing aids, cochlear implants, personal FM communication systems) to enhance hearing, and by taking full consideration of the fundamentals of speech production and of the transmission of speech sounds in the real-world environments of the child, such as at home and at school. A good understanding of the acoustics of speech communication is therefore essential to promote the most effective rehabilitation strategies.

■ The Acoustics of Speech Communication

The process of speech communication is mediated through the vocal-auditory channel and involves a minimum of three components (**Fig. 2.2**): a talker, an environment (or transmission medium, such as a living room or classroom), and a listener. Factors governing the produc-

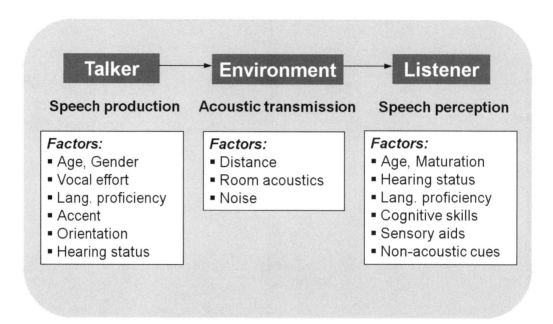

Fig. 2.2 Factors involved in human speech communication.

tion of speech include age, gender, vocal effort, language proficiency, and the accent of the talker and his or her orientation with respect to the listener. Before reaching the listener, speech sounds are modified by the acoustic transmission properties of the surrounding environment, including the effect of distance, early wall or ceiling reflections, late reverberation, and other room acoustic effects. Speech sounds may also be masked by interfering noise sources or competing signals. Auditory factors governing speech perception include age, hearing status, language proficiency and cognitive skills of the listener, the use of sensory aids or other assistive hearing devices, and the availability of nonacoustic cues (e.g., lip reading). In conversational speech, each individual in turn assumes the role of talker and of listener, and this process may involve many different individuals within a group (e.g., children in a classroom). Note that hearing loss may also affect speech production due to the loss of proper acoustic feedback or delays in language acquisition.

Production of Speech Sounds

The acoustic production of speech sounds involves several physiological systems and structures. The respiratory system provides the initial aerodynamic energy during the expiratory phase of breathing. The expiratory airflow in turn makes it possible to activate two distinct sound generation processes or acoustic sources: phonation for voiced sounds and turbulent noise for voiceless sounds (Fucci & Lass, 1999). These acoustic sources are then shaped or filtered by the resonant cavities of the vocal tract to produce a set of roughly 40 basic speech sounds or phonemes in English. The source-filter model of acoustic speech production is summarized in **Fig. 2.3**.

Voiced sounds originate at the larynx as quasi-periodic modulations of glottal airflow caused by fast successive opening and closing of the vocal folds during the process of phonation. Voiced sounds are characterized by a fundamental frequency or F0 at the inverse of the period of vocal fold vibration, and by a series of discrete harmonic components at integer multiples of the fundamental (i.e., at frequencies 2 × F0, 3 × F0, 4 × F0, etc.). Typical F0 values are in the range 100 to 140 Hz for adult males and 180 to 240 Hz for adult females. Children's F0 decreases rapidly with age, typically from as high as 400 to 500 Hz in newborns, to around 300 Hz at 3 to 4 years, and 250 Hz at

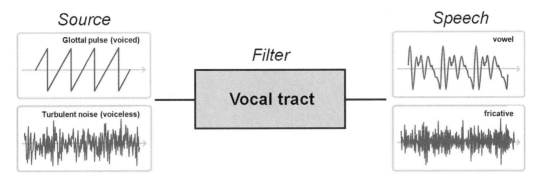

Fig. 2.3   Source-filter model of acoustic speech production.

10 years, before reaching gender-specific values at puberty and remaining relatively stable for several decades (Hixon, Weismer, & Hoit, 2008; Kent, 1997). Late in the lifespan, there is evidence that male F0 increases gradually, while female F0 decreases slightly.

Voiced sounds are filtered (or altered in a frequency-dependent manner) by the resonant cavities of the vocal tract before acoustic radiation into the surrounding environment. The resonant frequencies depend on the vocal tract geometry, as shaped by the position of the articulators at any given time. This results in sharp regions of frequency-selective amplification (or formants) altering the relative amplitude of the voice fundamental and harmonics. The different vowels are produced in this way by articulating different vocal tract shapes, which results in vowel-specific patterns of formant frequencies. Most of the acoustic energy is contained near the three lowest formants (F1, F2, and F3). Across vowels, F1 ranges from about 250 to 1,000 Hz, F2 from 800 to 2,800 Hz, and F3 from 2,000 to 3,600 Hz. Adult females typically have slightly higher (by about 10 to 20%) formant frequencies than adult males owing to their shorter vocal tract on average. Young children have even higher formant frequencies, decreasing toward adult values as physical development progresses. The production of nasal consonants (/m/, /n/, /ŋ/) is very similar to that of vowels except that the lowering of the velum flap to allow air passage to the nasal cavity and the associated closure of air passage through the mouth produce a more complex coupled acoustic resonant system. This system involves anti-formant frequencies, or regions of sharp frequency-selective attenuation, in addition to formants.

Nasal consonants are weaker in intensity than vowels due to the combined effects of the anti-formants and the damping by the soft mucus and cilia lining of the nasal passages. The dominant spectral feature of nasals is the so-called nasal murmur, a strong low-frequency formant around 250 to 300 Hz in adults (Kent, 1997).

Voiceless sounds are aperiodic noises created when the articulators are positioned to produce a major constriction (e.g., tongue elevated toward the alveolar ridge) within vocal tract or obstacle (e.g., teeth) to the expiratory airflow. This induces a turbulent airflow with associated acoustic noise. We can further distinguish between continuous voiceless sounds at the origin of the fricative consonants and transient voiceless sounds at the origin of stop consonants. Fricatives arise from continuous turbulent airflow through a static vocal tract constriction and typically last 100 to 175 ms across the different consonants. Stops are produced in two phases: a complete closure of the vocal tract by the articulators, creating a silent gap for approximately 50 to 90 ms, followed by a sudden release that generates a brief outburst of turbulent airflow and acoustic noise lasting about 10 to 25 ms. Unlike the case with voiced sounds, the acoustic energy of voiceless sounds is continuous in frequency, extending to 8,000 Hz or more. Voiceless sounds are filtered by the formants and antiformants of the vocal tract arising from the resonant properties and interaction of the air cavities on the two sides of the constriction point. The formants occur at higher frequencies than vowels and nasals. The place of constriction along the vocal tract determines the exact values of formants and the spectral shape of the resulting voiceless fricative (e.g.,

/f/, /θ/, /s/, /ʃ/) or stop (/p/, /t/, /k/) consonants. Production of the voiced fricatives (e.g., /v/, /ð/, /z/, /ʒ/) and stops (/b/, /d/, /g/) involves the vibration of the vocal folds in addition to the turbulent noise generation process, and thus they combine the characteristics of periodic and aperiodic sound.

Stops are relatively weak speech sounds, typically 12 to 24 dB less intense than vowels. Bilabials (/p/, /b/) are further characterized by a relatively flat frequency spectrum with some concentration of energy around 500 to 1,500 Hz and decreasing intensity above 5,000 Hz. Alveolars (/t/, /d/) have a broad concentration of energy around 3,000 to 5,000 Hz, and velars (/k/, /g/) typically show narrower peaks of energy in the range of 1,500 to 4,500 Hz (Ferrand, 2007; Hixon et al, 2008; Northern & Downs, 2002). However, their exact acoustic characteristics are very much influenced by the preceding and following vowels through the process of coarticulation. Fricatives are commonly categorized as sibilants (/s/, /z/, /ʃ/, /ʒ/) and nonsibilants (/f/, /v/, /θ/, /ð/). Sibilants are higher in intensity than nonsibilants by about 10 to 12 dB, and show fairly distinct spectral peaks, typically between 2,500 and 4,500 Hz for the palatals (/ʃ/, /ʒ/), and between 4,000 and 8,000 Hz for the alveolars (/s/, /z/) (Ferrand, 2007; Hixon et al, 2008; Northern & Downs, 2002). Nonsilibants are among the weakest speech sounds, characterized by relatively flat or rising frequency spectra with peaks of spectral energy occurring at very high frequencies, typically above 7,000 Hz for both the dentals (/θ/, /ð/) and labiodentals (/f/, /v/).

The acoustic characteristics of the individual speech sounds discussed so far, together with the prosodic features and the effects of coarticulation, are such that connected speech is a very dynamic, or time-varying, signal. There is a great deal of variation in acoustic energy, frequency distribution, and duration across the different phonemes, as clearly seen, for example, on the speech spectrogram for sentences (Borden et al, 2003; Hixon et al, 2008). Even with a constant vocal effort, the amplitude of speech varies over a range of about 30 dB from the weakest voiceless fricatives or stops to the loudest vowels, which are also usually the longest phonemes. The wide variation in the frequency distribution of acoustic energy is also clearly apparent on the speech spectrogram, with vowel and especially nasal energy mainly in the low to middle frequencies and

fricative energy extending over much higher frequencies. In addition to carrying the linguistic meaning of a message, connected speech conveys the personal characteristics and the emotional state of the talker. All these sources of information contribute to the accurate interpretation of spoken messages.

The long-term-average speech spectrum represents the overall contribution of all speech sounds in connected speech (**Fig. 2.4a**) and is often useful in estimating the impact of hearing loss or background noise on the audibility of speech cues, such as for the prescription of hearing aids. It is obtained by summing and averaging acoustic energy by frequency over a range of individuals and types of speech material. For normal vocal effort directly in front of the talker, the speech spectrum shows a broad peak of acoustic energy around 500 Hz, falling thereafter at a rate of about 4 to 6 dB per octave (doubling frequency). As expected, raising the vocal effort increases the overall speech level, typically by 20 dB from normal to shouting (**Fig. 2.4a**). Soft and whispered speech (not illustrated here) is 10 to 20 dB lower than normal speech. It is also clearly apparent in **Fig. 2.4a** that raising the vocal effort shifts energy toward higher frequencies. Consequently, there is a wider range of sound variation at high frequencies with changes in vocal effort than at low frequencies.

The orientation of the talker also affects the overall speech level and spectrum (**Fig. 2.4b**), due to the natural directivity of the human mouth and head baffle. More energy is emitted directly in front of a talker than toward the sides or to the rear. This results in about a 2- to 3-dB decrease in overall speech output toward the sides of the talker, and a 6-dB decrease to the rear, compared with speech output directly in front. However, the decrease is frequency dependent (**Fig. 2.4b**). At frequencies below about 1,000 Hz, the decrease due to orientation is only about 0 to 3 dB toward the sides and 3 to 6 dB to the rear. Speech output toward the sides and rear is more affected at higher frequencies. The loss of speech energy reaches 5 to 7 dB toward the sides and 10 to 18 dB to the rear in the frequency range of 1,500 to 6,000 Hz, compared with a talker directly in front. Altogether, these data indicate that voicing and vowel F1 information may be less affected by talker orientation at a fixed vocal effort, while vowel F2/F3 information and consonant energy may be significantly reduced, especially for speech emitted to the rear.

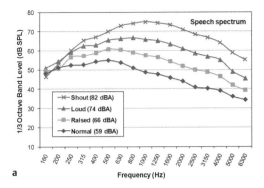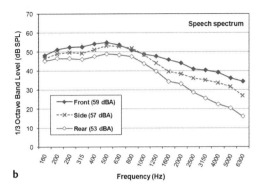

Fig. 2.4a,b Long-term-average speech spectrum in one-third octave bands. **(a)** Effect of vocal effort, one meter in front of talker. (Data from ANSI S3.5.) **(b)** Effect of talker orientation. (Human speech directivity data from Chu and Warnock (2002) applied to ANSI S3.5 speech spectrum at a normal vocal effort.)

Acoustic Transmission

In a free space, such as outdoors in an open area, sound level decreases away from the source at a rate of 6 dB for each doubling of distance (**Fig. 2.5a**) due to the geometric spreading of sound energy. In rooms, this rule applies only within a short distance from the source, such as a talker. Beyond this point, sound level decreases at a lower rate with distance due to room reflections (early and late reverberation) and stabilizes to a fairly uniform sound level far from the source (**Fig. 2.5a**). The decrease in sound level with distance depends on the sound absorption properties of the room surfaces (walls, floor, and ceiling) and objects within the room, which determine the proportion of sound absorbed rather than reflected back.

In a so-called dry room, characterized by highly absorptive surfaces (e.g., heavy carpet and drapes, soft furniture, acoustic ceiling tiles), the 6-dB decrease with doubling of distance will project over a longer distance from a talker than in a "live room" of the same size with surfaces that provide little sound absorption (e.g., hardwood, ceramic, or terrazzo floor; window panes; hard furniture). The speech level will also stabilize to a lower value in a dry room than in a live room (**Fig. 2.5a**). Vocal effort and orientation of the talker with respect to the listening position also affect the speech level in a given room (**Fig. 2.5b**). Raising vocal effort increases the speech level over all distances in a given direction away from the talker. In contrast, at a given vocal effort, the orientation of the talker mostly affects the

speech level in the vicinity of the talker. Due to the directivity of the human mouth (**Fig. 2.4b**), the speech level is lower at close range when the listener is to the side or rear of the talker rather than directly in front, but this effect gradually vanishes with increasing distance from the talker due to room reflections (**Fig. 2.5b**).

In noisy rooms, the characteristics of the talker and the room acoustic effects discussed above have important consequences for speech perception, as they control the signal-to-noise ratio (S/N) at the listening position. It is important, however, to distinguish between the early reflections reaching the listener, within about the first 50 ms after receiving the direct sound from the talker, which arrive soon enough to be integrated with the direct sound as the effective "signal," and the later-arriving reflections (or late reverberation), which are more dissociated from the direct sound and contribute additional "noise." In typical rooms, early reflections can add up to 9 dB in beneficial signal energy over the direct sound, significantly contributing to speech audibility and intelligibility, especially in situations where the talker is not facing the listener (Bradley, Sato, & Picard, 2003). Proper control of reverberation and background noise are thus important acoustic design factors to consider for good speech communication in rooms, and minimum performance requirements exist for the design of learning spaces, such as classrooms (ANSI/ASA S12.60–2010/Part I).

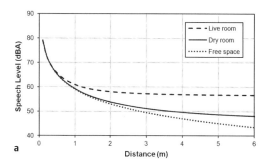 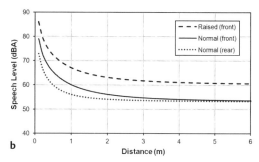

Fig. 2.5a,b Overall speech level as a function of distance from the talker in a small room. **(a)** Effect of room reverberation. **(b)** Effect of vocal effort and talker orientation.

Children with hearing loss typically require a higher S/N than children with normal hearing for similar speech perception performance, even when using properly fitted hearing aids or cochlear implants (see Chapters 3 and 4). Proper orientation and vocal effort by the talker, and appropriate listener distance in the vicinity of the talker will promote good acoustic transmission of speech. In some situations, special facilities may be required to further enhance the speech signal received by the child with hearing loss, even in properly designed acoustical spaces (see Chapter 8). One possible solution is the use of a personal FM transmission system, as often used in the classroom. A microphone near the teacher's mouth picks up the acoustic speech at a very high S/N, and the signal is transmitted wirelessly to the child's location, where it is received and transduced back as acoustic speech and channeled to the child via personal earphones or through sensory aids. This system effectively bypasses the room acoustic transmission effects of distance and reverberation, as well as the effects of talker orientation and vocal effort. The speech picked up is essentially independent of the talker's head and body motion, and the speech level can be controlled electronically at the listener's end. One important benefit of this technology is that it does not alter the acoustic conditions in the room for the other listeners. Sound field FM systems are also sometimes used. In this case, the speech at the receiving end is transmitted acoustically through the directional loudspeaker(s) placed close to the child. Special care must be exercised and expertise sought before using such technology since it can degrade the acoustic conditions for the other listeners, especially in rooms that are too reverberant. Chapter 8 discusses these and other approaches to ensure acoustic accessibility for the child.

Speech Perception

Sound reflections on the torso, diffraction effects of the head, and acoustic resonances of the pinna, concha cavity, and auditory canal all shape the sound signal reaching the human eardrum from the surrounding environment. The resulting transformations of sound to the eardrum, known as the head-related transfer functions (HRTFs), are highly directional and frequency dependent (Blauert, 1997). Consequently, the spectrum of the speech signal reaching the left and right eardrums depends on the angle of sound incidence with respect to the listener (**Fig. 2.6**). Most of the speech energy at the eardrum is contained in the fre-

quency range from 500 to 3,000 Hz, but there are important differences according to the angle of incidence. The overall speech level varies over a range of approximately 8 dB across angles in the horizontal plane, being highest for angles in the frontal-lateral side of the ear facing the source (azimuth angles 0 to 90°) and lowest for source angles on the opposite side of the ear (azimuth angles ≈ –90°) due to the head-shadow effect.

As shown in **Fig. 2.6**, spectral differences across angles of incidence are relatively small (0 to 7 dB) in the frequencies below 1,000 Hz, moderately large (7 to 12 dB) in the frequen-

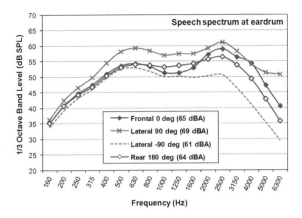

Fig. 2.6 Long-term-average speech spectrum at the listener's eardrum position for four directions of sound incidence (*azimuthal angle*): frontal (*0°*), lateral on the same side (*90°*) or the opposite side (*–90°*) as the source, and from the rear (*180°*). (Free-field to eardrum transfer functions from Shaw and Vaillancourt (1985) applied to ANSI S3.5 speech spectrum at a normal vocal effort.)

cies between 1,000 and 3,000 Hz, and quite large (12 to 22 dB) in the frequencies above 3,000 Hz. This indicates that voicing and vowel F1 information are little affected by the angle of sound incidence reaching the listener, while vowel F2/F3 information and consonant energy are much more variable. Front-rear differences are relatively small (less than 5 dB up to 6,000 Hz), with frontally received speech being more intense except in the range 800 to 1,600 Hz. In contrast, spectral differences are quite large between the ears for laterally received speech, favoring the ear facing the source by about 2 dB at 160 Hz, up to 20 to 25 dB in the range of 6,000 to 8,000 Hz.

In a given talker-listener communication situation, the spectral effects due to the orientation of the talker with respect to the listener position (**Fig. 2.4b**) compound with the spectral effects due to the orientation of the listener with respect to the talker position (**Fig. 2.6**). A most unfavorable situation may occur, for example, if a listener is oriented laterally at the rear of a talker. In this situation the speech signal reaching the opposite ear of the listener may be reduced by roughly 30 dB in the frequency range 4,000 to 6,000 Hz compared with the usual face-to-face communication arrangement. Even without considering the associated loss of visual cues, this high-frequency sound level reduction is 5 to 10 dB more than the talker can compensate for by raising his or her vocal effort from normal to a shout (**Fig. 2.4a**). In a child with unilateral or asymmetrical hearing loss, high-frequency cues important for vowel F2 contrasts (e.g., /i/-/u/) and consonant perception (e.g., /s/, /f/, /θ/) may be greatly reduced or rendered inaudible

in this situation, especially if the opposite ear is the better ear. Proper orientation of the talker and listener is important for maximizing audibility and ensuring accessibility to all speech sounds for children with hearing loss, as is the bilateral fitting of sensory aids to overcome head shadow effects.

It is important to realize, however, that the acoustic effects due to the orientation of the talker and listener are strongly apparent only in free space, where only the direct sound from the talker is reaching the listener, or in real rooms at a close range from the talker, where sound reflections are much weaker than the direct sound. At a distance from the talker in rooms, early reflections from walls, ceiling, and other surfaces provide useful speech signal energy from a range of angles of incidence around the listener, in addition to the direct sound from the talker. Such envelopment of speech information in real rooms from early reflections mitigates the acoustic effects due to talker-listener orientation.

As discussed previously, there are large frequency and intensity differences among the different speech sounds. The main frequency and intensity regions for vowels and consonants are summarized in **Fig. 2.7**. The speech area in this figure represents the frequency-intensity extent for speech produced at normal conversational levels. As illustrated, it spans a range of 30 dB in level, from 15 dB below to 15dB above the long-term speech spectrum at a normal vocal effort one meter in front of the talker (**Fig. 2.4a**). The upper limit thus represents the maximum level of the speech frequency components, whereas the lower limit represents the level below

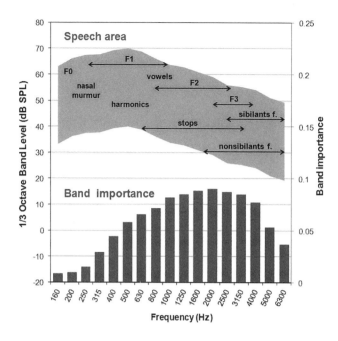

Fig. 2.7 Distribution of the different speech sounds across frequencies and levels in relation to the importance of the speech frequency bands for speech understanding.

which there is no useful speech information (Boothroyd, 2008). The speech area is shown on a vertical axis calibrated in sound pressure levels (dB SPL) to illustrate the relative strength of the different speech sounds on an absolute scale, but it is also often represented on a hearing level scale (dB HL) on an audiogram chart, where it is commonly referred to as the "speech banana" (Boothroyd, 2008; Northern & Downs, 2002).

The maximum acoustic energy around 500 Hz is related to the first formant of vowels, while higher vowel formants and especially consonant energy are weaker and higher in frequency. It is important to realize that not only is speech energy unevenly distributed across frequency (top of **Fig. 2.7**), but the relative information in speech is also frequency dependent (bottom of **Fig. 2.7**). As shown, the relative importance of the speech frequency bands for speech intelligibility is greatest in the range 1,000 to 3,000 Hz. About 70% of the speech information occurs above 1,000 Hz, with 25% above 3,000 Hz. Thus, while most of the acoustic energy in speech due to vowel F1 occurs in the frequencies below about 1,000 Hz, the major contribution to speech understanding is related to vowel F2 and consonant energy above 1,000 Hz.

In a child with normal hearing, the full extent of the speech area is above threshold, as shown in **Fig. 2.8**. All speech cues are audible

and accessible in this case, provided they are not masked by noise. In the case of child A, whose audiogram shows a moderately severe high-frequency hearing loss (**Fig. 2.1a**), low-frequency cues are audible, but high-frequency cues are below threshold and not accessible at a normal vocal effort. Shouted speech raises the speech area by around 20 to 25 dB at middle to high frequencies, which would increase the audibility of vowel F2 and consonant cues for this child, especially in the left ear; however, some speech sounds, such as the weakest fricatives (e.g., /f/, /θ/, /s/), will remain inaudible, especially in the right ear. In the case of child B, whose audiogram shows a profound hearing loss above 500 Hz (**Fig. 2.1b**), only a very small fraction of the speech area is audible at a normal vocal effort, in the right ear near 500 Hz, and no information is accessible in the left ear. Very little additional speech information would result from raising the vocal effort in this case. Consequently, the two children will likely require different audiologic interventions and fitting of sensory aids to ensure acoustic accessibility of all speech sounds in daily life. Boothroyd (2008) provides examples of the benefits of hearing aids and cochlear implants for speech audibility.

Access to acoustic information in relation to absolute hearing threshold is only one of several factors to consider in evaluating the

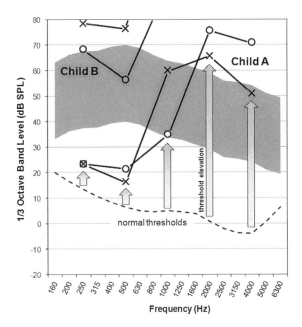

Fig. 2.8 The absolute hearing thresholds of the two children in **Fig. 2.1** in relation to the speech area at a normal vocal effort. Sound field data in dB SPL.

impact of hearing loss on speech understanding. Suprathreshold deficits can distort the speech cues even if audible, and external noise can mask speech information. Adequate linguistic and cognitive skills are also necessary, for example, to benefit from contextual information, as is access to visual and other nonacoustic cues in some cases.

Summary

A primary focus of audiologic intervention in children with hearing loss is to maximize the acoustic accessibility of all speech sounds in the different listening environments encountered in daily life. This requires full consideration of the production, transmission, and perception of speech between the talker(s) and the listening child. The following key points are noteworthy:

- Connected speech is made of many different sounds, voiced (periodic) and voiceless (aperiodic), with widely different frequency and amplitude characteristics, even at a constant vocal effort.
- The long-term-average speech spectrum represents the overall contribution of all speech sounds in connected speech. The normal speech spectrum peaks around 500 Hz and falls thereafter at a rate of about 4 to 6 dB per octave. Raising the vocal effort increases the overall speech level by up to 20 dB for shouted speech and shifts energy somewhat toward higher frequencies.

- The natural directivity of the human mouth is such that more energy is emitted directly in front of the talker than toward the sides or to the rear. Nondirect talker orientations can result in a loss of 3 to 6 dB in overall speech level at the listener's position, with considerably more losses at high frequencies (5 to 18 dB) than at low frequencies (0 to 6 dB).
- The orientation of the listener with respect to the incoming speech signal can result in an overall speech level variation of around 8 dB between the left and right eardrums due to direction-dependent torso reflections, head shadow effects, and acoustic resonances of the pinna and concha. Considerably more variation occurs at high frequencies (12 to 22 dB) than at middle (7 to 12 dB) or low frequencies (0 to 7 dB).
- The speech level decreases by 6 dB per each doubling of distance from a talker in free space. In rooms, this decrease occurs

only within a short distance from the talker. Further away, the level stabilizes due to sound reflections in the room. Early reflections reaching the listener within the first 50 ms after the direct sound can add up to 9 dB in beneficial speech signal energy, but late reverberation is detrimental to speech understanding. Early reflections are also beneficial in reducing the large sound level variations between the listener's ears in free space due to the orientation of the talker and listener.

- About 70% of the speech information is contained in the middle to high frequencies and is related to vowel F2 and consonant energy. Speech cues in this frequency range occur at a lower sound level compared with low-frequency voicing and vowel F1 information.
- Restoring the audibility of high-frequency speech cues in children with hearing loss is an important goal of rehabilitation. Minimizing head-shadow effects through proper talker-listener orientation, bilateral fittings of sensory aids, and other solutions is crucial to ensure acoustic accessibility of speech sounds in all situations.
- Suprathreshold deficits, linguistic and cognitive skills, external noise masking, and access to visual and nonacoustic cues are some of the other factors to consider in the treatment plan.

References

American National Standards Institute [ANSI]. (S12.60–2010). *Acoustical performance criteria, design requirements, and guidelines for schools, part 1: Permanent schools.* Melville, NY: Acoustical Society of America.

American National Standards Institute [ANSI]. (S3.5–1997 R2007). *Methods for the calculation of the speech intelligibility index.* New York: Acoustical Society of America.

American Speech-Language-Hearing Association (ASHA). (2011). Type, degree, and configuration of hearing loss. *Audiology Information Series 7976–16.* Retrieved from http://www.asha.org/uploadedFiles/AIS-Hearing-Loss-Types-Degree-Configuration.pdf

Blauert, J. (1997). *Spatial hearing: The psychophysics of human sound localization.* Cambridge, MA: The MIT Press.

Boothroyd, A. (2008). The acoustic speech signal. In J. R. Madell & C. Flexer (Eds.), *Pediatric audiology: Diagnosis, technology, and management* (pp. 161–169). New York: Thieme Medical Publishers.

Borden, G. J., Harris, K. S., & Raphael, L. J. (2003). *Speech science primer: Physiology, acoustics and perception of speech.* Baltimore, MD: Lippincott, Williams & Wilkins.

Bradley, J. S., Sato, H., & Picard, M. (2003). On the importance of early reflections for speech in rooms. *Journal of the Acoustical Society of America, 113*(6), 3233–3244.

Chu, W. T., & Warnock, A. C. C. (2002). Detailed directivity of sound fields around human talkers (Report IRC-RR-104). *NRC Institute for Research in Construction: Research Report.* Retrieved from http://www.nrc-cnrc.gc.ca/obj/irc/doc/pubs/rr/rr104/rr104.pdf

Ferrand, C. T. (2007). *Speech science: An integrated approach to theory and clinical practice.* Boston, MA: Pearson Education, Allyn & Bacon.

Fucci, D. J., & Lass, N. J. (1999). *Fundamentals of speech science.* Needham Heights, MA: Allyn & Bacon.

Hixon, T. J., Weismer, G., & Hoit, J. D. (2008). *Preclinical speech science: Anatomy, physiology, acoustics, and perception.* San Diego, CA: Plural.

Kent, R. D. (1997). *The speech sciences.* San Diego, CA: Singular.

Madell, J. R., & Flexer, C. (2008). *Pediatric audiology: Diagnosis, technology, and management.* New York: Thieme Medical Publishers.

Northern, J. L., & Downs, M. P. (2002). *Hearing in children.* Baltimore, MD: Lippincott Williams & Wilkins.

Shaw, E. A., & Vaillancourt, M. M. (1985). Transformation of sound-pressure level from the free field to the eardrum presented in numerical form. *Journal of the Acoustical Society of America, 78*(3), 1120–1123.

3 Optimizing Listening Potential through Acoustic Amplification

Teresa Y. C. Ching

Early language development is crucial for learning and paves the way for productive lives. In general, hearing children develop language and speech with little conscious effort, but children with hearing loss have difficulty doing so. After outlining the impact of hearing loss, this chapter examines candidacy for hearing aid amplification. Next, special considerations that apply to the provision of amplification for infants and young children are explained with reference to current evidence that guides best practice. Finally, methods for evaluation of the effectiveness of amplification are discussed together with recommendations for optimizing aural rehabilitation for children.

Impact of Hearing Loss and Candidacy for Hearing Devices

Impact of Hearing Loss

Sounds around us extend over a huge range of intensities, from below the normal threshold of hearing to above the normal level of discomfort or pain. Most of the time people with normal hearing can accommodate the range so that sounds are between their hearing thresholds and discomfort levels. However, this becomes difficult for people with hearing loss because they lose sensitivity for low-intensity sounds, yet perceive high-intensity sounds at close to normal loudness levels (Moore & Glasberg, 1986). The dynamic range is reduced with increasing hearing loss. Some sounds, including speech, may be inaudible or partly inaudible at many frequencies. Even when sounds are made audible through amplification, the ability of the impaired auditory system to separate or resolve the components in a complex sound (or auditory resolution) decreases as hearing loss increases. If we think of the auditory system as being made up of several channels or auditory filters, people with hearing loss show widened filter bandwidths (Moore, 1995, pp. 30–61). Consequently, spectral details of sounds will be smeared, such that /i/ and /u/ may sound similar to a child with severe hearing loss (see Chapter 2 for a detailed explanation of the relation between hearing loss and speech perception), because the individual formant peaks characterizing the respective vowel qualities could not be resolved and coded independently. There will also be more interactions between parts of the signal in different frequency ranges such that speech communication in noisy situations becomes difficult, and this difficulty increases with severity of hearing loss.

Effects of Hearing Loss on Language Development

The effect of a bilateral hearing loss on spoken language development in children has been reported in various studies that included samples of children with hearing loss identified after the first year of life, showing delays in language and literacy (see review by Moeller, Tomblin, Yoshinaga-Itano, Connor, & Jerger, 2007; and discussions in Chapter 1). Population studies in the United Kingdom (Kennedy et al, 2006) and in the Netherlands (Korver et al, 2010) that included children with hearing loss who were identified via universal newborn hearing screening and received intervention before 15 months of age fared no better. On average, the 44 children in the UK study and the 70 children in the Netherlands study performed below one standard deviation (SD) of the mean of normal-hearing children on measures of receptive and expressive language. A recent population study in Australia (Ching, Dillon, Marnane, et al, submitted) that included 255 children with hearing loss identified via newborn screening and who received intervention before 6 months of age indicated that the mean receptive and expressive language scores at 3 years of age were below one SD of the performance of children with normal hearing of the same age. The study calls for improved intervention strategies to take advantage of early detection and intervention to improve child outcomes.

The effect of a unilateral hearing loss on spoken language development and educational outcomes of children is less certain. Several studies on school-aged children recruited from clinical settings (Borg, Risberg, McAllister, Undermar, & Edquist, 2002; Sedey, Carpenter, & Stredler-Brown, 2002) and from school hearing screening records (Lieu, Tye-Murray, Karzon, & Piccirillo, 2010) revealed deficits in speech and language development. On the other hand, there were also reports that revealed no significant deficits (Keller & Bundy, 1980; Kiese-Himmel, 2002; Klee & Davis-Dansky, 1986; Tieri, Masi, Ducci, & Marsella, 1988). As no population-based studies on children with congenital unilateral hearing loss have been published, there is some uncertainty about the impact of untreated unilateral hearing loss on child outcomes. Nevertheless, it may be expected that binaural processes will suffer as a consequence of hearing loss of sufficient degree in the impaired ear that is untreated. This condition will make listening to speech in noisy and reverberant environments, such as classrooms, very difficult for the child.

Similar to the situation with unilateral hearing loss, it is also not clear whether the presence of a slight or mild hearing loss at birth adversely affects language development and educational outcomes of children. Research findings are contradictory, with some suggesting an adverse effect (Bess, Dodd-Murphy, & Parker, 1998; Tharpe, 2008) and others not (Wake et al, 2006).

The impact of congenital auditory neuropathy spectrum disorder (ANSD) on children's language development is not well understood. The presence of ANSD is characterized by elevated or abnormal auditory brainstem waveforms with evidence of cochlear outer hair cell function (Berlin, Morlet, & Hood, 2003). Children with ANSD can present with pure tone thresholds that vary from normal levels to profound degrees with wide-ranging configurations (Berlin et al, 2010; Sininger & Oba, 2001). Unlike people with sensorineural hearing loss, those with ANSD usually show normal frequency resolution and varying degrees of temporal disruption (Rance, 2005). Some children with ANSD demonstrate difficulties with speech understanding, which has been attributed to their reduced ability to perceive frequency and amplitude changes over time and to use amplitude envelope cues in speech. On the other hand, a recent population study on children with hearing impairment revealed that for a certain hearing threshold level, language outcomes at 3 years of age were not significantly different, on average, between children with ANSD and those without ANSD (Ching, Gardner-Berry, Day, Dillon, & Seeto, in preparation). The study recommended that children with ANSD should be provided with early intervention in the same way as children with sensorineural hearing loss.

Candidacy for Hearing Devices

A major goal of amplification is to provide an audible signal across as wide a frequency range as possible to maximize speech intelligibility while keeping overall loudness within a comfortable range. When a child is diagnosed with hearing loss, early provision of amplification supports development of communication between the child and the family, helps to avoid the negative effects of auditory deprivation (Hattori, 1993), and facilitates language development with educational intervention. Early auditory stimulation in both ears also enables development of neural connections that support binaural processing of sounds so that auditory functions, including localization and binaural suppression of noise, may be performed (Beggs & Foreman, 1980; Van Deun et al, 2010). Therefore, bilateral amplification should be provided to children with bilateral hearing impairment unless there is clear evidence that performance with two hearing aids is poorer than with one.

Once the degree of hearing loss can be estimated for at least one low (e.g., 500 Hz) and one high frequency (e.g., 2 kHz), amplification should be provided. For infants and young children, the estimation typically relies on auditory evoked potentials that provide frequency-specific information for each ear. Commonly used measures include auditory brainstem responses (Stapells, 2000), auditory steady-state responses (Rance et al, 2005) and electrocochleography (Wong, Gibson, & Sanli, 1997). These electrophysiological thresholds are reported in decibels nHL (normalized hearing level), the lowest stimulus level at which an electrophysiological response is present, relative to the lowest stimulus level at which adults with normal hearing report hearing the same stimuli. The electrophysiological thresholds must be converted into predicted behavioral thresholds for the infants by the use of correction figures (for a discussion, see Bagatto et al, 2005). Although the conversion can be done manually using published figures, it is more conveniently done using the hearing aid fitting software. Both the NAL-NL2 and DSL m[i/o] software allow direct entry of the observed electrophysiological thresholds and automatically convert them into predicted behavioral thresholds for calculating targets for amplification.

Because it is uncertain whether the presence of mild or minimal hearing loss has negative effects on a child's development, it is also not clear whether amplification reduces such effects. The same can be said for children with unilateral hearing loss. Therefore, decisions to fit hearing aids should be made on a case-by-case basis, taking into consideration the preferences of parents and the needs of the child. Where hearing thresholds on the impaired side show that loss is profound, the only technology that is likely to be effective is the use of wireless transmission from a microphone worn by a talker to a receiver worn by the child. This form of wireless transmission will provide the clearest speech no matter what degree of loss is present in the impaired ear. Even if hearing aids are not fitted to children with mild loss or unilateral hearing loss in their first few years of life, it is important to monitor their hearing status regularly because the hearing loss may progress to more severe degrees, or progress from unilateral to bilateral loss (Johansen, Hauch, Christensen, & Parving, 2004).

For children with average hearing thresholds exceeding 90 dB HL, it is generally recognized that performance with cochlear implants is superior to that with hearing aids (Archbold, Nikolopoulos, Lutman, & O'Donoghue, 2002; Mildner, Sindija, & Zrinski, 2006; Van Lierde, Vinck, Baudonck, De Vel, & Dhooge, 2005). Nonetheless, hearing aids provide stimulation to the auditory pathway prior to cochlear implantation, and the provision of early stimulation appears to increase children's ability to use binaural cues later in life (Van Deun et al, 2010). In fact, performance while wearing hearing aids is one of the factors to be considered before making the decision on whether to implant.

For children who receive a cochlear implant in one ear with residual hearing that can be aided in the other ear, a hearing aid should be fitted to the latter ear. There is ample evidence to indicate that a hearing aid in the other ear provides complementary speech cues (Ching & Incerti, 2012; Ching, van Wanrooy, & Dillon, 2007) and continued stimulation of the contralateral pathways of the auditory system. Acoustic amplification provides speech cues relating to fundamental frequency (Ching, 2011), which are important for acquiring suprasegmental and prosodic contrasts in speech and for perception of music (McDermott, 2011). Such information, however, is not well transmitted in current cochlear implant processing. For this reason, provision of low-frequency information via hearing aids complements the high-frequency information available through cochlear implants. For children with bilateral cochlear implants, those with prior experience of bimodal stimulation acquire better expressive language than those without such experience (Nittrouer & Chapman, 2009).

Children with ANSD are a special population for whom it is difficult to estimate the degree of pure-tone loss. For this reason, it has been general practice to delay intervention until reliable behavioral hearing thresholds can be obtained. As an estimated 60 to 90% of children with congenital ANSD have pure-tone loss of greater than 40 dB HL (Rance, 2005; Sininger & Oba, 2001), a delay in fitting amplification results in auditory deprivation that may have permanent adverse effects. In a recent population study that included children with ANSD who were fitted with hearing aids or provided with cochlear implants early in life (Ching, Gardner-Berry, et al, in preparation; Gardner-Berry, Ching, & Day, in preparation), the provision of early stimulation relied on the use of auditory evoked cortical potentials to determine the audibility of speech sounds in unaided and aided conditions. The evidence supports early amplification or cochlear implantation to restore audibility for children with or without ANSD.

▪ Pediatric Amplification

Special considerations apply to selection of hearing aid technology and fitting of hearing aids for infants and young children. They have smaller ears than adults do, they rely on auditory input to develop speech and language, they are not able to manually adjust their devices to optimize listening in different environments, and they are often not able to provide reliable verbal feedback about the effectiveness of amplification.

Once parents have made the decision for their child to be fitted with hearing aids, the style and size of device need to be selected. For infants and young children, behind-the-ear hearing aids are typically chosen for two reasons. First, a child's ears grow rapidly, especially over the first few years of life. The changing geometry of the ear canal necessitates frequent replacement of earmolds or devices to maintain a good fit, with earmolds being much less expensive to replace than in-the-ear devices that have to be custom-made for the user. Second, children often require certain hearing aid features, including directional microphones, direct audio input capability, and built-in receivers for wireless transmission, which are available only in behind-the-ear devices. The size of hearing aid to be fitted to a child depends largely on the degree of hearing loss, as the device must have maximum output that is sufficient to provide the gain required for adequate audibility.

The more severe the hearing loss, the higher the maximum output required, and typically the larger the hearing aid. For safety purposes, hearing devices fitted to children should have tamper-resistant battery doors to minimize the risk of battery ingestion.

The use of devices by children is typically mediated by parents or caregivers. Indeed, a recent study (Gilliver, Ching, & Sjahalam-King, submitted) revealed that parents felt that they were ill equipped for this role because they could not tell whether hearing aids were functioning properly, nor could they troubleshoot when they suspected a malfunction in the devices. Parents also expressed anxiety about supporting maximal hearing aid use during their child's first few years of life and yearned for better support with understanding. Consistent with other studies (Elfenbein, 2000; McCracken, Young, & Tattersall, 2008; Moeller, Hoover, Peterson, & Stelmachowicz, 2009; Sjoblad, Harrison, Roush, & McWilliam, 2001), strategies for device retention, troubleshooting, and counseling are required. A recent population study of children who were identified via newborn hearing screening in Australia shows consistent use of devices at 6 months after initial intervention, and by the time the children were 3 years of age, the hearing devices were used for more than 75% of the children's waking hours (Marnane & Ching, in preparation).

Hearing Aid Prescription for Children

The two most widely used prescriptive procedures for children are the Desired Sensation Level (DSL, Scollie et al, 2005; Seewald, Cornelisse, & Ramji, 1997) procedure and the National Acoustic Laboratories (NAL, Byrne, Dillon, Ching, Katsch, & Keidser, 2001; Dillon, Keidser, Ching, Flax, & Brewer, 2011) procedure. The DSL procedure prescribes more low-frequency gain than the NAL procedure for flat hearing loss, and more high-frequency gain than the NAL procedure for sloping loss (Byrne et al, 2001). Overall gain is higher for the DSL procedures than for the NAL procedure, across a range of input levels (Ching, Johnson, et al, in press). In choosing between prescriptions, the question to be addressed is whether the procedure that provides higher gain or the one associated with greater audibility leads to bet-

ter outcomes, and whether overall loudness is maintained at a comfortable level.

A comprehensive study performed in both Canada and Australia used a counterbalanced crossover design to compare the performance and preference of school-aged children when they used the NAL-NL1 versus the DSL [i/o] prescription (Ching, Scollie, Dillon, & Seewald, 2010). Despite a difference in overall gain of around 10 to 20 dB between prescriptions when applied in hearing aids (Ching et al, 2010), speech intelligibility was equally good for the two prescriptions (Scollie et al, 2010b). On average, identification of consonants in nonsense syllables presented in quiet was close to perfect, and the sentence reception threshold in noise was almost as good as for normal-hearing peers. There was, nonetheless, a tendency for children to prefer the

NAL-NL1 when listening in noisy real-world situations and the DSL [i/o] when listening in quiet situations or when listening to speech at low levels (Scollie et al, 2010a). There was also a tendency for children to prefer the prescription that they had prior experience with. The study demonstrated that the effect of prescription on children's speech perception was not significant. However, the choice of prescription may be important for children's development of speech and language when amplification is provided from the first few months of life. This question was addressed in a recent population study that randomly assigned hearing aid prescriptions to children for first fitting after diagnosis (Ching, Dillon, Hou, et al, in press). In that study, the speech, language, and functional development of 218 children were measured at 3 years of age. Despite the higher gains provided by the DSL compared with the NAL procedure, the choice of prescription for fitting was not significantly related to the development of auditory comprehension or expressive communication by children. As indicated in a comprehensive review of evidence on the effect of prescription on young children (Ching, 2012), amplification should be provided to children with hearing loss at an early age, using either the NAL or the DSL prescription.

Hearing Aid Technology for Children

Children rely on amplified auditory input to develop speech and language, and to acquire knowledge about the world around them. They need to hear speech at higher sensation levels than adults (Byrne, 1983; Nozza, Rossman, & Bond, 1991), and they need a higher signal-to-noise ratio than adults to understand speech in noisy environments (Gravel, Fausel, Liskow, & Chobot, 1999). **Table 3.1** gives a summary of features that are important for infants and young children.

Table 3.1 Amplification goals and hearing aid features

Age	Primary goals	Features
0–2 years	• Listening comfort • Ensure audibility • Support communication with family • Facilitate speech and language development	• Small behind-the-ear hearing aids • Wide dynamic range compression • Flexibility, multiple channels • Multiple listening programs • Feedback cancellation • Automatic switchable directional microphones • Tamper-proof battery door • Friction hook securely glued or screwed in place • Hearing aid retainers
2–5 years	• All of the above • Support communication in educational and play settings	• All of the above • Direct audio input • Telecoil to facilitate use of FM and telephone, if needed • Frequency lowering, if needed
5–11 years	• All of the above • Hear teacher and peers in school setting • Support communication with peers in social settings, sports • Support use of telephone	• All of the above • Telecoil to facilitate use of FM and telephone • Options for in-the-ear hearing aids, open fits
Young adulthood	• All of the above • Support communication in complex situations and listening environments	• All of the above • Options for in-canal devices

Wide Dynamic Range Compression

To achieve audibility with amplification, the wide range of real-world input levels needs to be compressed into the reduced dynamic range of an impaired ear. If the same amount of gain for low-level sounds to be audible is applied to high-level sounds, loudness discomfort may occur in many instances. Whereas adults can manipulate a volume control to ensure that input sounds over a range of levels are always amplified to achieve a preferred listening level, infants and young children are not able to do so. And yet they have as much need as an adult user of hearing aids to listen at a comfortable level with amplification. For this reason, an automated feature in hearing aids that gradually reduces gain as the input level rises above a middle range, and increases gain as the input level decreases below the middle range, would be essential for children. Wide dynamic range compression (WDRC) does precisely this.

WDRC not only ensures comfortable listening at all times, which is of utmost importance if devices are to be worn consistently, it also is beneficial for speech acquisition and functional performance in real life. There is evidence to suggest that WDRC is superior to linear amplification for perception of speech presented at low levels, horizontal localization at low levels, and functional performance in real life (Ching, Hill, Van Wanrooy, & Agung, 2004). Better perception of speech at low levels is crucial for children, as they rely on overhearing and incidental learning for acquiring speech and language (Akhtar, 2005). A comprehensive review of evidence on WDRC for children (Ching, 2012) left no doubt that it should be provided in hearing aids for infants and children.

Directional Microphones

Young children with hearing loss, like similar adults, have much difficulty understanding speech in noisy situations. There is evidence to suggest that children need a higher signal-to-noise ratio (S/N) than adults to perceive speech (Gravel et al, 1999; Nozza et al, 1991). They possibly need it even more often than adults because they are still acquiring language through hearing and have little or no ability to draw on contextual information and world knowledge to enhance speech perception as adults do.

The only feature in modern hearing aids that improves signal-to-noise ratio in noisy places is the directional microphone. However, young children have long been denied access to directional microphones because of disadvantages linked to fixed directionality. These include increased pickup of wind noise and reduced audibility of sounds coming from behind or from the sides. As a result, conventional wisdom has it that fixed directionality should not be used for children. Manual switching between microphone modes from omni to directional is also not viable; an astute observer/caregiver would have to be super-vigilant of the child hearing-aid user to switch between modes as called for by the changing environment (Moeller, Donaghy, Beauchaine, Lewis, & Stelmachowicz, 1996). With advances in technology, however, many hearing aids will automatically enable/disable directional microphones (i.e., switch from omni to directional mode) based on analysis of the environment they are in. Because young children are not able to operate manual switches, and it is not practical for a vigilant adult to continually observe the changing listening environments and needs of a child, an automatic switching arrangement in devices for young children is necessary. Benefits from an automatically switching directionality are possible as long as the switching mechanism chooses directional mode more often when speech is from the front and omnidirectional mode more often when speech is from the side or from the rear.

There is evidence from a study of hearing-impaired and normal-hearing children between 11 and 78 months of age showing that young children orient toward the dominant talker approximately 40% of the time in real-world environments (Ching, O'Brien, et al, 2009). This behavior allows directional advantage in situations that may be difficult for the child. From physical principles, directional microphones will offer an improved S/N to a child when the child is looking at the sound source within a distance that is not too much greater than the critical distance of the room, and if there is noise or reverberation in the environment. Quantification of the effect of directional microphones in real-life environments suggests that an advantage of about 3 dB is obtainable in these situations (Ching, O'Brien, et al, 2009). There are, nonetheless, potential disadvantages when the child is looking away from the primary talker (Ricketts & Galster, 2008). In those circumstances, even though sounds from the side or from behind will be attenuated by directional microphones, the compressor in a hearing aid with WDRC will increase gain for these sounds so that the net decrease is only about half of that associated with a directional microphone acting alone.

Children with normal binaural processing abilities are able to improve speech perception in noise when the location of noise is separated from the location of speech (Ching, van Wanrooy, Dillon, & Carter, 2011; Litovsky, 2005). This ability requires the child to use input from both ears effectively to reduce the effect of noise masking. Many children with hearing loss, however, demonstrate a deficit in this binaural processing ability. For these children, the provision of directional microphone capabilities in their hearing aids is crucial to enable them to hear speech in noise. As revealed in a comprehensive review of evidence on directional microphones for children (Ching, 2012), the current evidence supports the use of automatically switchable directionality in hearing aids for infants and young children to enable them to monitor the environments around them as well as to enhance the S/N in noisy situations when they look at the talker of interest.

Feedback Management

Whenever the real-ear-aided gain of a hearing aid exceeds the attenuation of the signal as it leaks from the ear canal, out past the earmold, and to the hearing aid microphone, feedback oscillation (whistling) is likely. Feedback is a particular problem for infants and young children because they are often in positions where reflecting surfaces are in close proximity to the head, such as lying down or leaning against a supporting body or object, and also because children's ear canals rapidly change in shape and size over their first few years of life, resulting in less-than-ideal fitting. Once feedback oscillation occurs, it reduces the amplification that the hearing aid can provide to external sounds, may mask perception of other sounds, and may be annoying to the child and to those in the vicinity.

Feedback oscillation must therefore be prevented. First and foremost is the need to ensure that earmolds provide a good fit, and to replace them as often as is necessary. Coating the ear-mold with gel is helpful in minimizing leakage. If oscillation does not disappear even after a good fit is ensured, conventional feedback management may be applied by reducing gain in the hearing aid. This may be implemented either on a broadband basis or only in frequency regions where the oscillation occurs.

Most advanced hearing aids now include a feedback cancellation algorithm that automatically detects feedback oscillation and takes measures to suppress it. Feedback cancellation enables the achievement of higher gain, and so can directly improve the audibility of speech. Even though it may produce some distortions or extraneous sounds when it is actively applied aggressively to prevent oscillation, these artifacts are not as bad as the feedback oscillation they are preventing. Feedback cancellation should routinely be enabled in hearing aids for young children unless the loss is moderate such that feedback oscillation is unlikely to be a problem.

Fitting and Verification of Hearing Aids

Determining hearing thresholds is the first step toward hearing aid fitting. Because a newborn has smaller ears than an average adult, and because transducers of earphones are calibrated so that an average adult with normal hearing has thresholds of 0 dB HL, the calibration will not be appropriate for an infant with normal hearing. As a child grows, the length and volume of the ear canal change. These changes impact hearing assessment as well as the hearing aid fitting method chosen. Ear canal length is directly related to the resonant frequency of the unaided ear canal and, hence, to the frequency of the peak of the real-ear, unaided gain curve. On average, the resonant frequency is around 5 to 6 kHz at birth and decreases to around 3 kHz by the age of 2 to 3 years, close to the resonance of 2.7 kHz that applies to the average adult (Kruger, 1987). If stimuli are presented via supra-aural headphones, the infant's very-high-frequency canal resonance will make hearing thresholds worse than they really are at 3 kHz (Voss & Herrmann, 2005). The volume of the ear canal increases as the child grows. If stimuli are presented via an insert earphone, a higher sound pressure level (SPL) will be present in the infant's ear than in the adult's ear at all frequencies. The infant will therefore appear to have less hearing loss than the adult at all frequencies. Hearing thresholds (in dB HL) may therefore appear to change during the first few years of a child's life just because of changes in the size of the child's ears (Moodie, Sinclair, Fisk, & Seewald, 2000). Both the DSL and the NAL procedures effectively resolve the issue of changing ear geometry. The DSL procedure expresses hearing thresholds in terms of dB SPL in the ear canal (Seewald & Scollie, 2003), whereas the NAL procedure expresses thresholds in terms of equivalent adult hearing level (Ching & Dillon, 2003).

Consideration of ear canal acoustics is essential not only for determining hearing thresholds, but also for specifying the gain-frequency response targets for fitting. The changing resonant characteristics of a child's unaided ear canal over time require that prescriptive targets be specified in terms of real-ear-aided gain (REAG) rather than real-ear insertion gain if the amplified levels at a child's eardrum are to provide consistent stimulation to the auditory system as the child grows. A REAG target specifies the increase in signal level when the ear is aided relative to the level of the signal in the sound field, irrespective of the gain provided by the unaided ear canal. The REAG can be expressed as the sum of the real ear–coupler difference (RECD) and the gain measured in a coupler (CG), that is, REAG = RECD + CG. For a certain audiogram, individual coupler gain targets to achieve a prescribed REAG can be derived once the RECD of the ear is known. For a given REAG, higher coupler gains will be required as RECD decreases with age-related growth in the size of the ear canal. If measurement of individual RECD is not possible, published age-appropriate values may be used. Both the DSL and the NAL procedures incorporate age-appropriate RECDs in their fitting software and provide REAG and CG targets for fitting.

Using the REAG-CG approach for fitting, verification can be achieved by adjusting and measuring the hearing aids in an HA2-2cc coupler to match prescriptive targets (Bagatto et al, 2005; King, 2010). Other methods have also been used, including the measurement of aided thresholds and calculations of audibility. Measurements of aided thresholds have poor reliability, are susceptible to circuit and amplified room noise, and are very time consuming to measure, even for children who are able to provide reliable behavioral responses (Hawkins, 2004). Visual displays of aided speech audibility show how much of an assumed speech spectrum is audible to a child when hearing aids are worn. Calculated audibility or measures of aided thresholds do not ensure that the amplification is optimally effective for an individual (Byrne & Ching, 1997). Therefore, evaluation of the effectiveness of amplification is crucial.

■ Evaluation of Effectiveness of Amplification

Effective amplification makes speech audible in a way that enables a hearing-impaired child to extract the most information possible from the audible signal. Making speech audible is undoubtedly central to effective amplification, but maximizing audibility will not always optimize speech intelligibility. There is evidence to suggest that predicting speech intelligibility from calculated audibility results in an overestimation for children (Scollie, 2008) and adults with severe hearing loss (Ching, Dillon, & Byrne, 1998). Especially in frequency regions where hearing loss is severe or profound, greater audibility leads to little or no improvement in speech intelligibility but an increase in loudness. The latter is a concern when loudness gives rise to discomfort, resulting in reduced usage of the device. The budget for loudness is limited in the impaired ear due to the reduced dynamic range associated with the impairment. More effective audibility is likely to result from amplification characteristics that furnish more loudness to frequency regions where audibility contributes more to speech intelligibility than to other regions, while keeping the overall loudness within the range of comfortable listening (Ching, Dillon, Katsch, & Byrne, 2001).

In the fitting of hearing aids to adults or older children, it is common to ask for verbal feedback and then fine-tune their devices accordingly. When one is fitting hearing aids to infants and young children, however, reliable verbal feedback on the quality of amplification is often not possible. Although prescriptions meet amplification needs on average, individuals may differ in preferred gain and frequency response, and in their perceptions of aided speech intelligibility and sound quality (Byrne, 1986; Leijon, Lindkvist, Ringdahl, & Israelsson, 1990). Previous studies have revealed that about one-third to one-quarter of children functioned more effectively in real life when they used hearing aids that provided either more or less low-frequency emphasis than the targets prescribed for fitting (Ching, Hill, & Dillon, 2008). Furthermore, advances in signal processing features in hearing aids need to be evaluated for their effectiveness in children. When there are changes in hearing thresholds that call for modifications of fitting, it is also necessary to check that the amplification is optimal for the child.

How to Evaluate

A range of methods are available for evaluation of the effectiveness of amplification (Bagatto, Moodie, Seewald, Bartlett, & Scollie, 2011; Stelmachowicz, 1999), including speech tests (Bess et al, 1996), loudness ratings (Kawell, Kopun, & Stelmachowicz, 1988), paired-comparison judgments (Ching, Hill, Birtles, & Beecham, 1999; Eisenberg & Levitt, 1991), subjective reports by parents and teachers (for a summary, see Ching & Hill, 2007; also Bagatto et al, 2011), and objective methods using electrophysiological measurements. As indicated in a comprehensive review of evidence (Ching, 2012), effectiveness of amplification for children is best determined by evaluating aided performance using subjective reports and objective electrophysiological measures. **Table 3.2** shows the age range for which different types of evaluation methods apply.

Table 3.2 Evaluation tools

Tools		Children < 3 years	Children 3–5 years	Children ≥ 6 years
Subjective	Laboratory/ ideal conditions		Speech tests (limited by language ability)	Speech perception tests (limited by language ability) Loudness rating Paired-comparison judgment
	Real-world environments	Parents' report Teachers' report	Parents' report Teachers' report	Parents' report Teachers' report Self-report
Objective	Laboratory conditions	Cortical auditory evoked potential	Cortical auditory evoked potential	Cortical auditory evoked potential

Subjective Evaluation: Report Tools

The performance of hearing aids (or cochlear implants or both) can be evaluated by asking the parent, the teacher, and the child—when he or she is old enough to provide information—about how much the devices help in real life. Of the report measures published to date, the Parents' Evaluation of Aural/Oral Performance of Children (PEACH, Ching & Hill, 2007), the Infant-Toddler Meaningful Auditory Integration Scale (IT-MAIS, Zimmerman-Phillipps, Osberger, & Robbins, 1998), and the Meaningful Auditory Integration Scale (MAIS, Robbins, Renshaw, & Berry, 1991) have been shown to be significantly correlated with other measures of hearing function or speech and language ability.

PEACH is a functional assessment scale that is based on a systematic use of parents' observations of their child functioning in real-world quiet and noisy situations. Extensive normative data, including information on test–retest reliability, inter-rater reliability, critical difference scores, internal consistency, and subscale scores, are available for children between 1 month and 4 years of age (Ching & Hill, 2007; Ching et al, 2008). A form with items suitable for teachers (Teachers' Evaluation of Aural/Oral Performance of Children, TEACH) and a form for self-report by older children (Self Evaluation of Listening Function, SELF) are also available. All forms are freely downloadable (www.outcomes.nal.gov.au). There is evidence to show that the PEACH scores correlate with standardized measures of children's language development (Ching, Dillon, Day, & Crowe, 2007) at 3 years of age and with objective measures of audibility based on evoked cortical responses in infants (Golding et al, 2007). For comparisons of the relative effectiveness of different amplification conditions, the difference in PEACH scores correlates with the difference in TEACH scores and with preference judgments obtained from children (Ching et al, 2008).

There are also reports on correlations between the IT-MAIS scores and the latency of evoked cortical responses in children with ANSD (Sharma, Cardon, Henion, & Roland, 2011) and with speech babbling in infants (Kishon-Rabin, Taitelbaum-Swead, Ezrati-Vinacour, & Hildesheimer, 2005). There is also evidence showing that the MAIS scores correlate with monosyllable word identification scores for children with cochlear implants (Robbins, Svirsky, Osberger, & Pisoni, 1998).

Alternative approaches to the use of standardized questionnaires are to set listening goals for individuals based on parents' expectations (Family Expectations Worksheet, Palmer & Mormer, 1999; Client-Oriented Scale of Improvement—Child Version, www.nal.gov.au). In these instances, the milestones of normal-hearing children (Developmental Index of Audition and Listening [DIAL], Palmer & Mormer, 1999) may be used as a guide.

Objective Electrophysiological Measure

Objective electrophysiological testing has been used extensively for hearing assessment of infants, and its results often form the basis for predicting hearing thresholds for fitting hearing aids to infants and young children. An objective method for evaluating the appropriateness of amplification is to use cortical auditory evoked potentials (CAEPs). This method allows speech sounds to be used as stimuli and records electrophysiological responses from the cortical region. CAEPs can be reliably recorded in infants and young children in response to speech stimuli under aided and unaided conditions (Cone-Wesson & Wunderlich, 2003), and their presence has been correlated with auditory perception and normal receptive language at 1 year of age (Kurtzberg, 1989). In a recent study of 28 aided infants and children ages 6 weeks to 3 years and 5 months (Golding et al, 2007), the presence or absence of CAEPs to three speech stimuli that have spectral peaks in the low, middle, and high frequency regions was compared with observed auditory behaviors solicited using the PEACH questionnaire (Ching & Hill, 2007). A positive correlation between the number of detected CAEPs and the age-corrected PEACH score was found. The results suggest that detection of

CAEPs to speech stimuli is a valid measure of aided functional performance in infants and young children.

There are several reasons why this objective method of CAEP testing is valuable for evaluation of the effectiveness of amplification for young children. First, initial hearing aid fitting is often based on hearing thresholds estimated from electrophysiological test results. Such estimates may result in under-amplification even when prescriptive targets derived from the predicted hearing thresholds have been well matched. An absence of CAEP responses under aided conditions would suggest that the hearing aid may not provide sufficient gain for audibility in some frequency regions. If these test outcomes are consistent with other information about the child, hearing aid gain frequency responses should be adjusted.

Second, if every effort has been made to fine-tune a child's hearing aid and there is still an absence of CAEP response with aiding, this is a particularly important piece of information to contribute to a referral or decision about cochlear implantation. Because current evidence clearly attests to the importance of implantation within the first year of life (Ching, Dillon, et al, 2009) to facilitate speech and language development, there should be no delays in referral for cochlear implant candidacy evaluation if the optimal listening opportunity can be afforded only by the use of a cochlear implant.

Third, in some cases of ANSD, CAEP responses may be detected when auditory brainstem responses (ABRs) are abnormal or absent (Hood, 1999; Rance, Cone-Wesson, Wunderlich, & Dowell, 2002). A case study of an infant who had repeatable CAEPs to speech stimuli presented at conversational levels demonstrated the inaccuracy of the severity of hearing loss suggested by ABR results and could have led to over-amplification had hearing aids been adjusted on the basis of the estimated thresholds (Pearce, Golding, & Dillon, 2007). A recent population study suggests that children diagnosed with ANSD would benefit from amplification in the same way as those without ANSD (Ching, Gardner-Berry, et al, in preparation), so long as the amplification is guided by detection of speech sounds as evidenced by CAEP responses. This approach of using CAEP responses to evaluate hearing requirements will minimize the risk of damage to the outer hair cells by amplified sound (Stredler-Brown, 2002).

The presence of CAEPs to speech stimuli provides physiological evidence that the stimuli have arrived at the cortex and are potentially audible to the infant with hearing aids fitted (Korczak, Kurtzberg, & Stapells, 2005). Detection is the first step in the cognitive processes associated with discrimination of speech. Without sound detectability, a child cannot be expected to develop spoken language.

In summary, each child should receive an evaluation of outcomes after amplification is provided to validate benefits or assist with fine tuning. Evaluations should also be performed after introduction of new features or technology that supports hearing aid amplification, and at different ages or stages of development when amplification needs increase in complexity. For all children, regular monitoring of progress should be undertaken and evaluation of the effectiveness of amplification should be an integral part of the process of aural rehabilitation.

The ultimate goal of aural rehabilitation is that the child with hearing loss develops good speech and language abilities. Even though attainment of this goal relies on a range of factors, some of which are not directly related to hearing (Ching, Dillon, Marnane, et al, submitted), optimizing hearing is a first and necessary step. Given consistent usage of hearing devices, stimulating auditory input, and effective educational intervention, children with hearing loss may be expected to have access to the same opportunities as their normal-hearing peers.

◼ Acknowledgments

I am grateful to Harvey Dillon, Alison King, and Kirsty Gardner-Berry for sharing their thoughts on some of the issues discussed in this chapter.

References

Akhtar, N. (2005). The robustness of learning through overhearing. *Developmental Science, 8*(2), 199–209.

Archbold, S. M., Nikolopoulos, T. P., Lutman, M. E., & O'Donoghue, G. M. (2002). The educational settings of profoundly deaf children with cochlear implants compared with age-matched peers with hearing aids: Implications for management. *International Journal of Audiology, 41*(3), 157–161.

Bagatto, M., Moodie, S., Scollie, S., Seewald, R., Moodie, S., Pumford, J., & Liu, R. (2005). Clinical protocols for hearing instrument fitting in the Desired Sensation Level method. *Trends in Amplification, 9*(4), 199–226.

Bagatto, M. P., Moodie, S. T., Seewald, R. C., Bartlett, D. J., & Scollie, S. D. (2011). A critical review of audiological outcome measures for infants and children. *Trends in Amplification, 15*(1), 23–33.

Beggs, W. D. A., & Foreman, D. L. (1980). Sound localization and early binaural experience in the deaf. *British Journal of Audiology, 14*(2), 41–48.

Berlin, C. I., Hood, L. J., Morlet, T., Wilensky, D., Li, L., Mattingly, K. R., . . . Frisch, S. A. (2010). Multi-site diagnosis and management of 260 patients with auditory neuropathy/dyssynchrony (auditory neuropathy spectrum disorder). *International Journal of Audiology, 49*(1), 30–43 10.3109/14992020903160892.

Berlin, C. I., Morlet, T., & Hood, L. J. (2003). Auditory neuropathy/dyssynchrony: Its diagnosis and management. *Pediatric Clinics of North America, 50*(2), 331–340, vii–viii.

Bess, F. H., Chase, P. A., Gravel, J. S., Seewald, R. C., Stelmachowicz, P. G., Tharpe, A. M., & Hedley-Williams, A. (1996). Amplification for infants and children with hearing loss. *American Journal of Audiology, 5*(1), 53–68.

Bess, F. H., Dodd-Murphy, J., & Parker, R. A. (1998). Children with minimal sensorineural hearing loss: Prevalence, educational performance, and functional status. *Ear and Hearing, 19*(5), 339–354.

Borg, E., Risberg, A., McAllister, B., Undermar, B. M., & Edquist, G. (2002). Language development in hearing-impaired children: Establishment of a reference material for a "Language test for hearing-impaired children," LATHIC. *International Journal of Pediatric Otorhinolaryngology, 65*, 15–26.

Byrne, D. (1983). Word familiarity in speech perception testing of children. *Australian and New Zealand Journal of Audiology, 5*(2), 77–80.

Byrne, D. (1986). Effects of frequency response characteristics on speech discrimination and perceived intelligibility and pleasantness of speech for hearing-impaired listeners. *Journal of the Acoustical Society of America, 80*(2), 494–504.

Byrne, D., & Ching, T. Y. C. (1997). Optimising amplification for hearing impaired children: I. Issues and procedures. *Australian Journal of Education of the Deaf, 3*(1), 21–28.

Byrne, D., Dillon, H., Ching, T. Y. C., Katsch, R., & Keidser, G. (2001). NAL-NL1 procedure for fitting nonlinear hearing aids: Characteristics and comparisons with other procedures. *Journal of the American Academy of Audiology, 12*(1), 37–51.

Ching, T. Y. C. (2011). Acoustic cues for consonant perception with combined acoustic and electric hearing in children. *Seminars in Hearing, 32*(1), 32–41.

Ching, T. Y. C. (2012). Hearing aids for children. In L. Wong & L. Hickson (Eds.), *Evidence based practice in audiologic intervention* (pp. 93–118). San Diego: Plural Publishing.

Ching, T. Y. C., & Dillon, H. (2003). Prescribing amplification for children: Adult-equivalent hearing loss, real-ear aided gain, and NAL-NL1. *Trends in Amplification, 7*(1), 1–9.

Ching, T. Y. C., Dillon, H., & Byrne, D. (1998). Speech recognition of hearing-impaired listeners: Predictions from audibility and the limited role of high-frequency amplification. *Journal of the Acoustical Society of America, 103*(2), 1128–1140.

Ching, T. Y. C., Dillon, H., Day, J., & Crowe, K. (2007). The NAL study on longitudinal outcomes of hearing-impaired children: Interim findings on language of early and later-identified children at 6 months after hearing aid fitting. Paper presented at the A Sound Foundation Through Early Amplification: Fourth International Conference, Stafa, Switzerland.

Ching, T. Y. C., Dillon, H., Day, J., Crowe, K., Close, L., Chisholm, K., & Hopkins, T. (2009). Early language outcomes of children with cochlear implants: Interim findings of the NAL study on longitudinal outcomes of children with hearing impairment. *Cochlear Implants International, 10*(Suppl. 1), 28–32.

Ching, T. Y. C., Dillon, H., Hou, S., Zhang, V., Day, J., Crowe, K., . . . Thomson, J. (Early online). A randomised controlled comparison of NAL and DSL prescriptions for young children: Hearing aid characteristics and performance outcomes at 3 years of age. *International Journal of Audiology.*

Ching, T. Y. C., Dillon, H., Katsch, R., & Byrne, D. (2001). Maximizing effective audibility in hearing aid fitting. *Ear and Hearing, 22*(3), 212–224.

Ching, T. Y. C., Dillon, H., Marnane, V., Hou, S., Day, D., Seeto, M., . . . Hopkins, K. (Submitted). Outcomes of early- and late-identified children at 3 years of age: Findings from a prospective population-based study. *Ear and Hearing.*

Ching, T. Y. C., Gardner-Berry, K., Day, J., Dillon, H., & Seeto, M. (In preparation). Outcomes of children with auditory neuropathy spectrum disorder at 3 years of age. *International Journal of Audiology.*

Ching, T. Y. C., & Hill, M. (2007). The Parents' Evaluation of Aural/Oral Performance of Children (PEACH) scale: Normative data. *Journal of the American Academy of Audiology, 18*(3), 220–235.

Ching, T. Y. C., Hill, M., Birtles, G., & Beecham, L. (1999). Clinical use of paired comparisons to evaluate hearing aid fitting of severely/profoundly hearing impaired children. *Australian and New Zealand Journal of Audiology, 21*(2), 51–63.

Ching, T. Y. C., Hill, M., & Dillon, H. (2008). Effect of variations in hearing-aid frequency response on real-life functional performance of children with severe or profound hearing loss. *International Journal of Audiology, 47*(8), 461–475.

Ching, T. Y. C., Hill, M., Van Wanrooy, E., & Agung, K. (2004). The advantages of wide-dynamic-range compression over linear amplification for children. *National Acoustic Laboratories Annual Report, 2003/2004,* 45–49.

Ching, T. Y. C., & Incerti, P. (2012). Bimodal fitting or bilateral cochlear implantation? In L. Wong & L. Hickson (Eds.), *Evidence based practice in audiologic intervention* (pp. 213–233). San Diego: Plural Publishing.

Ching, T. Y. C., Johnson, E. E., Hou, S., Dillon, H., Zhang, V., Burns, L., . . . Flynn, C. (Submitted). A comparison of NAL and DSL prescriptive methods for paediatric hearing aid fitting: Estimates of loudness and speech intelligibility. *International Journal of Audiology.*

Ching, T. Y. C., O'Brien, A., Dillon, H., Chalupper, J., Hartley, L., Hartley, D., . . . Hain, J. (2009). Directional effects on infants and young children in real life: Implications for amplification. *Joural of Speech, Language, and Hearing Research, 52*(5), 1241–1254.

Ching, T. Y. C., Scollie, S. D., Dillon, H., & Seewald, R. (2010). A cross-over, double-blind comparison of the NAL-NL1 and the DSL v4.1 prescriptions for children with mild to moderately severe hearing loss. *International Journal of Audiology, 49*(Suppl. 1), S4–S15 10.3109/14992020903148020.

Ching, T. Y. C., Scollie, S. D., Dillon, H., Seewald, R., Britton, L., & Steinberg, J. (2010). Prescribed real-ear and achieved real-life differences in children's hearing aids adjusted according to the NAL-NL1 and the DSL v.4.1 prescriptions. *International Journal of Audiology, 49*(Suppl. 1), S16–S25.

Ching, T. Y. C., van Wanrooy, E., & Dillon, H. (2007). Binaural-bimodal fitting or bilateral implantation for managing severe to profound deafness: A review. *Trends in Amplification, 11*(3), 161–192.

Ching, T. Y. C., van Wanrooy, E., Dillon, H., & Carter, L. (2011). Spatial release from masking in normal-hearing children and children who use hearing aids. *Journal of the Acoustical Society of America, 129*(1), 368–375.

Cone-Wesson, B., & Wunderlich, J. (2003). Auditory evoked potentials from the cortex: Audiology applications. *Current Opinion on Otolaryngology and Head Neck Surgery, 11*(5), 372–377.

Dillon, H., Keidser, G., Ching, T. Y. C., Flax, M., & Brewer, S. (2011). The NAL-NL2 prescription procedure. *Focus (San Francisco, CA), 40,* 1–10.

Eisenberg, L. S., & Levitt, H. (1991). Paired comparison judgments for hearing aid selection in children. *Ear and Hearing, 12*(6), 417–430.

Elfenbein, J. (2000). Batteries required: Instructing families on the use of hearing instruments. In R. Seewald (Ed.), *A sound foundation through early amplification: Proceedings of an international conference* (pp. 141–149). Stafa, Switzerland: Phonak.

Gardner-Berry, K., Ching, T. Y. C., & Day, J. (In preparation). Cortical evoked potentials and outcomes of children with auditory neuropathy spectrum disorders at 3 years of age. *International Journal of Audiology.*

Gilliver, M., Ching, T. Y. C., & Sjahalam-King, J. (Submitted). When expectation meets experience: Parents' recollections and experiences of a child with hearing impairment. *International Journal of Audiology.*

Golding, M., Pearce, W., Seymour, J., Cooper, A., Ching, T., & Dillon, H. (2007). The relationship between obligatory cortical auditory evoked potentials (CAEPs) and functional measures in young infants. *Journal of the American Academy of Audiology, 18*(2), 117–125.

Gravel, J. S., Fausel, N., Liskow, C., & Chobot, J. (1999). Children's speech recognition in noise using omnidirectional and dual-microphone hearing aid technology. *Ear and Hearing, 20*(1), 1–11.

Hattori, H. (1993). Ear dominance for nonsense-syllable recognition ability in sensorineural hearing-impaired children: Monaural versus binaural amplification. *Journal of the American Academy of Audiology, 4*(5), 319–330.

Hawkins, D. B. (2004). Limitations and uses of the aided audiogram. *Seminars in Hearing, 25*(1), 51–62.

Hood, L. J. (1999). A review of objective methods of evaluating auditory neural pathways. *Laryngoscope, 109*(11), 1745–1748.

Johansen, I. R., Hauch, A. M., Christensen, B., & Parving, A. (2004). Longitudinal study of hearing impairment in children. *International Journal of Pediatric Otorhinolaryngology, 68*(9), 1157–1165.

Kawell, M. E., Kopun, J. G., & Stelmachowicz, P. G. (1988). Loudness discomfort levels in children. *Ear and Hearing, 9*(3), 133–136.

Keller, W. D., & Bundy, R. S. (1980). Effects of unilateral hearing loss upon educational achievement. *Child: Care, Health and Development, 6*(2), 93–100.

Kennedy, C. R., McCann, D. C., Campbell, M. J., Law, C. M., Mullee, M., Petrou, S., . . . Stevenson, J. (2006).

Language ability after early detection of permanent childhood hearing impairment. *New England Journal of Medicine, 354*(20), 2131–2141.

Kiese-Himmel, C. (2002). Unilateral sensorineural hearing impairment in childhood: Analysis of 31 consecutive cases. *International Journal of Audiology, 41*(1), 57–63.

King, A. M. (2010). The national protocol for paediatric amplification in Australia. *International Journal of Audiology, 49*(Suppl. 1), S64–S69.

Kishon-Rabin, L., Taitelbaum-Swead, R., Ezrati-Vinacour, R., & Hildesheimer, M. (2005). Prelexical vocalization in normal hearing and hearing-impaired infants before and after cochlear implantation and its relation to early auditory skills. *Ear and Hearing, 26*(4, Suppl.), 17S–29S.

Klee, T. M., & Davis-Dansky, E. (1986). A comparison of unilaterally hearing-impaired children and normal-hearing children on a battery of standardized language tests. *Ear and Hearing, 7*(1), 27–37.

Korczak, P. A., Kurtzberg, D., & Stapells, D. R. (2005). Effects of sensorineural hearing loss and personal hearing aids on cortical event-related potential and behavioral measures of speech-sound processing. *Ear and Hearing, 26*(2), 165–185.

Korver, A. M. H., Konings, S., Dekker, F. W., Beers, M., Wever, C. C., Frijns, J. H. M., & Oudesluys-Murphy, A. M.; DECIBEL Collaborative Study Group. (2010). Newborn hearing screening vs. later hearing screening and developmental outcomes in children with permanent childhood hearing impairment. *JAMA, 304*(15), 1701–1708 [Journal article].

Kruger, B. (1987). An update on the external ear resonance in infants and young children. *Ear and Hearing, 8*(6), 333–336.

Kurtzberg, D. (1989). Cortical event-related potential assessment of auditory system function. *Seminars in Hearing, 10,* 252–262.

Leijon, A., Lindkvist, A., Ringdahl, A., & Israelsson, B. (1990). Preferred hearing aid gain in everyday use after prescriptive fitting. *Ear and Hearing, 11*(4), 299–305.

Lieu, J. E. C., Tye-Murray, N., Karzon, R. K., & Piccirillo, J. F. (2010). Unilateral hearing loss is associated with worse speech-language scores in children. *Pediatrics, 125*(6), e1348–e1355 10.1542/peds.2009-2448.

Litovsky, R. Y. (2005). Speech intelligibility and spatial release from masking in young children. *Journal of the Acoustical Society of America, 117*(5), 3091–3099.

Marnane, V., & Ching, T. Y. C. (In preparation). How often do early- and late-identified children use their hearing devices: Findings from a longitudinal population study. *International Journal of Audiology.*

McCracken, W., Young, A., & Tattersall, H. (2008). Universal newborn hearing screening: Parental reflections on very early audiological management. *Ear and Hearing, 29*(1), 54–64.

McDermott, H. (2011). Benefits of combined acoustic and electric hearing for music and pitch perception. *Seminars in Hearing, 32*(1), 103–114.

Mildner, V., Sindija, B., & Zrinski, K. V. (2006). Speech perception of children with cochlear implants and children with traditional hearing aids. *Clinical Linguistics & Phonetics, 20*(2-3), 219–229.

Moeller, M. P., Donaghy, K. F., Beauchaine, K. L., Lewis, D. E., & Stelmachowicz, P. G. (1996). Longitudinal study of FM system use in nonacademic settings: Effects on language development. *Ear and Hearing, 17*(1), 28–41.

Moeller, M. P., Hoover, B., Peterson, B., & Stelmachowicz, P. G. (2009). Consistency of hearing aid use in infants with early-identified hearing loss. *American Journal of Audiology, 18*(1), 14–23.

Moeller, M. P., Tomblin, J. B., Yoshinaga-Itano, C., Connor, C. M., & Jerger, S. (2007). Current state of knowledge: Language and literacy of children with hearing impairment. *Ear and Hearing, 28*(6), 740–753.

Moodie, K. S., Sinclair, S. T., Fisk, T., & Seewald, R. (2000). Individualized hearing instrument fitting for infants. In R. Seewald (Ed.), *A Sound Foundation through Early Amplification: Proceedings of an international conference* (pp. 213–217). Stafa, Switzerland: Phonak.

Moore, B. C. (1995). *Perceptual consequences of cochlear damage.* New York: Oxford University Press Inc.

Moore, B. C., & Glasberg, B. R. (1986). A comparison of two-channel and single-channel compression hearing aids. *Audiology, 25*(4-5), 210–226.

Nittrouer, S., & Chapman, C. (2009). The effects of bilateral electric and bimodal electric–acoustic stimulation on language development. *Trends in Amplification, 13*(3), 190–205.

Nozza, R. J., Rossman, R. N. F., & Bond, L. C. (1991). Infant-adult differences in unmasked thresholds for the discrimination of consonant-vowel syllable pairs. *Audiology, 30*(2), 102–112.

Palmer, C., & Mormer, E. (1999). Goals and expectations of the hearing aid fitting. *Trends in Amplification, 4*(2), 61–71.

Pearce, W., Golding, M., & Dillon, H. (2007). Cortical auditory evoked potentials in the assessment of auditory neuropathy: Two case studies. *Journal of the American Academy of Audiology, 18*(5), 380–390.

Rance, G. (2005). Auditory neuropathy/dys-synchrony and its perceptual consequences. *Trends in Amplification, 9*(1), 1–43.

Rance, G., Cone-Wesson, B., Wunderlich, J., & Dowell, R. C. (2002). Speech perception and cortical event related potentials in children with auditory neuropathy. *Ear and Hearing, 23*(3), 239–253.

Rance, G., Roper, R., Symons, L., Moody, L. J., Poulis, C., Dourlay, M., & Kelly, T. (2005). Hearing threshold estimation in infants using auditory steady-state responses. *Journal of the American Academy of Audiology, 16*(5), 291–300.

Ricketts, T. A., & Galster, J. (2008). Head angle and elevation in classroom environments: Implications for amplification. *Speech, Language, and Hearing Research, 51*(2), 516–525.

Robbins, A. M., Renshaw, J. J., & Berry, S. W. (1991). Evaluating meaningful auditory integration in profoundly hearing-impaired children. *American Journal of Otology, 12*(Suppl.), 144–150.

Robbins, A. M., Svirsky, M. A., Osberger, M. J., & Pisoni, D. B. (1998). Beyond the audiogram: The role of functional assessments. In F. H. Bess (Ed.), *Children with hearing impairments: Contemporary trends* (pp. 105–124). Nashville, TN: Vanderbilt Bill Wilkerson Center Press.

Scollie, S. D. (2008). Children's speech recognition scores: The Speech Intelligibility Index and proficiency factors for age and hearing level. *Ear and Hearing, 29*(4), 543–556.

Scollie, S. D., Ching, T. Y. C., Seewald, R., Dillon, H., Britton, L., Steinberg, J., & Corcoran, J. (2010a). Evaluation of the NAL-NL1 and DSL v4.1 prescriptions for children: Preference in real world use. *International Journal of Audiology, 49*(Suppl. 1), S49–S63.

Scollie, S. D., Ching, T. Y. C., Seewald, R. C., Dillon, H., Britton, L., Steinberg, J., & King, K. A. (2010b). Children's speech perception and loudness ratings when fitted with hearing aids using the DSL v.4.1 and the NAL-NL1 prescriptions. *International Journal of Audiology, 49*(Suppl. 1), S26–S34.

Scollie, S., Seewald, R., Cornelisse, L. E., Moodie, S., Bagatto, M., Laurnagaray, D., ... Pumford, J. (2005). The Desired Sensation Level multistage input/output algorithm. *Trends in Amplification, 9*(4), 159–197.

Sedey, A. L., Carpenter, K., & Stredler-Brown, A. (2002). Unilateral hearing loss: What do we know, what should we do? Paper presented at the National Symposium on Hearing in Infants, Breckenridge, CO.

Seewald, R., Cornelisse, L. E., & Ramji, K. V. (1997). DSL v4.1 for Windows: A software implementation of the Desired Sensation Level (DSL [i/o]) method for fitting linear gain and wide-dynamic-range compression hearing instruments. Users' manual. London, Ontario: University of Western Ontario Hearing Health Care Research Unit.

Seewald, R. C., & Scollie, S. D. (2003). An approach for ensuring accuracy in pediatric hearing instrument fitting. *Trends in Amplification, 7*(1), 29–40.

Sharma, A., Cardon, G., Henion, K., & Roland, P. (2011). Cortical maturation and behavioral outcomes in children with auditory neuropathy spectrum disorder. *International Journal of Audiology, 50*(2), 98–106.

Sininger, Y. S., & Oba, S. (2001). Patients with auditory neuropathy: Who are they and what can they hear? In Y. S. Sininger & A. Starr (Eds.), *Auditory neuropathy: New perspective on hearing disorders* (pp. 15–35). San Diego, CA: Singular, Thomson Learning.

Sjoblad, S., Harrison, M., Roush, J., & McWilliam, R. A. (2001). Parents' reactions and recommendations after diagnosis and hearing aid fitting. *American Journal of Audiology, 10*(1), 24–31.

Stapells, D. R. (2000). Frequency-specific evoked potential audiometry in infants. In R.C. Seewald (Ed.), *A sound foundation through early amplification: Proceeedings of an international conference* (pp. 13–32). Stafa, Switzerland: Phonak AG.

Stelmachowicz, P. G. (1999). Hearing aid outcome measures for children. *Journal of the American Academy of Audiology, 10*(1), 14–25, quiz 66.

Stredler-Brown, A. (2002). Developing a treatment program for children with auditory neuropathy. *Seminars in Hearing, 23*(3), 239–249.

Tharpe, A. M. (2008). Unilateral and mild bilateral hearing loss in children: Past and current perspectives. *Trends in Amplification, 12*(1), 7–15.

Tieri, L., Masi, R., Ducci, M., & Marsella, P. (1988). Unilateral sensorineural hearing loss in children. *Scandinavian Audiology. Supplementum, 30,* 33–36.

Van Deun, L., van Wieringen, A., Scherf, F., Deggouj, N., Desloovere, C., Offeciers, F. E., ... Wouters, J. (2010). Earlier intervention leads to better sound localization in children with bilateral cochlear implants. *Audiology & Neuro-Otology, 15*(1), 7–17.

Van Lierde, K. M., Vinck, B. M., Baudonck, N., De Vel, E., & Dhooge, I. (2005). Comparison of the overall intelligibility, articulation, resonance, and voice characteristics between children using cochlear implants and those using bilateral hearing aids: A pilot study. *International Journal of Audiology, 44*(8), 452–465.

Voss, S. E., & Herrmann, B. S. (2005). How does the sound pressure generated by circumaural, supra-aural, and insert earphones differ for adult and infant ears? *Ear and Hearing, 26*(6), 636–650.

Wake, M., Tobin, S., Cone-Wesson, B., Dahl, H. H., Gillam, L., McCormick, L., ... Williams, J. (2006). Slight/mild sensorineural hearing loss in children. *Pediatrics, 118*(5), 1842–1851.

Wong, S. H. W., Gibson, W. P. R., & Sanli, H. (1997). Use of transtympanic round window electrocochleography for threshold estimations in children. *American Journal of Otolaryngology, 18*(5), 632–636.

Zimmerman-Phillipps, S., Osberger, M. J., & Robbins, J. M. (1998). Infant-Toddler: Meaningful Auditory Integration Scale (IT-MAIS). In W. Eastabrooks (Ed.), *Cochlear implants for kids* (pp. 379–386). Washington, DC: AG Bell Association for the Deaf.

4 Optimizing Listening Potential through Cochlear Implants

Maximizing the child's auditory potential is the cornerstone of a solid rehabilitation program. As discussed in the previous chapter, the overwhelming majority of children with hearing loss have sufficient residual hearing to benefit from acoustic amplification. Recent newborn screening follow-up studies suggest that approximately 10 to 15% of children are identified with profound hearing loss, while another 10 to 15% have severe hearing loss (Watkin & Baldwin, 2011). Prior to the advent of pediatric cochlear implantation in the 1990s, despite limited access to acoustic information, many children with profound hearing loss and intensive rehabilitation developed spoken language skills through the use of hearing aids. However, it has been well documented that cochlear implants provide such children with greater access to auditory cues, so that many can acquire spoken language skills comparable to those of their normal-hearing peers (Hayes, Geers, Treiman, & Moog, 2009; Nicholas & Geers, 2006; Niparko et al, 2010; Svirsky, Teoh, & Neuburger, 2004). Essentially, cochlear implants have become standard care for children with severe to profound hearing loss who derive limited benefit from hearing aids.

This chapter presents recent developments in cochlear implant technology and practices, including current trends in candidacy evaluation and decision making for children at different ages and stages of development. Programming of the speech processor and ongoing audiologic management of children are presented. The chapter also includes a brief description of other implantable technologies.

▒ Cochlear Implants

Several cochlear implant systems are currently available (see suggested manufacturers' websites at end of the chapter), and all have the common goal to bypass the damaged cochlea and directly stimulate auditory nerve fibers that deliver information to higher levels of the auditory system and brain for auditory processing and, ultimately, speech understanding. Temporal bone studies suggest that the degree of nerve fiber survival in sensorineural hearing loss varies greatly, from 10 to 70% of the rate in the normal healthy cochlea (Hinojosa & Marion, 1983; Nadol, Young, & Glynn, 1989). Some of the variation in auditory abilities observed in users of cochlear implants may be associated with etiology. However, at this time there is no clear evidence of an association between etiology or larger populations of nerve fibers and auditory processing with a cochlear implant. For both adults (Friedland, Venick, & Niparko, 2003; Gomaa et al, 2003; Rubinstein, Parkinson, Tyler, & Gantz, 1999) and children, duration of deafness (i.e., for children, age of implantation) and preoperative hearing levels or speech understanding seem to be the best predictors of auditory outcomes with a cochlear implant (Nicholas & Geers, 2006; Niparko et al, 2010; Tyler et al, 2000).

Cochlear implantation involves the surgical insertion of a receiver stimulator in the mastoid bone and the placement of an electrode array in the scala tympani of the cochlea, where it generally rests against the outer cochlear wall, as shown by temporal bone studies (Almond & Brown, 2009). The internal cochlear implant receiver stimulator communicates with an externally worn transmitter, held in place on the head by a magnet (**Fig. 4.1**). The transmitter is coupled to a speech processor that encodes speech and environmental acoustic information that is delivered to the electrode array. Like acoustic hearing aids, cochlear implant devices vary according to manufacturer, with differences in physical characteristics, such as the number and spacing of electrodes in the electrode array, and in speech processing algorithms. Due to ongoing changes in technology, a discussion of these parameters is beyond the scope of this chapter. For additional details, readers can consult the manufacturers' websites listed at the end of the chapter.

The speech processor is custom programmed (see programming section below) for each individual to deliver the appropriate level of electrical current to the internal device. As noted, cochlear implant systems vary in several parameters, such as the number of electrodes, speech encoding algorithms, and processing speed. However, in all systems, electrodes are arranged to capitalize on the tonotopic properties of the normal cochlea, where high-frequency tuning occurs at the basal end, while low-frequency tuning is found at the apical end. This principle is key to an understanding of the basic functioning of a cochlear implant. Unlike acoustic hearing instruments, a cochlear implant does not amplify speech sounds to make them audible for individuals with residual hearing. Rather, as shown in **Fig. 4.1**, a cochlear implant delivers information to points along an electrode array; this information is sent to the auditory nerve fibers and interpreted by the brain as sounds. Despite rapid progress in cochlear implant technology since devices were first approved for children in the United States in 1990, the representation of fine temporal structure that contributes to speech understanding, particularly in difficult acoustic conditions, remains one of the greatest challenges in the field (Wilson & Dorman, 2009).

The goal of pediatric cochlear implantation is identical to that for acoustic amplification: to provide children with the best possible access to sound in order to make spoken language acquisition possible. Continued research and development in cochlear implant technology can be expected to improve the quality of auditory information provided through implant devices. Cochlear implant manufacturers' websites provide useful, up-to-date information on technological advances, as well as the specific technical characteristics of different implant systems (see the suggested websites at the end of the chapter).

Cochlear Implant Evaluation

A large volume of evidence is available about the auditory benefits of cochlear implantation for children with severe to profound hearing loss (NHS National Institute for Health and Clinical Excellence, 2009; Thoutenhoofd et al, 2005). Cochlear implantation has now become a standard intervention, and candidacy decisions for children who derive little or no benefit from acoustic amplification and who otherwise have typical development are generally relatively straightforward. Typically,

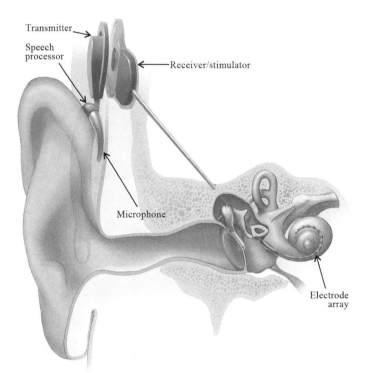

Fig. 4.1 Schematic of a cochlear implant device. (Used with permission from National Institutes of Health, NIH Medical Arts.)

regulatory bodies, such as the United States Food and Drug Administration (FDA), establish candidacy criteria that include a minimum chronological age of 12 months (although some children are now implanted younger); profound hearing loss of 90 dB or greater for children age 12 to 24 months, or severe to profound loss for children over 24 months of age; and no medical or radiologic contraindications. Manufacturer and FDA or other country-specific guidelines can be consulted for specific indications for different devices. Candidacy evaluations may vary slightly from one cochlear implant program to another, but there are many similarities. Most cochlear implant centers adopt a team approach to care, and a comprehensive interdisciplinary evaluation is performed to assess candidacy-related issues in multiple domains and to provide parents with information.

Audiologic. Most children undergo a trial period with acoustic hearing aids before proceeding to a cochlear implant unless the indications are very clear—for example, in the case of meningitis, where ossification of the cochlea is a concern in delaying surgery. Children followed audiologically in centers where both acoustic amplification and cochlear implant surgery are provided undergo a fairly seamless transition in terms of audiologic management; others may be transferred specifically to a cochlear implant center for the audiologic component of the evaluation. In addition to obtaining audiometric information on each ear, preferably behavioral confirmation of the results from evoked potential testing, audiologic assessment to determine cochlear implant candidacy involves speech recognition measures, if the child is old enough to perform the testing. Parent questionnaires that probe auditory functioning can provide useful information for young children.

Communication. A language assessment that varies in content depending on the age and stage of the child is conducted by a clinician/teacher. In some cases, information on language and communication functioning may be combined with audiologic results to help determine whether cochlear implantation is likely to provide additional benefits for children where candidacy is less certain, for example, those with residual hearing (as discussed below). For all children, the comprehensive assessment serves as baseline information used in evaluating future progress with the cochlear implant. For children with additional developmental disabilities (see below and Chapter 7), an assessment of the child's potential to develop oral language and communication skills more broadly provides both the parents and

cochlear implant team with useful information in decision making.

Medical and radiologic. Through the medical evaluation, the otologist (cochlear implant surgeon) aims to assess the child's medical status, as well as the structural characteristics of the auditory system. As discussed in Chapter 1, malformations of inner ear structures are present in 20% or more of children with sensorineural hearing loss (Coticchia, Gokhale, Waltonen, & Sumer, 2006). High-resolution computed tomography, frequently in combination with magnetic resonance imaging, is routinely used to assess the status of the inner ear structures prior to implantation (Buchman, Adunka, Zdanski, & Pillsbury, 2011). Surgeons can use this information in counseling families and discussing the prognosis and potential challenges for a given child with parents and rehabilitation specialists. For example, a deficient or absent cochlear nerve may be a contra-indication to cochlear implantation. An ossified cochlea may influence the choice of internal implant device. For a discussion of medical and surgical aspects of cochlear implantation, refer to Tucci and Pilkington (2009) and Buchman et al (2011).

Psychosocial. Pediatric cochlear implant teams frequently include a social worker or psychologist, or both, to assist with assessing child and parent readiness and needs. Cognitive-related information relative to the child's overall functioning may also be obtained as this information can be important in helping parents understand their child's areas of strengths and any non-hearing-related difficulties. For some parents, the costs of the cochlear implant and ongoing upkeep can be problematic, and a family support worker can assist in guiding families to additional resources.

Other considerations. The child's particular circumstances typically determine the need for further assessment and consultation with other specialists, including neurologists, developmental pediatricians, and mental health providers. Additional medical specialists (e.g., cardiologists) may also be involved depending on the presence of complex medical conditions that place the child at risk for complications during surgery. In addition, for children of school age, members of the child's educational team should be involved in the candidacy process. For some older children, referral for cochlear implantation may in fact be initiated by the specialized educator of the hearing-impaired/speech-language pathologist, who provides regular intervention to the child in the school system.

Candidacy Decisions

Although most candidacy decisions are relatively clear from an audiologic and medical point of view, for some parents the decision can be difficult (Johnston et al, 2008; Most & Zaidman-Zait, 2003). Even when the need for cochlear implantation is relatively apparent to parents who have opted for spoken language, research with families indicates that the cochlear implant process can be an emotionally charged and difficult period (Hyde, Punch, & Komesaroff, 2010; Johnston et al, 2008). Some parents may require considerable support and time to adapt to this change in their child's care, while others will be anxious to proceed with surgery as quickly as possible.

Some teams have adopted decision-making instruments, such as the Children's Cochlear Implant Profile (CHIP), which includes a list of 10 factors or adaptations (Hellman et al, 1991), or the Nottingham Children's Implant Profile (NChip) (Nikolopoulos, Dyar, & Gibbin, 2004), to systematically consider factors that are important in pediatric candidacy decisions. For example, the CHIP assists the team in evaluating candidacy by taking into account chronological age, duration of deafness, medical or radiologic anomalies, other developmental disabilities, functional hearing levels, speech and language abilities, family structure and support, family expectations, educational environment, and postimplant support services available. Using an adapted version of the CHIP, Daya et al (1999) calculated a graded profile analysis score that was found to be significantly associated with the rate of speech perception in children. Such tools can be useful in team decisions and also in counseling families about postimplantation expectations. More recently, as bilateral cochlear implants have become more standard care, the decision regarding two surgeries can also be a difficult one for some parents (Ramsden, Papaioannou, Gordon, James, & Papsin, 2009). In particular, when children are already functioning well with one implant, families may need support in weighing the potential benefits associated with a second implant (Fitzpatrick, Jacques, & Neuss, 2011; Johnston, Durieux-Smith, O'Connor, et al, 2009).

Early Cochlear Implantation

There is a large body of evidence documenting that children who receive cochlear implants during the preschool years can develop spoken language skills (Fitzpatrick, Crawford, Ni, & Durieux-Smith, 2011; Nicholas & Geers, 2006; Niparko et al, 2010). These studies and other research documenting longer-term results show that some children attain skills commensurate with their hearing peers. Similar to children who use acoustic amplification, a myriad of child and family factors can impact spoken language acquisition in children with cochlear implants (Geers, Strube, Tobey, Pisoni, & Moog, 2011; Nicholas & Geers, 2006; Niparko et al, 2010). One of the most important documented factors predicting outcomes in these children is age at implantation. Since the 1990s, several studies have reported preferential results for children receiving implants at earlier ages (Fryauf-Bertschy, Tyler, Kelsay, Gantz, & Woodworth, 1997; Kirk et al, 2002; Nicholas & Geers, 2006).

Earlier studies established the benefits for children implanted at age 2 or 3 compared with those implanted in the later preschool years, and more recent work has shifted to examining the effects of age at implantation even in children implanted before their first birthday (Vlastarakos et al, 2010). For example, an Australian study reported faster growth rates for 19 children implanted before 12 months of age compared with children implanted between 12 and 24 months. The rate of language growth for the early-implanted children was comparable to that of peers with normal hearing (Dettman, Pinder, Briggs, Dowell, & Leigh, 2007). Other studies have not shown clear evidence for early versus late implantation (Fitzpatrick et al, 2012; Moog & Geers, 2003) for children implanted during the preschool years, but the results may depend on how early children receive access to sound. There is also no clear evidence of a critical age for optimal results, but earlier age at implantation and consequently early access to hearing is supported by research in neuroplasticity and critical auditory stimulation periods, as discussed in the first chapter of this book (Gordon & Harrison, 2005; Sharma, Dorman, & Kral, 2005; Sharma, Dorman, Spahr, & Todd, 2002).

Candidacy Questions for Special Subgroups of Children

The recommendation to proceed from acoustic amplification to cochlear implant surgery is usually not complicated for clinical teams treating a "typical" child who has limited access to acoustic information from hearing aids. However, candidacy decisions can be rather complex for special subgroups of children. These subgroups include children with residual hearing who demonstrate some benefit from hearing aids, children who are late identified or did not have access to implants in the early years (e.g., new immigrants), older children and adolescents who were not audiologic candidates in the early years, and children with complex medical or additional developmental disabilities (Fitzpatrick et al, 2009; Olds, Fitzpatrick, Steacie, McLean, & Schramm, 2007; Wiley & Meinzen-Derr, 2009). A review of studies from 2000 to 2007 in the United States suggests that children of diverse backgrounds and socioeconomic status may not be appropriately represented in cochlear implant populations (Belzner & Seal, 2009). Despite the overall trend toward earlier cochlear implantation, research has shown that a substantial number of children will continue to receive cochlear implants well beyond their first birthday (Fitzpatrick & Brewster, 2008). Primary reasons for late implantation are progressive hearing loss, the presence of other disabilities that may contribute to delayed decisions about the usefulness of cochlear implants, and delays in surgery due to other health complications (Fitzpatrick, Johnson, & Durieux-Smith, 2011; McCracken & Turner, 2012).

Children with Residual Hearing

The question of how much hearing is too much has received attention in the literature (Eisenberg, Martinez, Sennaroglu, & Osberger, 2000; Fitzpatrick et al, 2009; Leigh, Dettman, Dowell, & Sarant, 2011). Children with residual hearing who have some access to open-set speech recognition may receive cochlear implants at later ages due to uncertainty about the additional benefits of cochlear implants over acoustic hearing aids (Fitzpatrick, McCrae, & Schramm, 2006; Fitzpatrick et al, 2009). Studies suggest that children with average hearing levels in the severe range and open-set speech understanding, although not considered candidates in the 1990s, may derive greater benefit from cochlear implants than from acoustic hearing aids (Dettman et al, 2004; Fitzpatrick et al, 2006; Leigh et al, 2011). However, there appears to be some difference in the interpretation of implant candidacy for children with residual hearing (Dettman et al, 2004; Fitzpatrick et al, 2009).

In several studies, equivalent or functional equivalent hearing levels have been calculated for children with cochlear implants, with the results compared with those obtained for children with acoustic amplification. As early as 1994, Boothroyd and Eran (1994) estimated that children with cochlear implants functioned like children using conventional amplification with average hearing loss of 88 dB HL (hearing level). Since then, there have been advances in technology and earlier age of implantation. For example, Blamey et al (2001) concluded that children with implants and an average hearing loss of 106 dB HL performed on speech perception, production, and language measures like children with hearing aids with an average hearing loss of 78 dB HL. There is little research that directly compares children with severe loss who use hearing aids with similar groups using cochlear implants. In a large UK survey of parents and teachers of children with and without cochlear implants, Stacey, Fortnum, Barton, and Summerfield (2006) reported that spoken language and educational outcomes for children with cochlear implants were comparable to those for nonimplanted children with average hearing levels in the range of 80 to 104 dB HL. The study reported equivalent hearing levels ranging from 68 to 82 dB HL specifically for auditory performance.

Results for children with implants have led some authors to suggest that pediatric candidacy criteria can be expanded to include severe hearing loss (Gordon, Twitchell, Papsin, & Harrison, 2001; Leigh et al, 2011). Leigh et al (2011) proposed guidelines for candidacy decisions based on a study of 142 children ages 4 to 16 years with average hearing levels ranging from 28 to 125 dB HL, 62 of whom used hearing aids and 80 of whom used cochlear implants. Based on speech recognition test scores, equivalent average thresholds were calculated for open-set phonemes and sentences.

The study concluded that cochlear implantation can be recommended for children with a pure-tone average of 75 to 90 dB HL, with the understanding that there is a 75% chance of improvement in outcomes over hearing aids. According to the study, hearing aids remain the technology of choice for children with pure-tone average thresholds better than 75 dB HL. In a Canadian study, clinicians expressed uncertainty and differing views related to the appropriateness of cochlear implants for children with hearing loss in the 70 to 90 dB HL range. Clinicians were more likely to take additional information into account for these borderline cases, including spoken language skills, progress in intervention, and social and academic functioning (Fitzpatrick et al, 2009).

The clinician/teacher who follows the child and family on an ongoing basis in diverse learning environments is well positioned to provide input into candidacy issues. In our research, clinicians emphasized the need to consider functional abilities as much as hearing abilities measured from tests. Audiologists and clinicians/teachers underscored the importance of assessment beyond speech recognition tests to examine distance hearing and overall ease of listening in real-world environments and for school-age children functioning in the classroom (Fitzpatrick et al, 2009). In this research, the notion of team input and decision making, although important for all children receiving cochlear implants, was underscored as a critical component of the evaluation process for these children. Not only is the decision a challenging one for cochlear implant teams, parents of these children also find the decision difficult (Hyde et al, 2010). The precise hearing level for an individual child at which a cochlear implant can provide more acoustic information than conventional hearing aids remains uncertain; therefore, knowledge from experienced clinicians/teachers must be applied to the decision-making process. The case presented below in the section on "late-implanted children" (Group 2) provides a clinical example of why children with residual hearing sometimes receive implants at a later age.

Late-Implanted Children

Group 1. Another group of children for whom candidacy decisions can be difficult are those who arrive from other countries or from circumstances where cochlear implantation was not an option in the early years. Complicating the situation, these children frequently have had little or no experience even with hearing aids and may have had limited access to rehabilitation services. Not only are the children experiencing a new beginning, but the family faces a variety of other challenges in the new culture (Rhoades, 2010; Rhoades, Price, & Perigoe, 2004; Xu, 2007). As previously indicated, age at implantation has been identified as a critical determinant of spoken language outcomes. Research has generally shown poorer results for children who are late implanted (Kirk et al, 2002; McConkey Robbins, Koch, Osberger, Zimmerman-Phillips, & Kishon-Rabin, 2004; Stacey et al, 2006). This is not surprising given the information presented in Chapter 1 related to neural plasticity and critical auditory learning periods. Exceptions regarding late implantation are children who, as discussed in a subsequent section, had sufficient residual hearing and the benefit of auditory experience prior to implantation and who have developed auditory skills with a cochlear implant.

Group 2. Another group of late-implanted children are those who were not obvious candidates during the preschool years because they benefited from acoustic amplification and learned spoken language. This group of children were born in the 1990s, before cochlear implantation criteria had expanded to include the majority of children with severe to profound hearing loss. Studies have shown that these children developed spoken language and, in many cases, became competent communicators (Eriks-Brophy et al, 2012; Goldberg & Flexer, 2001). However, given their limited access, particularly to high-frequency components of the acoustic signal (Boothroyd, 2008), results may not be comparable to current expectations, particularly in relation to speech intelligibility, speech perception, and overall auditory functioning. Fitzpatrick and Brewster (2008) documented that more than half the children implanted in Canada in 2005 were over age 3 years. As cochlear implantation became standard practice, more of these children received implants at later ages. While studies show that their speech reception outcomes are not generally comparable to those of early-implanted children or adults with postlinguistic deafness, they have derived auditory benefits from their cochlear implants (Arisi et al, 2010; Fitzpatrick, Séguin, & Schramm, 2004; Schramm, Fitzpatrick, & Séguin, 2002; Waltzman, Roland, & Cohen, 2002). These children present particular

challenges because the overarching question is: Will an implant provide more auditory information despite a critical period of suboptimal auditory stimulation? The following example briefly illustrates the potential benefits that cochlear implantation has provided to some adolescents.

Sarah was a 15-year-old girl with a severe to profound hearing loss, identified at age 2 years, whose parents had worked very diligently to help her develop spoken language skills. She attended a regular education program and continued to develop and improve spoken language skills throughout the school years. By the time she reached age 13, cochlear implantation for children with Sarah's degree of hearing loss had become common practice in her local area, and her parents wondered whether she would benefit. Despite her intelligible speech and age-appropriate vocabulary and language skills as measured on language tests (see below), the parents were concerned that Sarah had to expend incredible effort to keep up in school and that she did not fully participate in discussions at the dinner table, for example, and in general avoided group activities. They were referred to the cochlear implant program for a full assessment. Sarah received a cochlear implant and, although it took a little time for her to adapt to the new sounds, she wore it on a full-time basis. She made a decision to discontinue hearing aid use shortly after receiving the implant, stating that it interfered with the quality of sound from her implant. Three months after implantation she reported much more successful use of her cell phone, and her parents noticed an increase in conversations in the car and, over all, more participation at home with them and her two siblings.

Auditory Neuropathy

Children with auditory neuropathy spectrum disorder (ANSD) present special challenges for cochlear implant teams. Briefly, these children present a clinical profile that differs audiologically from cochlear hearing loss. Typical audiologic profiles for ANSD have been described in the literature (Starr, Picton, Sininger, Hood, & Berlin, 1996; Starr, Sininger, & Pratt, 2000):

- Hearing loss with a sensorineural pattern of mild to profound degree
- Presence of otoacoustic emissions (OAEs) (energy produced by outer hair cells)
- Cochlear microphonics (generated from polarization and depolarization of hair cells) present and larger than normal in auditory brainstem response (ABR) recording
- Absent or abnormal ABR regardless of degree of hearing loss
- Poor speech recognition levels relative to the audiometric hearing levels
- No acoustic (middle ear muscle) reflex

An estimated 5 to 10% of children with permanent hearing loss present with an audiologic profile consistent with ANSD (Rance & Starr, 2011). Audiometric results in children with ANSD can be highly variable from one test

session to another, and a minority of children even appear to present with normal hearing levels (Berlin, Morlet, & Hood, 2003). In some individuals, OAEs disappear but the reason remains unknown (Rance et al, 1999; Starr et al, 2000). Further complicating decision making is that spontaneous improvement has been reported in a minority of cases (Raveh, Buller, Badrana, & Attias, 2007). Furthermore, for these children, ABR results cannot be used to predict auditory thresholds, making decisions about cochlear implantation difficult for younger children. Therefore, behavioral measurements and careful observation of functional auditory behavior are extremely important.

Since individuals frequently have more difficulty with speech recognition than would be anticipated based on audiogram results, their performance, even when equipped with hearing technology, may not be in line with general expectations for children with hearing loss (Rance & Barker, 2008; Rance, Barker, Sarant, & Ching, 2007). Cochlear implantation may be indicated even for children whose audiometric levels are not in the severe to profound range. The uncertainty surrounding these children means that cochlear implantation may not occur as early as in typical cochlear hearing losses. In 2008, a team of experts in auditory neuropathy assembled to develop comprehensive guidelines for the identification and follow-up care of children with ANSD (Guidelines for Identification and Management of Infants and Young Children with Auditory Neuropathy Spectrum Disorder, 2008).

Research has shown that for some individuals who derive limited benefit from hearing aids, cochlear implants are highly successful in directly stimulating the auditory nerve, such that users achieve speech recognition comparable to those with sensory hearing loss (Gibson & Sanli, 2007; Madden, Hilbert, Rutter, Greinwald, & Choo, 2002; Rance & Barker, 2008). However, it appears that the ability to achieve synchronicity in the auditory system may depend on the site of lesion (neuropathy), and results can be variable; some fail to achieve neural synchronization, for example, when ANSD is associated with cochlear nerve deficiency (Teagle et al, 2010). Various potential lesion sites have been identified, including inner hair cells, hair cell synapses, and the auditory nerve (Rance & Starr, 2011).

Complicating outcomes for children with ANSD is that many are affected by other developmental disabilities, and it is sometimes difficult to conclude whether limited auditory progress is due to the quality of sound through the cochlear implant or to the presence of other disabilities. The next case example features a child with auditory neuropathy who did not receive a cochlear implant until age 2 years, as ANSD was not identified through newborn hearing screening. The child, who otherwise presented with no developmental concerns, followed a trajectory in auditory and spoken language development consistent with that of peers with sensory hearing loss and, by school age, demonstrated speech and language skills comparable to peers with normal hearing.

Child with Auditory Neuropathy—Case Example

(Case example contributed by Deirdre Neuss, Children's Hospital of Eastern Ontario.)

Jenny is a 6-year-old girl identified with bilateral profound hearing loss with evidence of ANSD. Her hearing disorder was not identified until she was almost 2 years of age because she passed newborn hearing screening tests using OAEs. In the absence of risk factors for hearing loss, no other testing was conducted. Jenny's parents, however, had been concerned about her hearing for some time and were seen in the audiology clinic several times, but inconsistent audiometric results were obtained, making a definitive diagnosis difficult. OAEs were present at testing; ANSD was confirmed based on ABR results and further testing. Hearing aids were fitted and she was enrolled in weekly auditory-verbal therapy sessions. Little progress was made with hearing aids, and a cochlear implant was recommended within a couple of months. Although starting late and having developed essentially no spoken language prior to implantation, Jenny soon learned to detect and meaningfully process sounds with her implant. With excellent input from her family, she developed listening and spoken language comparable to children with a cochlear hearing loss. She received a second cochlear implant at age 4½ years. She carries on open-set conversations with ease and continues to advance her listening skills. As shown by the language assessments summarized in **Table 4.1**, despite late access to hearing, Jenny's speech and language results at age 5 were comparable to those of her age mates with normal hearing.

Children with Additional Developmental Disabilities

Another group of children who require special consideration related to cochlear implant decision making are those with disabilities in addition to hearing loss. Intervention practices with these children are discussed in Chapter 7, but the topic is mentioned here because the presence of other disabilities can be a factor affecting candidacy decisions. A survey of Canadian centers indicated that children with additional disabilities were not generally implanted until around 2000 (Fitzpatrick & Brewster, 2008), and other researchers have also reported an increase in implantation in children with additional developmental disabilities (Meinzen-Derr, Wiley, Grether, & Choo, 2011; Wiley, Jahnke, Meinzen-Derr, &

Table 4.1 Speech and language results obtained for child with auditory neuropathy spectrum disorder on standardized norm-referenced tests at age 5 years, 2 months

Test measure	Standard score
Goldman-Fristoe Test of Articulation (GFTA)	89
PLS Auditory Comprehension	99
PLS Expressive Communication	116
CELF-P Linguistic Concepts	12
CELF-P Basic Concepts	10
CELF-P Sentence Structure	8
CELF-P Recalling Sentences in Context	7
CELF-P Formulating Labels	13
CELF-P Word Structure	10

Abbreviations: PLS, Preschool Language Scale (standard scores for PLS and GFTA between 85 and 100 are considered within the average range); CELF-P, Clinical Evaluation of Language Fundamental—Preschool (standard scores between 7 and 13 are within the average range).

Choo, 2005). This represents a change in practice compared to the early years of cochlear implantation. The availability of objective measures for programming speech processors coupled with the expected auditory benefits of cochlear implantation, even when spoken language understanding may not be achieved, have likely contributed to this growing trend. In addition, as cochlear implantation became more mainstream, parents became more aware of the potential for auditory benefits even when spoken language was not an expected outcome.

As the example shows, decision making for children with additional disabilities may be more difficult and may take longer (McCracken & Turner, 2012). A recent study examining late cochlear implantation found that 18 of 43 children received a cochlear implant more than 12 months after hearing loss identification (Fitzpatrick, Johnson, et al, 2011). While the majority of implantation delays were due to progressive or late-onset hearing loss, four of these children experienced delays due to the presence of other severe disabilities. Although the disability itself did not constitute a reason for the delay, it resulted in more time for definitive confirmation of severe to profound hearing loss, uncertainty about the potential

benefits of cochlear implants, and possible delays due to complex health issues. All of these issues can affect parent and clinician decisions.

Outcomes reported for children with additional disabilities are quite variable, and in some studies appear to be associated with the extent of cognitive delay (Edwards, 2007; Holt & Kirk, 2005; Olds, Fitzpatrick, Schramm, & McLean, 2006; Wiley, Meinzen-Derr, & Choo, 2008). In a recent study of 15 children with cochlear implants who had additional disabilities, children were matched based on cognitive level to peers with normal hearing (Meinzen-Derr et al, 2011). Children with cochlear implants were found to have significant receptive and expressive language delays with greater discrepancies between language scores and cognitive functioning than their cognitively matched peers.

A review of our clinical data on children with severe developmental delay with implant experience ranging from almost 2 years to 8 years found that 8 of 13 children continued to use the device. As shown in **Fig. 4.2**, the majority of the children demonstrated some improvement after implantation in auditory functioning based on the MAIS or IT-MAIS auditory behavior questionnaire. However,

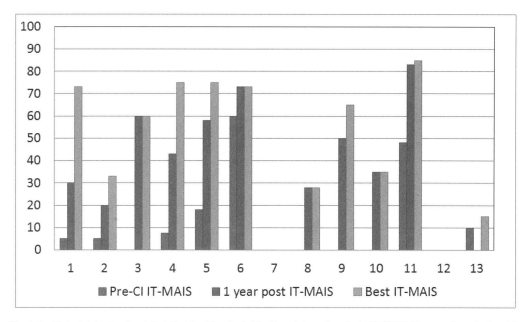

Fig. 4.2   Clinical data showing Infant Toddler-Meaningful Auditory Integration Scale (IT-MAIS) (% correct) results for children with cochlear implants and severe developmental disabilities. Child 7 and 12 obtained 0% at all test intervals.

none of the children made gains in open-set speech recognition or developed spoken language skills. Qualitative research with parents suggests that, despite the more limited gains relative to typically developing peers, parents perceive numerous benefits, even in children with complex and severe developmental disabilities. Research has found that parents reported some communication progress post-implantation and noted benefits related to connectedness, social interaction, and environmental awareness (Olds et al, 2007; Wiley et al, 2005). Parents also indicated that they would make the same decision to have their child implanted if presented with the choice again. Case examples of children with additional disabilities who received cochlear implants are presented in Chapter 7.

Bilateral Implant Decisions

In the first 15 years or so of cochlear implantation, unilateral implantation was standard care for individuals with severe to profound hearing loss. More recently, bilateral cochlear implants, like bilateral hearing aids, have become the preferred choice for all children as well as for adults in some centers. Regardless of whether acoustic, electric, or combined stimulation is used, it is generally well recognized that binaural hearing offers advantages for the overwhelming majority of individuals with hearing loss (Dunn, Yost, Noble, Tyler, & Witt, 2006). However, in some health systems, decisions on bilateral implants have been largely governed by the availability of additional funding for the devices and clinical resources (Fitzpatrick, Jacques, et al, 2011; Summerfield, Lovett, Bellenger, & Batten, 2010). The benefits of bilateral implantation have been widely described and include, notably, localization and improved speech understanding in the presence of noise. Several systematic reviews provide support for the benefits of bilateral implantation in both children and adults (Brown & Balkany, 2007; Ching, van Wanrooy, & Dillon, 2007; Johnston, Durieux-Smith, Angus, O'Connor, & Fitzpatrick, 2009; Murphy & O'Donoghue, 2007).

As bilateral implantation has become more integrated into clinical care, simultaneous implantation, or short delays between the first and second implants have been widely advocated to ensure that both ears receive optimal auditory stimulation from the very beginning (Gordon & Papsin, 2009; Papsin & Gordon, 2008). Decision making may be more difficult for parents of children (or for children themselves) who received a unilateral implant prior to the widespread availability of bilateral implants. Until recently, most children received unilateral implants, and many of them have been or are being considered for sequential implantation. In these cases, age at implantation seems to be a major determinant of binaural benefits, although some researchers argue that while bilateral benefits may be observed, true binaural integration is not likely when bilateral implantation is performed later in life (Gordon, Papsin, & Harrison, 2006; Gordon, Valero, van Hoesel, & Papsin, 2008). Research from laboratory studies and from real-world observations seems to indicate that even children with long delays between first and second implants can derive substantial benefits from two implants (Fitzpatrick, Jacques, et al, 2011; Peters, Litovsky, Parkinson, & Lake, 2007; Zeitler et al, 2008). There is some evidence that age at first implant may be an important predictor of outcome (Peters et al, 2007). The following case provides a clinical example of a child who received considerable benefit from a second implant despite a more than 5-year delay between implants. It is important to note that this child had substantial residual hearing prior to cochlear implantation

Child with Delay between Sequential Cochlear Implants

(Case example contributed by Rosemary Somerville, Children's Hospital of Eastern Ontario, Ottawa.)

Justin was referred to audiology through newborn hearing screening at 1 month of age and was diagnosed with bilateral moderate to severe hearing loss through ABR and OAE testing. He received hearing aids within 3 weeks and was enrolled in an auditory-verbal program, where he made good progress in developing spoken language. Behavioral audiometry results at 1 year (**Fig. 4.3a**) continued to show a moderate to severe hearing loss, but by 2 years of age, hearing thresholds had deteriorated to severe to profound levels in both ears (**Fig. 4.3b**). Further follow-up showed enlarged vestibular aqueduct syndrome consistent with a diagnosis of Pendred syndrome. At age 2 years, Justin received a unilateral cochlear implant (standard care at the time) and continued to progress well. As a child from a bilingual home, he learned to speak both languages. At school entry, speech and language results were at or above age-appropriate levels.

Justin's residual hearing continued to deteriorate, and he received a second cochlear implant 5 years after the first one. On the day of activation of his new implant, using the new implant only, his auditory skills were limited to identifying words in a closed-set task based on number of syllables—for example, "ice cream cone" versus "sandwich"—and he was able to understand a few simple open-set familiar phrases, such as "What's your name?" He received intensive intervention aimed at developing his auditory skills with the new implant. As shown in **Table 4.2**, after 1 month Justin was showing high-level auditory skills on speech recognition testing, and within 6 months these skills were aligned with those following the first implant. His family also reported subjective benefits, such as an overall greater ease of listening.

Although there is good evidence for improved speech perception in the midst of noise (Ching et al, 2007; Johnston, Durieux-Smith, Angus, et al, 2009; Peters et al, 2007), the evidence for localization from two implants, at least in everyday environments, is less compelling (Fitzpatrick, Jacques, et al, 2011; Galvin, Mok, Dowell, & Briggs, 2008). In interviews with parents of 14 children who received a second implant at various times (up to 9.6 years) after the first implant, parents reported one of the most important advantages of bilateral implants to be overall greater ease of listening and less fatigue. An additional benefit for many parents was knowing that they had provided the very best technology for their children and were taking advantage of the neuroplasticity of the auditory system (Fitzpatrick, Jacques, et al, 2011). Interestingly, families also report more subtle benefits, such as the availability of a backup device in the event that the original one fails and comfort in the knowledge that their children had been provided with the best available access to sound.

There is a general consensus that the decision to undertake bilateral implantation should

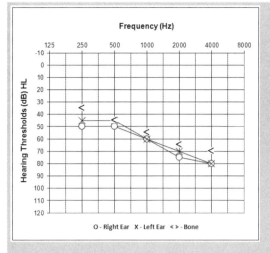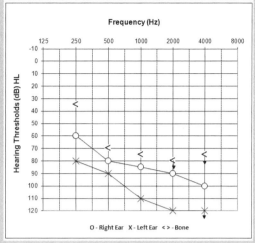

Fig. 4.3a,b **(a)** Audiometric thresholds at 1 year of age. **(b)** Audiometric thresholds at 2 years of age shortly before the first cochlear implantation.

be made when there has been a clear determination of lack of binaural benefit from the use of a hearing aid in the nonimplanted ear. Several studies have documented considerable benefits from bimodal hearing, that is, combined cochlear implant and hearing aid use. Ching et al (2007) and Schafer et al (2007) provide reviews of the benefits of bimodal hearing and bilateral implants. In the early days of cochlear implantation, most children had such limited hearing that little consideration was generally given to using acoustic amplification in the nonimplanted ear. However, in recent years, with expanded criteria, more children with residual hearing are being implanted, and consideration should always be given to whether binaural benefits can be derived from acoustic devices (Ching, Incerti, Hill, & van Wanrooy, 2006; Perreau, Tyler, Witt, & Dunn, 2007; Schafer et al, 2007).

Table 4.2 Speech recognition results at 1, 3, and 6 months postimplantation using a second implant only for a child with a 5-year delay between first and second implants; all tests were administered using recorded material

Test	1 month postimplantation	3 months postimplantation	6 months postimplantation
PBK	72%	92%	100%
MLNT	96%	92%	—
HINT (quiet) HINT (noise) + 10 dB S/N	98% —	100% —	100% 80%
GASP sentences	100%	100%	—

Abbreviations: PBK, Phonetically Balanced Kindergarten Test; MLNT, Multisyllabic Lexical Neighborhood Test; HINT, Hearing in Noise Test; S/N, signal-to-noise ratio; GASP, Glendonald Auditory Screening Procedure.

Hybrid Cochlear Implants

The documentation of cochlear implant advantages even for individuals with substantial residual hearing, has led to a growing interest in the use of "hybrid" devices. These devices combine electrical and acoustic information in the same ear (von Ilberg, Baumann, Kiefer, Tillein, & Adunka, 2011). Wilson and Dorman (2008) provide a review of the various techniques, including the use of shorter cochlear implant electrode arrays to preserve low-frequency hearing, to achieve electroacoustic stimulation in the same ear. Electroacoustic stimulation has been shown to provide advantages for listening in quiet and in noise and for perception of music. Essentially, these devices provide individuals with access to low-frequency sound under about 1,000 Hz through acoustic devices, and electrical stimulation in the high frequencies, and this arrangement has been shown to be advantageous when low-frequency hearing is present (Gantz & Turner, 2003; Gifford, Dorman, McKarns, & Spahr, 2007). The use of natural or amplified low-frequency hearing seems to help the listener perceive differences in these frequencies, which is not easily achieved through full electrical stimulation. These studies suggest that even a small amount of low-frequency information can provide important acoustic cues that can facilitate speech recognition in noise and improve music perception. Therefore, for individuals with residual hearing in the low frequencies, preservation of hearing can offer advantages for speech understanding. Interest has therefore grown in the preservation of low-frequency hearing during the surgical procedure to allow maximal use of bimodal hearing devices (Gantz, Turner, Gfeller, & Lowder, 2005; Gstoettner et al, 2006; Skarzynski & Lorens, 2010). Skarzynski and Lorens (2010) recently published data for 15 children with residual hearing who showed significant improvement in speech recognition scores in quiet and in noise after receiving a device that permitted combined electroacoustic stimulation.

In the interest of providing optimal hearing access, an array of choices of hearing aids, cochlear implants, or combined types of stimulation currently exist. The various combinations are listed in **Table 4.3** and can be summarized as (1) two hearing aids, (2) two cochlear implants, (3) one cochlear implant and one hearing aid in opposite ears, (4) cochlear implant combined with acoustic amplification in same ear and cochlear implant only in the opposite ear, (5) cochlear implant with acoustic aid in same ear and hearing aid only in opposite ear, and (6) both cochlear implant and acoustic aid in each ear. It is important that the clinician guiding the family work closely with clinical audiology teams to ensure familiarity with the various combinations of hearing devices, invest in learning and assisting the family with appropriate troubleshooting, and offer the family support in their decisions.

Table 4.3   Combinations of hearing technology

Right ear	Left ear
Hearing aid	Hearing aid
Cochlear implant	Cochlear implant
Cochlear implant	Hearing aid
Cochlear implant combined with hearing aid	Hearing aid
Cochlear implant combined with hearing aid	Cochlear implant
Cochlear implant combined with hearing aid	Cochlear implant combined with hearing aid

▓ Audiologic Management of Children with Cochlear Implants

Speech Processor Programming

All cochlear implant systems offer a choice of speech processing strategies, and new strategies are continuously under development (Wilson & Dorman, 2008, 2009). Wilson and Dorman (2009) describe two categories of speech processing strategies: envelope extraction strategies and fine structure strategies. Envelope strategies have different characteristics that are identified under various manufacturer names, such as continuous interleaved sampling, advanced combination encoder, spectral peak, and HiResolution. Fine structure processing strategies were introduced more recently and are aimed at better reproducing the fine structure information in speech and environmental sounds to improve speech recognition. See Wilson and Dorman (2009) for a review of common speech processing strategies. Characteristics of the different strategies vary and can be manipulated through programming of the processor. They include such aspects as number of active channels (sites of stimulation), rate of stimulation, and pulse width, as well as speech processor gain and volume. In addition, for some devices, different types of microphones can be selected to optimize sound. Generally, manufacturers provide default parameters, but these may require manipulation and adjustment by the audiologist to customize the program for an individual user to achieve optimal results.

Behavioral programming of speech processor (mapping). Essentially, the programming of a speech processor involves selecting a speech processing strategy and then mapping a range of acoustic sound from near 0 to 100 dB into an electric dynamic range of about 10 dB (Wilson & Dorman, 2009). The actual programming or "mapping" of a speech processor is carried out using techniques employed in conducting hearing assessments. The audiologist attempts to determine the levels of electrical current that allow the child to perceive an adequate range of sound while ensuring that sounds are comfortable. Fitting techniques with young children may include both behavioral and objective methods. Behavioral

testing is often much like obtaining a standard audiogram from a child using visual reinforcement or play audiometry with young children. Cochlear implant speech processors, like hearing aids, also provide multiple programming options such that different "listening" programs with different speech processing strategies can be created, or multiple versions of the same processing strategy but with variations in different parameters can be entered in the processor.

Objective speech processor programming. In the early years of cochlear implantation, programming of the speech processor was entirely dependent on the child's behavioral responses to electrical stimulation. A variety of objective programming techniques have been developed that can assist the audiologist in achieving optimal speech processor tuning. Neural response measurements (electrically evoked whole nerve action potentials) permit measurement of the action potentials from the auditory nerve in response to electrical stimulation. These measurements can be performed using various manufacturers' software and may provide confirmation of a response to stimulation and guide the audiologist in estimating comfort levels for the child (Hughes, 2006; Hughes, Brown, Abbas, Wolaver, & Gervais, 2000). Electrically evoked brainstem response audiometry can also provide information about the response of the auditory nerve and portions of the brainstem to electrical stimulation and can be particularly helpful in cases where action potentials cannot be elicited (Brown et al, 2000). In addition, the use of electrically evoked stapedius reflex thresholds, which involves measurement of a stapedial reflex to electrical stimulation, has been found useful for estimating comfort levels for electrical stimulation in the programming of individuals who cannot provide reliable behavioral responses (Hodges et al, 1997). These measures can be used to confirm and estimate responses, and they can be combined with behavioral measures to customize the device for each child.

Using well-programmed implant(s), children can be expected to access all of the sounds of the speech spectrum. If this is not achieved, various parameters of the speech processor can be manipulated to optimize hearing. For young children, programming of the speech processor may need to take place over several sessions and include both behavior and objective programming techniques for an optimal program to be achieved. The use of multiple programs can help establish appropriate levels for young children, for example by including a series of progressively louder programs that can be carefully used while parents and clinicians/educators observe the child's reactions to sounds. Sound field audiometry can be combined with these behavioral observations to gauge whether children are detecting sounds at expected levels, and may provide guidance regarding the need to augment electrical stimulation levels. However, sound field results should be interpreted with caution as they do not provide information about processing abilities but are limited to the softest level of sound a child detects with the cochlear implant processor worn with the recommended settings. A typical sound field audiogram for a child with bilateral cochlear implants is shown in **Fig. 4.4**.

Ongoing Audiologic Management of the Cochlear Implant

Generally, cochlear implant clinics maintain a program of regular follow-up to ensure that the child is receiving appropriate sound information through the implant device. These visits are typically more frequent for young children in the early stages of fitting the speech processor and obtaining optimal levels of electrical current. Consequently, input from the child's clinician/teacher can be of critical importance in the early months of device programming as the child is becoming adjusted to the new sounds. Since the therapist and family work closely together on a regular basis, including between scheduled audiology visits, they may be the first to observe changes in the child's audi-tory skills, discomfort with certain sounds, or general lack of progress, all of which can signal the need for adjustment of the speech processor program. During the early years of cochlear implantation, programming or "mapping" was generally required frequently to accommodate changes in threshold levels. Newer systems have become more sophisticated in the way that sound is electrically processed, and there appear to be less dramatic changes in current level requirements for most children. However, clinicians/teachers and parents who interact regularly with the child should alert audiologists to any concerns based on their observation of their child.

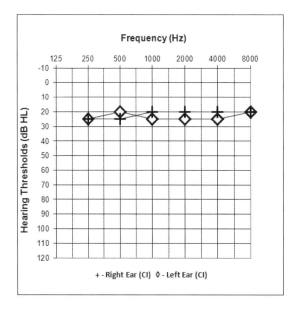

Fig. 4.4 Example of typical detection thresholds obtained with each cochlear implant.

Device failure is also a concern and may not be immediately evident to young children who are just learning to hear. Improvements in implant design by manufacturers are expected to result in a higher cumulative survival rate for implant devices. However, the survival rate can also be affected by a manufacturing defect in a particular device or an uncommon device malfunction. Therefore, the question of proper internal device functioning should be raised after external equipment issues have been ruled out whenever there are notable declines in auditory performance. An additional concern that has arisen since cochlear implantation was first implemented is the increased risk of meningitis in children who use cochlear implants (Biernath et al, 2006; Mancini et al, 2008).

Validation of Results

Similar to hearing aids, it is important to verify that the cochlear implant system is functioning optimally and also to validate results with the implant. Here the role of the clinician/teacher is critical in ensuring that the child is processing sounds adequately with the cochlear implant. Speech recognition measures are commonly used to quantify the auditory benefit from a cochlear implant, and several speech recognition (also called speech perception) tests, both closed- and open-set measures, have been developed to assess children preimplantation and to document auditory progress. Closed-set measures provide the listener with a specific set of responses—for example, a set of 12 pictures—whereas open-set measures provide no response set and the listener repeats what is heard. These tests, presented at selected audiometric levels in a sound suite, generally involve lists of phonemes, words, or sentences and are generally selected according to on the individual's cognitive and performance levels. For young children, or those with very little or no vocabulary, where speech recognition tests cannot be administered, several auditory questionnaires (some of which are described in Chapter 3) are useful in determining auditory access with cochlear implants. One widely used test in cochlear implant evaluations is the Meaningful Auditory Integration Scale (MAIS, Robbins, Renshaw, & Berry, 1991) or the version developed for younger children, the Infant-Toddler Meaningful Integration Scale (IT-MAIS, Zimmerman-Phillips, Robbins, & Osberger, 2000). This questionnaire, administered to parents, probes 10 auditory behaviors, such as the child's ability to respond to environmental sounds and to respond to his or her name in quiet and in noise. Another widely used questionnaire developed specifically for use with young children is the LittlEARS auditory questionnaire, a 35-item caregiver report that assesses auditory behaviors in the first 2 years of exposure to hearing (Coninx et al, 2009; Tsiakpini et al, 2004). Information gleaned from these tools or speech perception tests, combined with observation and assessment of the child's auditory and communicative functioning, is useful in monitoring progress and constructing the child's rehabilitation program.

Variability in outcomes has been reported across cochlear implant studies for both children and adults. Ultimately, the goal for children is to equip them with sufficient "hearing" to develop spoken language skills. Our data for a clinical sample show that children receiving cochlear implants at a mean age of 26 months who receive auditory and spoken language stimulation can expect on average to achieve age-appropriate speech and language scores on average at age 4 to 5 years (Fitzpatrick et al, 2011). For example, on expressive language testing, children in this study received a mean score of 88 (the mean standard score for the test is 100), which is within the expected range for peers with normal hearing. However, performance on these language tests was highly variable, with standard scores ranging from 50 to 140. The highest scores illustrate the tremendous potential for some children with early cochlear implantation; the lower scores serve as a reminder that many other factors interact to determine performance and that many of these children are functioning with restricted hearing and language skills in comparison to their peers with normal hearing. The range of outcomes supports that many children continue to require specific and focused intensive auditory and spoken language stimulation to become competent oral communicators.

The keen observations of an experienced clinician/teacher are even more important with very young children who cannot reliably perform speech recognition testing and who have insufficient vocabulary for testing. As noted previously, as a first step, concerns about lack of response or slower auditory development should be addressed through reprogramming of the speech processor and further assessment through objective and behavioral testing.

Given the continuous updates in technology, children can be expected to receive new speech processors or speech processing programs at various times during their rehabilitation program, and these new technologies may require a period of adjustment and encouragement. Good baseline information about children's auditory abilities is important in assessing whether hearing with the new strategy or device is comparable or improved. Collaboration and communication between audiologists, clinicians/teachers, and parents are essential in ensuring optimal hearing access.

Enhancing Listening with Cochlear Implants

Ensuring access to hearing throughout the child's daily activities is crucial to hearing and to spoken language. One of the major limitations of cochlear implants (Wilson & Dorman, 2009) and acoustic hearing aids involves understanding speech in competing noise and in group situations (Crandell & Smaldino, 2000). Therefore, an essential part of audiologic management involves the fitting of classroom audio distribution systems (e.g., remote microphone systems) to enhance speech understanding in the classroom setting (Flexer, 2004). Chapter 8 in this book describes in detail the rationale, technical aspects, and specific applications of these different devices for children with hearing loss, including those with cochlear implants. Before children enter school, audiologists may also recommend remote microphone systems for use in nursery and day care, and in some cases for home listening. Decisions are generally made on a case-by-case basis, taking into account the individual child's learning environment, as well as the family's particular circumstances. Remote microphone systems are, however, routinely recommended for children once they enter the school system, given the limitations related to distance hearing and hearing in noise (Flexer, 2004). Various applications and the advantages of remote microphone technology are discussed in detail in Chapter 8.

Other Implantable Devices

Bone-Anchored Hearing Aid

In the past 20 years, implantable technologies other than cochlear implants have become an option for certain hearing disorders.

The majority of children with permanent hearing loss have sensorineural loss, but a small number present with permanent bilateral conductive hearing loss. Historically, individuals with bilateral conductive hearing loss were fitted with bone conduction, rather than air conduction, hearing aids (as discussed in Chapter 3). Bone conduction hearing devices are designed to bypass the damaged external and middle ear systems to transmit mechanical vibrations directly to the cochlea. Traditional bone conduction hearing aids were held in place by a headband and were very uncomfortable, particularly for young children, and conduction between the bone vibrator and the skull (mastoid bone) was sometimes inefficient. These traditional instruments have largely been replaced by the implantable bone-anchored hearing aid (Baha). The Baha consists of a bone-anchored (using a 4-mm titanium screw) implant, a speech processor worn externally on the head, and an abutment that connects the implant and the processor. Through a process called osseointegration, the titanium screw is anchored to the skin (Hodgetts, 2011).

Initially, only individuals with permanent bilateral conductive hearing loss, such as that associated with bilateral atresia, were candidates for a Baha. Candidacy has expanded to include individuals with mixed hearing loss who cannot wear conventional acoustic hearing aids (for example, individuals with chronic ear discharge) and individuals with unilateral hearing loss, including conductive, mixed, and sensorineual types of loss (Hodgetts, 2011). Typically, young children are not candidates for Baha surgery until they reach 5 years of age, due to the increased risk related to the thinness of the developing skull (Snik, Leijendeckers, Hol, Mylanus, & Cremers, 2008). For children under age 10, a two-stage Baha surgery procedure is generally recommended in which the implant is first installed and the Baha abutment is installed a few months after the first surgery (Buchman et al, 2011; Snik et al, 2005). Prior to surgery, young children can be fitted with a Baha Softband, a set-up where the Baha is attached to a small plastic disk secured by an elastic headband. The Baha Softband offers an alternative to a conventional bone conduction hearing aid and delivers vibrations via the skin (subcutaneously) to the cochlea. Direct bone conduction as provided by the Baha implant is recommended as soon as it is medically feasible (Hodgetts, 2011). For further details regarding candidacy, as well as fitting and verification procedures for the Baha, refer to Hodgetts (2011).

Other Implantable Devices

Two other implantable devices used rarely in young children but that may be encountered occasionally in work with older children and adolescents include the middle ear implant and the auditory brainstem implant (Otto, Brackmann, & Hitselberger, 2004).

Middle ear implant. The middle ear implant is indicated for individuals who have mixed or sensorineural hearing loss of moderate to severe degree and who cannot use conventional acoustic hearing aids for medical reasons (e.g., recurring external otitis media) (Dumon et al, 2009). At the time of this writing, the middle ear implant has been approved only for use in adults. The system includes an internal device that resembles a cochlear implant but without electrodes. Instead, it uses a floating mass transducer, which is attached to the malleus and vibrates the middle ear ossicles. This provides more direct stimulation to the cochlea than a conventional acoustic device. The device is coupled to an external processor (Leutje et al, 2002).

Auditory brainstem implant. Individuals who lose hearing in both ears due to neurofibromatosis type II, a genetic condition associated with bilateral acoustic neuromas, may be candidates for an auditory brainstem implant. This pathology can cause partial or total obliteration (destruction) of the auditory nerve such that cochlear implantation is ineffective. Although acoustic information through the auditory brainstem implant is much more limited than through cochlear implants, research suggests that the device provides individuals with some speech recognition, facilitates speech reading, and provides individuals with improved contact with the auditory environment (Colletti et al, 2005; Otto, Brackmann, Hitselberger, Shannon, & Kuchta, 2002). It has also been recommended that auditory brainstem implants be considered for patients who have bilateral cochlear aplasia and cochlear injuries or other conditions preventing their benefiting from cochlear implants (Cervera-Paz & Manrique, 2005; Colletti et al, 2004).

▨ Summary

This chapter discussed means of providing children with access to hearing when conventional acoustic hearing aids are not sufficient or not appropriate for the degree or nature of the individual's hearing loss. Considerable technological progress has led to many more possibilities for children with hearing loss, including the use of unilateral and, more recently, bilateral cochlear implants, as well as cochlear implants combined with acoustic hearing devices in one or both ears. Over all, pediatric cochlear implantation has resulted in possibilities for auditory access and spoken language that were just emerging 20 years ago. However, despite the tremendous progress in device and processing strategies, gaps remain between the hearing abilities of children with cochlear implants and those of their peers with normal hearing. Accordingly, children and their families continue to require considerable support in developing adequate spoken language. Later chapters discuss how to support parents and eventually children themselves in maximizing auditory and spoken language potential. These chapters highlight the outcomes that are possible through application of the best technology and the best available evidence to the audiologic rehabilitation process.

■ Acknowledgments

We are grateful to the clinicians at the Children's Hospital of Eastern Ontario for contribution of clinical data and to Nathalie Wakil for assisting with the preparation and analysis of clinical data presented in this chapter.

■ Cochlear Implant Manufacturer Websites

Advanced Bionics Corporation, www.advancedbionics.com

Cochlear Corporation, www.cochlear.com

Med-El Corporation, www.medel.com

Neurelec, www.neurelec.com

■ References

Almond, M., & Brown, D. J. (2009). The pathology and etiology of sensorineural hearing loss and implications for cochlear implantation. In J. K. Niparko (Ed.), *Cochlear implants: Principles and practices* (2nd ed., pp. 43–87). Philidelphia, PA: Lippincott Williams & Wilkins.

Arisi, E., Forti, S., Pagani, D., Todini, L., Torretta, S., Ambrosetti, U., & Pignataro, L. (2010). Cochlear implantation in adolescents with prelinguistic deafness. *Otolaryngology—Head and Neck Surgery, 142*(6), 804–808.

Belzner, K. A., & Seal, B. C. (2009). Children with cochlear implants: A review of demographics and communication outcomes. *American Annals of the Deaf, 154*(3), 311–333.

Berlin, C. I., Morlet, T., & Hood, L. J. (2003). Auditory neuropathy/dyssynchrony: Its diagnosis and management. *Pediatric Clinics of North America, 50*(2), 331–340, vii–viii.

Biernath, K. R., Reefhuis, J., Whitney, C. G., Mann, E. A., Costa, P., Eichwald, J., & Boyle, C. (2006). Bacterial meningitis among children with cochlear implants beyond 24 months after implantation. *Pediatrics, 117*(2), 284–289.

Boothroyd, A. (2008). The acoustic speech signal. In J. R. Madell & C. Flexer (Eds.), *Pediatric audiology: Diagnosis, technology, and management* (pp. 159–167). New York: Thieme Medical Publishers.

Boothroyd, A., & Eran, O. (1994). Auditory speech perception capacity of child implant users expressed as equivalent hearing loss. *Volta Review, 96*(5), 151–167.

Brown, C. J., Hughes, M. L., Luk, B., Abbas, P. J., Wolaver, A. A., & Gervais, J. P. (2000). The relationship between EAP and EABR thresholds and levels used to program the nucleus 24 speech processor: Data from adults. *Ear and Hearing, 21*(2), 151–163.

Brown, K. D., & Balkany, T. J. (2007). Benefits of bilateral cochlear implantation: A review. *Current Opinion in Otolaryngology and Head & Neck Surgery, 15*(5), 315–318.

Buchman, C. A., Adunka, O. F., Zdanski, C. J., & Pillsbury, H. C. (2011). Medical considerations for infants and children with hearing loss: The otologists' perspective. In R. Seewald & A.-M. Tharpe (Eds.), *Comprehensive handbook of pediatric audiology* (pp. 137–153). San Diego, CA: Plural Publishing, Inc.

Cervera-Paz, F. J., & Manrique, M. J. (2005). Traditional and emerging indications in cochlear and auditory brainstem implants. *Revue de Laryngologie—Otologie—Rhinologie, 126*(4), 287–292.

Ching, T. Y., Incerti, P., Hill, M., & van Wanrooy, E. (2006). An overview of binaural advantages for children and adults who use binaural/bimodal hearing devices. *Audiology & Neuro-Otology, 11*(Suppl. 1), 6–11.

Ching, T. Y., van Wanrooy, E., & Dillon, H. (2007). Binaural-bimodal fitting or bilateral implantation for managing severe to profound deafness: A review. *Trends in Amplification, 11*(3), 161–192.

Colletti, V., Carner, M., Miorelli, V., Guida, M., Colletti, L., & Fiorino, F. (2005). Auditory brainstem implant (ABI): New frontiers in adults and children. *Otolaryngology—Head and Neck Surgery, 133*(1), 126–138.

Colletti, V., Fiorino, F. G., Carner, M., Miorelli, V., Guida, M., & Colletti, L. (2004). Auditory brainstem implant as a salvage treatment after unsuccessful cochlear implantation. *Otology Neurotology, 25*(4), 485–496, discussion 496.

Coninx, F., Weichbold, V., Tsiakpini, L., Autrique, E., Bescond, G., Tamas, L., . . . Brachmaier, J. (2009). Validation of the LittlEARS Auditory Questionnaire in children with normal hearing. *International Journal of Pediatric Otorhinolaryngology, 73*(12), 1761–1768.

Coticchia, J. M., Gokhale, A., Waltonen, J., & Sumer, B. (2006). Characteristics of sensorineural hearing loss in children with inner ear anomalies.

American Journal of Otolaryngology, 27(1), 33–38.

Crandell, C. C., & Smaldino, J. J. (2000). Classroom acoustics for children with normal hearing and with hearing impairment. *Language, Speech, and Hearing Services in Schools, 31,* 362–370.

Daya, H., Figueirido, J. C., Gordon, K. A., Twitchell, K., Gysin, C., & Papsin, B. C. (1999). The role of a graded profile analysis in determining candidacy and outcome for cochlear implantation in children. *International Journal of Pediatric Otorhinolaryngology, 49*(2), 135–142.

Dettman, S. J., D'Costa, W. A., Dowell, R. C., Winton, E. J., Hill, K. L., & Williams, S. S. (2004). Cochlear implants for children with significant residual hearing. *Archives of Otolaryngology—Head and Neck Surgery, 130*(5), 612–618.

Dettman, S. J., Pinder, D., Briggs, R. J., Dowell, R. C., & Leigh, J. R. (2007). Communication development in children who receive the cochlear implant younger than 12 months: Risks versus benefits. *Ear and Hearing, 28*(Suppl. 1), 11S–18S.

Dumon, T., Gratacap, B., Firmin, F., Vincent, R., Pialoux, R., Casse, B., & Firmin, B. (2009). Vibrant Soundbridge middle ear implant in mixed hearing loss: Indications, techniques, results. *Revue de Laryngologie—Otologie—Rhinologie, 130*(2), 75–81.

Dunn, C. D., Yost, W., Noble, W. G., Tyler, R. S., & Witt, S. A. (2006). Advantages of binaural hearing. In S. B. Waltzman & J. T. J. Roland (Eds.), *Cochlear implants* (pp. 205–221). New York: Thieme Medical Publishers.

Edwards, L. C. (2007). Children with cochlear implants and complex needs: A review of outcome research and psychological practice. *Journal of Deaf Studies and Deaf Education, 12*(3), 258–268.

Eisenberg, L. S., Martinez, A. S., Sennaroglu, G., & Osberger, M. J. (2000). Establishing new criteria in selecting children for a cochlear implant: Performance of "platinum" hearing aid users. *Annals of Otology, Rhinology, and Laryngology, 185*(12, Suppl. 185), 30–33.

Eriks-Brophy, A., Durieux-Smith, A., Olds, J., Fitzpatrick, E., Duquette, C., & Whittingham, J. (2012). Communication, academic, and social skills of young adults with hearing loss. *Volta Review, 112*(1), 5–35.

Fitzpatrick, E., & Brewster, L. (2008). Pediatric cochlear implantation in Canada: Results of a survey. *Canadian Journal of Speech-Language Pathology and Audiology, 32*(1), 29–35.

Fitzpatrick, E., McCrae, R., & Schramm, D. (2006). Cochlear implantation in children with residual hearing [Electronic]. *BMC Ear Nose and Throat Journal 6*(7).

Fitzpatrick, E., Olds, J., McCrae, R., Durieux-Smith, A., Gaboury, I., & Schramm, D. (2009). Pediatric cochlear implantation: How much hearing is too much? *International Journal of Audiology, 48,* 101–107.

Fitzpatrick, E., Séguin, C., & Schramm, D. (2004). Cochlear implantation in adolescents and adults with prelinguistic deafness: Outcomes and candidacy issues. *International Congress Series, 1273,* 269–272.

Fitzpatrick, E. M., Crawford, L., Ni, A., & Durieux-Smith, A. (2011). A descriptive analysis of language and speech skills in 4- to 5-yr-old children with hearing loss. *Ear and Hearing, 32*(5), 605–616.

Fitzpatrick, E. M., Jacques, J., & Neuss, D. (2011). Parental perspectives on decision-making and outcomes in pediatric bilateral cochlear implantation. *International Journal of Audiology, 50*(10), 679–687.

Fitzpatrick, E. M., Johnson, E., & Durieux-Smith, A. (2011). Exploring factors that affect the age of cochlear implantation in children. *International Journal of Pediatric Otorhinolaryngology, 75*(9), 1082–1087.

Fitzpatrick, E. M., Olds, J., Gaboury, I., McCrae, R., Schramm, D., & Durieux-Smith, A. (2012). Comparison of outcomes in children with hearing aids and cochlear implants. *Cochlear Implants International, 13*(1), 5–15.

Flexer, C. (2004). Classroom amplification systems. In R. J. Roeser & M. P. Downs (Eds.), *Auditory disorders in school children* (pp. 284–305). New York: Thieme Medical Publishers.

Friedland, D. R., Venick, H. S., & Niparko, J. K. (2003). Choice of ear for cochlear implantation: The effect of history and residual hearing on predicted postoperative performance. *Otology Neurotology, 24*(4), 582–589.

Fryauf-Bertschy, H., Tyler, R. S., Kelsay, D. M., Gantz, B. J., & Woodworth, G. G. (1997). Cochlear implant use by prelingually deafened children: The influences of age at implant and length of device use. *Journal of Speech, Language, and Hearing Research, 40*(1), 183–199.

Galvin, K. L., Mok, M., Dowell, R. C., & Briggs, R. J. (2008). Speech detection and localization results and clinical outcomes for children receiving sequential bilateral cochlear implants before four years of age. *International Journal of Audiology, 47*(10), 636–646.

Gantz, B. J., & Turner, C. W. (2003). Combining acoustic and electrical hearing. *Laryngoscope, 113*(10), 1726–1730.

Gantz, B. J., Turner, C. W., Gfeller, K. E., & Lowder, M. W. (2005). Preservation of hearing in cochlear implant surgery: Advantages of combined electrical and acoustical speech processing. *Laryngoscope, 115*(5), 796–802.

Geers, A. E., Strube, M. J., Tobey, E. A., Pisoni, D. B., & Moog, J. S. (2011). Epilogue: Factors contributing to long-term outcomes of cochlear implantation in early childhood. *Ear and Hearing, 32*(Suppl. 2), 84S–92S.

Gibson, W. P., & Sanli, H. (2007). Auditory neuropathy: An update. *Ear and Hearing, 28*(2, Suppl.), 102S–106S.

Gifford, R. H., Dorman, M. F., McKarns, S. A., & Spahr, A. J. (2007). Combined electric and contralateral acoustic hearing: Word and sentence recognition with bimodal hearing. *Journal of Speech, Language, and Hearing Research, 50*(4), 835–843.

Goldberg, D. M., & Flexer, C. (2001). Auditory-verbal graduates: Outcome survey of clinical efficacy. *Journal of the American Academy of Audiology, 12*(8), 406–414.

Gomaa, N. A., Rubinstein, J. T., Lowder, M. W., Tyler, R. S., & Gantz, B. J. (2003). Residual speech perception and cochlear implant performance in postlingually deafened adults. *Ear and Hearing, 24*(6), 539–544.

Gordon, K. A., & Harrison, R. V. (2005). Hearing research forum: Changes in human central auditory development caused by deafness in early childhood. *Hearsay, 17*, 28–34.

Gordon, K. A., & Papsin, B. C. (2009). Benefits of short interimplant delays in children receiving bilateral cochlear implants. *Otology Neurotology, 30*(3), 319–331.

Gordon, K. A., Papsin, B. C., & Harrison, R. V. (2006). An evoked potential study of the developmental time course of the auditory nerve and brainstem in children using cochlear implants. *Audiology & Neuro-Otology, 11*(1), 7–23.

Gordon, K. A., Twitchell, K. A., Papsin, B. C., & Harrison, R. V. (2001). Effect of residual hearing prior to cochlear implantation on speech perception in children. *Journal of Otolaryngology, 30*(4), 216–223.

Gordon, K. A., Valero, J., van Hoesel, R., & Papsin, B. C. (2008). Abnormal timing delays in auditory brainstem responses evoked by bilateral cochlear implant use in children. *Otology Neurotology, 29*(2), 193–198.

Gstoettner, W. K., Helbig, S., Maier, N., Kiefer, J., Radeloff, A., & Adunka, O. F. (2006). Ipsilateral electric acoustic stimulation of the auditory system: Results of long-term hearing preservation. *Audiology & Neuro-Otology, 11*(Suppl. 1), 49–56.

Guidelines for Identification and Management of Infants and Young Children with Auditory Neuropathy Spectrum Disorder. (2008). Retrieved from http://www.childrenscolorado.org/pdf/Guidelines%20for%20Auditory%20Neuropathy%20-%20BDCCH.pdf.

Hayes, H., Geers, A. E., Treiman, R., & Moog, J. S. (2009). Receptive vocabulary development in deaf children with cochlear implants: Achievement in an intensive auditory-oral educational setting. *Ear and Hearing, 30*(1), 128–135.

Hellman, S. A., Chute, P. M., Kretschmer, R. E., Nevins, M. E., Parisier, S. C., & Thurston, L. C. (1991). The development of a Children's Implant Profile. *American Annals of the Deaf, 136*(2), 77–81.

Hinojosa, R., & Marion, M. (1983). Histopathology of profound sensorineural deafness. *Annals of the New York Academy of Sciences, 405*, 459–484.

Hodges, A. V., Balkany, T. J., Ruth, R. A., Lambert, P. R., Dolan-Ash, S., & Schloffman, J. J. (1997). Electrical middle ear muscle reflex: Use in cochlear implant programming. *Otolaryngology—Head and Neck Surgery, 117*(3 Pt 1), 255–261.

Hodgetts, B. (2011). Other implantable devices: Bone-anchored hearing aids. In R. Seewald & A.-M. Tharpe (Eds.), *Comprehensive handbook of pediatric audiology* (pp. 585–598). San Diego, CA: Plural Publishing, Inc.

Holt, R. F., & Kirk, K. I. (2005). Speech and language development in cognitively delayed children with cochlear implants. *Ear and Hearing, 26*(2), 132–148.

Hughes, M. L. (2006). Fundamentals of clinical ECAP measures in cochlear implant. Part 1: Use of the ECAP in speech processor programming. *Audiology Online.* Retrieved from http://www.audiologyonline.com/articles/article_detail.asp?article_id=1569.

Hughes, M. L., Brown, C. J., Abbas, P. J., Wolaver, A. A., & Gervais, J. P. (2000). Comparison of EAP thresholds with MAP levels in the nucleus 24 cochlear implant: Data from children. *Ear and Hearing, 21*(2), 164–174.

Hyde, M., Punch, R., & Komesaroff, L. (2010). Coming to a decision about cochlear implantation: Parents making choices for their deaf children. *Journal of Deaf Studies and Deaf Education, 15*(2), 162–178 10.1093/deafed/enq004.

Johnston, J. C., Durieux-Smith, A., Angus, D., O'Connor, A., & Fitzpatrick, E. (2009). Bilateral paediatric cochlear implants: A critical review. *International Journal of Audiology, 48*(9), 601–617.

Johnston, J. C., Durieux-Smith, A., O'Connor, A., Benzies, K., Fitzpatrick, E. M., & Angus, D. (2009). The development and piloting of a decision aid for parents considering sequential bilateral cochlear implantation for their child with hearing loss. *Volta Review, 109*(2–3), 121–141.

Johnston, J. C., Durieux-Smith, A., Fitzpatrick, E., O'Connor, A., Benzies, K., & Angus, D. (2008). An assessment of parents' decision-making regarding paediatric cochlear implants. *Canadian Journal of Speech-Language Pathology and Audiology, 32*(4), 169–182.

Kirk, K. I., Miyamoto, R. T., Lento, C. L., Ying, E., O'Neill, T., & Fears, B. (2002). Effects of age at implantation in young children. *Annals of Otology, Rhinology & Laryngology,* (Suppl. 189), 69–73.

Leigh, J., Dettman, S., Dowell, R., & Sarant, J. (2011). Evidence-based approach for making cochlear implant recommendations for infants with residual hearing. *Ear and Hearing, 32*(3), 313–322 10.1097/AUD.0b013e3182008b1c.

Leutje, D. M., Brackmann, D., Balkany, T. J., Maw, J., Baker, R. S., Kelsall, D., . . . Arts, A. (2002). Phase III clinical trial results with the Vibrant Soundbridge: A prospective controlled multicenter study. *Otolaryngology–Head and Neck Surgery, 126*(2), 97–107.

Madden, C., Hilbert, L., Rutter, M., Greinwald, J., & Choo, D. (2002). Pediatric cochlear implantation in auditory neuropathy. *Otology & Neurotology, 23*(2), 163–168.

Mancini, P., D'Elia, C., Bosco, E., De Seta, E., Panebianco, V., Vergari, V., & Filipo, R. (2008). Follow-up of cochlear implant use in patients who developed bacterial meningitis following cochlear implantation. *Laryngoscope, 118*(8), 1467–1471.

McConkey Robbins, A., Koch, D. B., Osberger, M. J., Zimmerman-Phillips, S., & Kishon-Rabin, L. (2004). Effect of age at cochlear implantation on auditory skill development in infants and toddlers. *Archives of Otolaryngology and Head and Neck Surgery, 130*(5), 570–574.

McCracken, W., & Turner, O. (2012). Deaf children with complex needs: Parental experience of access to cochlear implants and ongoing support. *Deafness & Education International, 14*(1), 22–35.

Meinzen-Derr, J., Wiley, S., Grether, S., & Choo, D. I. (2011). Children with cochlear implants and developmental disabilities: A language skills study with developmentally matched hearing peers. *Research in Developmental Disabilities, 32*(2), 757–767.

Moog, J. S., & Geers, A. E. (2003). Epilogue: Major findings, conclusions and implications for deaf education. *Ear and Hearing, 24*(Suppl. 1), 121S–125S.

Most, T., & Zaidman-Zait, A. (2003). The needs of parents of children with cochlear implants. *Volta Review, 103*(2), 99–113.

Murphy, J., & O'Donoghue, G. M. (2007). Bilateral cochlear implantation: An evidence-based medicine evaluation. *Laryngoscope, 117*(8), 1412–1418.

Nadol, J. B., Jr., Young, Y. S., & Glynn, R. J. (1989). Survival of spiral ganglion cells in profound sensorineural hearing loss: Implications for cochlear implantation. *Annals of Otology, Rhinology, and Laryngology, 98*(6), 411–416.

NHS National Institute for Health and Clinical Excellence. (2009). *Cochlear implants for children and adults with severe to profound deafness.* Retrieved from http://www.nice.org.uk/TA166

Nicholas, J. G., & Geers, A. E. (2006). Effects of early auditory experience on the spoken language of deaf children at 3 years of age. *Ear and Hearing, 27*(3), 286–298.

Nicholas, J., & Geers, A. E. (2007). Will they catch up? The role of age at cochlear implantation in the spoken language development of children with severe to profound hearing loss. *Journal of Speech, Language and Hearing Research, 50*, 1048–1062.

Nikolopoulos, T. P., Dyar, D., & Gibbin, K. P. (2004). Assessing candidate children for cochlear implantation with the Nottingham Children's Implant Profile (NChIP): The first 200 children. *Journal of Pediatric Otorhinolaryngology, 68*(2), 127–135.

Niparko, J. K., Tobey, E. A., Thal, D. J., Eisenberg, L. S., Wang, N. Y., Quittner, A. L., & Fink, N. E.; CDaCI Investigative Team. (2010). Spoken language development in children following cochlear implantation. *Journal of the American Medical Association, 303*(15), 1498–1506.

Olds, J., Fitzpatrick, E., Schramm, D., & McLean, J. (2006). *Outcome of cochlear implantation in children with complex disabilities.* Paper presented at the 4th Widex Congress of Pediatric Audiology, Ottawa, Canada.

Olds, J., Fitzpatrick, E. M., Steacie, J., McLean, J., & Schramm, D. (2007). *Parental perspectives of outcome after cochlear implantation in children with complex disabilities.* Paper presented at the International Conference on Cochlear Implants in Children, Charlotte, NC.

Otto, S. R., Brackmann, D. E., & Hitselberger, W. E. (2004). Auditory brainstem implantation in 12- to 18-year-olds. *Archives of Otolaryngology and Head and Neck Surgery, 130*(5), 656–659.

Otto, S. R., Brackmann, D. E., Hitselberger, W. E., Shannon, R. V., & Kuchta, J. (2002). Multichannel auditory brainstem implant: Update on performance in 61 patients. *Journal of Neurosurgery, 96*(6), 1063–1071.

Papsin, B. C., & Gordon, K. A. (2008). Bilateral cochlear implants should be the standard for children with bilateral sensorineural deafness. *Current Opinion in Otolaryngology & Head & Neck Surgery, 16*(1), 69–74.

Perreau, A. E., Tyler, R. S., Witt, S., & Dunn, C. (2007). Selection strategies for binaural and monaural cochlear implantation. *American Journal of Audiology, 16*(2), 85–93.

Peters, B. R., Litovsky, R., Parkinson, A., & Lake, J. (2007). Importance of age and postimplantation experience on speech perception measures in children with sequential bilateral cochlear implants. *Otology & Neurotology, 28*(5), 649–657.

Ramsden, J. D., Papaioannou, V., Gordon, K. A., James, A. L., & Papsin, B. C. (2009). Parental and program's decision making in paediatric simultaneous bilateral cochlear implantation: Who says no and why? *International Journal of Pediatric Otorhinolaryngology, 73*(10), 1325–1328 10.1016/j.ijporl.2009.05.001.

Rance, G., & Barker, E. J. (2008). Speech perception in children with auditory neuropathy/dyssynchrony managed with either hearing aids or cochlear implants. *Otology & Neurotology, 29*(2), 179–182.

Rance, G., Barker, E. J., Sarant, J. Z., & Ching, T. Y. C. (2007). Receptive language and speech production in children with auditory neuropathy/dyssynchrony type hearing loss. *Ear and Hearing, 28*(5), 694–702.

Rance, G., Beer, D. E., Cone-Wesson, B., Shepherd, R. K., Dowell, R. C., King, A. M., . . . Clark, G. M. (1999). Clinical findings for a group of infants and young children with auditory neuropathy. *Ear and Hearing, 20*(3), 238–252.

Rance, G., & Starr, A. (2011). Auditory neuropathy/dys-synchrony type hearing loss. In R. Seewald & A.-M. Tharpe (Eds.), *Comprehensive handbook of pediatric audiology* (pp. 225–242). San Diego, CA: Plural Publishing, Inc.

Raveh, E., Buller, N., Badrana, O., & Attias, J. (2007). Auditory neuropathy: Clinical characteristics and therapeutic approach. *American Journal of Otolaryngology, 28*(5), 302–308.

Rhoades, E. A. (2010). Core constructs of family therapy. In E. A. Rhoades & J. Duncan (Eds.), *Auditory-verbal practice: Toward a family-centered approach* (pp. 137–163). Springfield, IL: Charles C Thomas Publisher, Ltd.

Rhoades, E. A., Price, F., & Perigoe, C. B. (2004). The changing American family & ethnically diverse children with hearing loss and multiple needs *Volta Review, 104*(4, monograph), 285–305.

Robbins, A. M., Renshaw, J. J., & Berry, S. W. (1991). Evaluating meaningful auditory integration in profoundly hearing-impaired children. *American Journal of Otology, 12*(Suppl.), 144–150.

Rubinstein, J. T., Parkinson, W. S., Tyler, R. S., & Gantz, B. J. (1999). Residual speech recognition and cochlear implant performance: Effects of implantation criteria. *American Journal of Otology, 20*(4), 445–452.

Schafer, E. C., Amlani, A. M., Seibold, A., & Shattuck, P. L. (2007). A meta-analytic comparison of binaural benefits between bilateral cochlear implants and bimodal stimulation. *Journal of the American Academy of Audiology, 18*(9), 760–776.

Schramm, D., Fitzpatrick, E., & Séguin, C. (2002). Cochlear implantation for adolescents and adults with prelinguistic deafness. *Otology & Neurotology, 23*(5), 698–703.

Sharma, A., Dorman, M. F., & Kral, A. (2005). The influence of a sensitive period on central auditory development in children with unilateral and bilateral cochlear implants. *Hearing Research, 203*(1-2), 134–143.

Sharma, A., Dorman, M. F., Spahr, A. J., & Todd, N. W. (2002). Early cochlear implantation in children allows normal development of central auditory pathways. *The Annals of Otology, Rhinology, and Laryngology, 189*(Suppl.), 38–41.

Skarzynski, H., & Lorens, A. (2010). Electroacoustic stimulation in children. In P. Van de Heyning & A. Kleine Punte (Eds.), *Cochlear implants and hearing preservation: Advances in otorhinolaryngology* (Vol. 67, pp. 135–143). Basel: Karger.

Snik, A. F. M., Leijendeckers, J., Hol, M., Mylanus, E. A. M., & Cremers, C. W. R. J. (2008). The bone-anchored hearing aid for children: Recent developments. *International Journal of Audiology, 47*(9), 554–559.

Snik, A. F. M., Mylanus, E. A. M., Proops, D. W., Wolfaardt, J. F., Hodgetts, W. E., Somers, T., . . . Tjellstrom, A. (2005). Consensus statements on the BAHA system: Where do we stand at present? *Annals of Otology, Rhinology, and Laryngology, 114*(12, Suppl. 195), 1–12.

Stacey, P. C., Fortnum, H. M., Barton, G. R., & Summerfield, A. Q. (2006). Hearing-impaired children in the United Kingdom, I: Auditory performance, communication skills, educational achievements, quality of life, and cochlear implantation. *Ear and Hearing, 27*(2), 161–186.

Starr, A., Picton, T. W., Sininger, Y. S., Hood, L. J., & Berlin, C. I. (1996). Auditory neuropathy. *Brain, 119*(Pt. 3), 741–753.

Starr, A., Sininger, Y. S., & Pratt, H. (2000). The varieties of auditory neuropathy. *Journal of Basic and Clinical Physiology and Pharmacology, 11*(3), 215–230.

Summerfield, A. Q., Lovett, R. E., Bellenger, H., & Batten, G. (2010). Estimates of the cost-effectiveness of pediatric bilateral cochlear implantation. *Ear and Hearing, 31*(5), 611–624 10.1097/AUD.0b013e3181de40cd.

Svirsky, M. A., Teoh, S. W., & Neuburger, H. (2004). Development of language and speech perception in congenitally, profoundly deaf children as a function of age at cochlear implantation. *Audiology & Neuro-Otology, 9*(4), 224–233.

Teagle, H. F. B., Roush, P. A., Woodard, J. S., Hatch, D. R., Zdanski, C. J., Buss, E., & Buchman, C. A. (2010). Cochlear implantation in children with auditory neuropathy spectrum disorder. *Ear and Hearing, 31*(3), 325–335 10.1097/AUD.0b013e3181ce693b.

Thoutenhoofd, E. D., Archbold, S. M., Gregory, S., Lutman, M. E., Nikolopoulos, T. P., & Sach, T. H. (2005). *Paediatric cochlear implantation: Evaluating outcomes.* London: Whurr Publishers Ltd.

Tsiakpini, L., Weichbold, V., Kuehn-Inacker, H., Coninx, F., D'Haese, P., & Almandin, S. (2004). *LittlEARS Auditory Questionnaire.* Innsbruck, Austria: MED-EL.

Tucci, D. L., & Pilkington, T. M. (2009). Medical and surgical aspects of cochlear implantation. In J. K. Niparko (Ed.), *Cochlear implants: Principles and practices* (2nd ed.) (pp. 161–186). Philidelphia, PA: Lippincott Williams & Wilkins.

Tyler, R. S., Kelsay, D. M., Teagle, H. F., Rubinstein, J. T., Gantz, B. J., & Christ, A. M. (2000). 7-year speech perception results and the effects of age, residual hearing and preimplant speech perception in prelingually deaf children using the Nucleus and

Clarion cochlear implants. *Advances in Oto-Rhino-Laryngology, 57,* 305–310.

Vlastarakos, P. V., Proikas, K., Papacharalampous, G., Exadaktylou, I., Mochloulis, G., & Nikolopoulos, T. P. (2010). Cochlear implantation under the first year of age—the outcomes: A critical systematic review and meta-analysis. *International Journal of Pediatric Otorhinolaryngology, 74*(2), 127–132.

von Ilberg, C. A., Baumann, U., Kiefer, J., Tillein, J., & Adunka, O. F. (2011). Electric-acoustic stimulation of the auditory system: A review of the first decade. *Audiology & Neuro-Otology, 16*(Suppl. 2), 1–30.

Waltzman, S. B., Roland, J. T., Jr, & Cohen, N. L. (2002). Delayed implantation in congenitally deaf children and adults. *Otology & Neurotology, 23*(3), 333–340.

Watkin, P. M., & Baldwin, M. (2011). Identifying deafness in early childhood: Requirements after the newborn hearing screen. *Archives of Disorders in Childhood, 96,* 62–66.

Wiley, S., Jahnke, M., Meinzen-Derr, J., & Choo, D. (2005). Perceived qualitative benefits of cochlear implants in children with multi-handicaps. *International Journal of Pediatric Otorhinolaryngology, 69*(6), 791–798.

Wiley, S., & Meinzen-Derr, J. (2009). Access to cochlear implant candidacy evaluations: Who is not making it to the team evaluations? *International Journal of Audiology, 48*(2), 74–79.

Wiley, S., Meinzen-Derr, J., & Choo, D. (2008). Auditory skills development among children with developmental delays and cochlear implants. *Annals of Otology, Rhinology, and Laryngology, 117*(10), 711–718.

Wilson, B. S., & Dorman, M. F. (2008). Cochlear implants: Current designs and future possibilities. *Journal of Rehabilitation Research and Development, 45*(5), 695–730.

Wilson, B. S., & Dorman, M. F. (2009). The design of cochlear implants. In J. K. Niparko (Ed.), *Cochlear implants: Principles and practices* (2nd ed.) (pp. 95–135). Philadelphia, PA: Lippincott Williams & Wilkins.

Xu, Y. (2007). Empowering culturally diverse families of children with disabilities: The double ABCX model. *Early Childhood Education Journal, 34*(6), 431–437.

Zeitler, D. M., Kessler, M. A., Terushkin, V., Roland, T. J., Jr, Svirsky, M. A., Lalwani, A. K., & Waltzman, S. B. (2008). Speech perception benefits of sequential bilateral cochlear implantation in children and adults: A retrospective analysis. *Otology & Neurotology, 29*(3), 314–325.

Zimmerman-Phillips, S., Robbins, A. M., & Osberger, M. J. (2000). Assessing cochlear implant benefit in very young children. *Annals of Otology, Rhinology, and Laryngology, 185*(Suppl.), 42–43.

5 Creating Optimal Listening and Learning Environments in the First Years

Newborn hearing screening has become a worldwide public health initiative, and as a result more children with permanent hearing loss are identified in the first few months or even days of life. For various reasons, some children are not identified with hearing loss until after the early infancy period, even when screening initiatives are in place. While parent guidance is advocated throughout the child's development, in these early stages the primary focus of intervention is on parent support and education rather than "therapy" with the child. Working closely with parents, direct intervention through embellished play activities is increased as the child grows. The premise of intervention as described in this book is that children can best develop listening and spoken language in naturally enriched family, play, and learning environments. This chapter focuses on optimizing listening and spoken language during the child's first 2 to 2½ years. We describe intervention practices with young children in which a family-oriented approach is applied and we emphasize parents' needs in the very early years. Specific parent guidance techniques and intervention strategies are elaborated. Practical aspects of intervention with young children are also described.

▪ Parent Guidance and Spoken Language Development

Family-Oriented Guidance

Parent guidance and support can be viewed as including three essential components: (1) information and education, (2) coaching to create an optimal listening and learning environment, and (3) teaching parents specific listening and language facilitation techniques (**Fig. 5.1**). In addition to the support that is provided specifically through the audiologic rehabilitation program, some parents can benefit from external supports in other areas when dealing with hearing loss–associated issues; several of these points are discussed in subsequent sections.

The following is an example of a child identified during infancy with a hearing loss.

Baby Simeon was born at 41 weeks' gestation without complications in a hospital setting to Canadian-born Korean parents. At birth, with parental consent, a newborn hearing screening test was conducted in the hospital using an otoacoustic emission screening procedure. The test, which yielded a pass/refer result, indicated that Simeon should be referred for a second screening. The parents were told that due to the screening test results, Simeon should be taken to a community screening clinic for a second test within the next month. The parents left the hospital with Simeon when he was 2 days old and the following week took him to a screening clinic in a community center a few blocks from their home. Again they were informed that the test gave a refer result and they were instructed to take him to their local children's hospital audiology program for a full audiologic evaluation. The referral and appointment were managed by the screening program. At 6 weeks of age, Simeon was seen for a battery of diagnostic tests and the pediatric audiologist informed the parents that their child presented with a severe to profound sensorineural hearing loss based on auditory brainstem response test results. On the same day, the parents saw an otolaryngologist at the hospital. A few days later, they met with a family support worker, who told them about the various intervention options for Simeon, ranging from programs with a focus on listening and spoken language acquisition (e.g., auditory-verbal therapy) to programs with an emphasis on visual communication (e.g., American Sign Language). The parents quickly opted to proceed with hearing aids. They wanted to do what was necessary to help Simeon learn to speak, and hearing loss

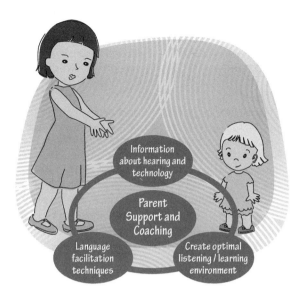

Fig. 5.1 Components of parent support and coaching.

was an entirely new phenomenon for them. They enrolled in the intervention program at their local hospital. Simeon received follow-up from a pediatric hearing team that included an otolaryngologist, audiologist, social worker, and listening and spoken language specialist. Binaural hearing aids were fitted within 3 weeks, and through weekly intervention sessions, the parents began learning about hearing loss and how to develop Simeon's auditory skills.

Scenarios similar to this one are repeated again and again for thousands of infants and their families. Historically, prior to screening, parents observed their children's development and went through a process of identifying or guessing about the hearing disorder themselves. In contrast, many of today's parents arrive in audiology clinics and are presented with the diagnosis without realizing that their child has a problem. While parents generally feel very positively about the benefits of early identification, it is important to realize that they have had no preparation time to confront the problem (Fitzpatrick, Graham, Durieux-Smith, Angus, & Coyle, 2007; Young & Tattersall, 2005; Young & Tattersall, 2007). Therefore, some parents may need time to work through the diagnosis, which can result in delays to amplification and intervention (Pipp-Siegel, Sedey, & Yoshinaga-Itano, 2002). According to parents, among the most important aspects of care at this critical time is the quality of communication with professionals and the availability of information (Fitzpatrick, Graham, et al, 2007; McCracken, Young, & Tattersall, 2008).

Studies show that parents have a variety of reactions and need considerable support throughout these early months (Fitzpatrick, Angus, Durieux-Smith, Graham, & Coyle, 2008; Young & Tattersall, 2007). However, this process of acceptance is not a short-term event and will continue for many families throughout much of the child's life (Luterman, 2006), particularly at periods of transition, such as a change in hearing status or amplification needs, as well as when the child starts preschool or elementary school, or moves from one school level or program to another.

Recognizing that parents are at different stages of understanding and managing their child's hearing loss is of prime importance for clinicians/teachers as they begin guiding parents in stimulating their child's language development. Throughout the early months of learning about their child's hearing loss, parents may need ongoing guidance and direction to engage in their child's development. Using a parent-validated questionnaire to measure stress, Meinzen-Derr, Lim, Choo, Buyniski, and Wiley (2008) found that caregivers of children with hearing loss had greater stress levels than those of children with normal hearing, and that health care–related concerns were especially high in the first 24 months following diagnosis. Not surprisingly, one particularly stressful period in the very early stages after confirmation of the hearing loss is related to receiving hearing aids or cochlear implants (Burger et al,

2005). For some parents, this event brings a stark realization that their child has a permanent disorder. Perhaps one of the greatest challenges for professionals is adapting their parent guidance approach to individual parents. It is important to recognize that some parents prefer an action-oriented approach from the beginning, as reflected in this mother's comments when she was interviewed about her needs after learning about her child's hearing disorder:

> But there's not a lot out there for people who just move on, so let's move beyond the psychosocial aspect, which I think is important for some people, but there are some people who just move beyond that really quickly and want to do other things.

It is important to be aware that different families will come to the rehabilitation process at different entry points and levels of readiness to begin intervention work. Parents of children with late-onset hearing loss may experience a different process of discovering hearing loss, particularly if the results from the first screening tests suggest normal hearing. As evidence is collected from newborn hearing screening initiatives, it is becoming increasingly clear that delayed onset of hearing loss is more prevalent than was initially documented (Fitzpatrick, 2011c; Lü et al, 2011; Watkin & Baldwin, 2011). Other families may have learned about the child's hearing loss later due to poor follow-up from universal newborn hearing screening (UNHS), a concern reported in some regions (Shulman et al, 2010). Others from countries where screening is not available may simply not have had access to early identification services.

Factors Affecting Families

There is a growing recognition that family engagement in the rehabilitation process is one of the most important determinants of outcomes. Parents have been described as the "essential partners" when the focus is on a spoken language intervention program for children with hearing loss (Simser, 1999). Accordingly, it is important that rehabilitation specialists take into account the individual family characteristics and social and cultural contexts that affect families' abilities in adverse situations (Rhoades, 2010a; Rhoades, Price, & Perigoe, 2004). We present brief examples of some of the factors that impact family engagement in the intervention program. While none of these factors is insurmountable or even necessarily a barrier, practitioners need to be sensitized to the potential influences on the family's acceptance and the adjustments required to follow intervention programs. For a more in-depth study of family-centered practice in developing spoken language, refer to Rhoades and Duncan (2010).

Socioeconomic Status

It has been well documented in the health literature that socioeconomic position is the single most important factor predicting health outcomes (Marmot & Wilkinson, 2006). In the hearing loss literature, socioeconomic status has been shown to be a determinant of outcomes in children with cochlear implants (Niparko et al, 2010). Other studies have found parent education level to be associated with better spoken language outcomes (Fitzpatrick, Durieux-Smith, Eriks-Brophy, Olds, & Gaines, 2007; Sininger, Grimes, & Christensen, 2010). In practical terms related to intervention, socioeconomic status can affect parents' abilities to purchase and maintain hearing aids or cochlear implants, to secure transportation to a clinic, to provide care for other children at home to enable them to attend audiology and intervention sessions, to make time to provide intensive stimulation at home for the child with hearing loss while caring for other children, and simply to "take a break" from day-to-day parenting. The demands of caring for a child with special needs can be more difficult for parents with limited financial resources or extended family support. Decisions about optimal child care and preschool placements can also be affected by family circumstances and resources. Concerns about income and other practical needs can supersede the very best intentions. Overall, the family's ability to provide technology and auditory and language stimulation need to be taken into consideration in developing a care program. Ideally, practitioners work with other resources, such as social workers and child agencies, to put additional supports in place.

Family Characteristics

Various family characteristics can influence the functioning of the family unit (Rhoades, 2010b). Children are born and grow up in families with very different compositions, and family composition can change throughout the child's developmental years. For example, children may be living with a single parent, with two parents but in two different homes, with grandparents, in a foster home, or with more than one adult, all of which potentially affect the quality and degree of language stimulation. Different arrangements can (although not necessarily will) impact the continuity of interactions and make common goal setting in language development more difficult to achieve (Bernstein & Eriks-Brophy, 2010).

Societies are becoming increasingly diverse from cultural and religious or philosophical perspectives. For example, families newly arrived in a country are often faced with challenges related to cultural adaptation and the burden of learning a new language. Clinicians/ teachers need knowledge about and sensitivity to cultural and related influences on parent–child interaction styles (Rhoades, 2010b). Customs, attitudes toward use of hearing technology, education, and child behavior practices can vary across cultures and even from one parent to another. Clinicians/teachers are therefore faced with the task of learning, adapting, and developing different techniques for different situations. Professionals have the challenge of responding to individual and diverse family needs to maximize the spirit of collaboration in helping parents learn about and realize their child's spoken language and overall communication potential. Rhoades (2008) and Rhoades and Duncan (2010) provide useful discussions of the issues facing families in minority linguistic and cultural situations and the need for culturally sensitive intervention.

Linguistic Situation

In today's multicultural societies, many children receiving intervention will be exposed to more than one language and come from families whose native language is not that of the clinician/educator or the region where they are growing up. In certain cultures, grandparents may be very intimately involved in the early education of the child, and in some cases the language of communication, or at least the dialect used, may differ (Simser, 1999). As described in Chapter 12, in some countries children may be in families where different languages are used by family members and nannies or other caregivers who are very involved in providing language stimulation for the child. In other situations, particularly bilingual countries, families may simply have a strong desire that their child be able to speak more than one mainstream language.

Historically, exposure to only the "mainstream" or school language was recommended for children, particularly those with severe and profound hearing loss, regardless of the language of the home. This was because late identification and limited access to hearing had such negative consequences for spoken language development that the acquisition of two languages was considered unattainable (Ling & Ling, 1978). The current view is that exposure to more than one language in early childhood does not delay language acquisition in typically developing children, and parents should talk to their children in the language that they themselves are most comfortable using, on the assumption that children will receive richer linguistic input (Paradis, Crago, Genesee, & Rice, 2003). With the availability of earlier and better-quality access to hearing, these theories are also generally applied to children with hearing loss. The situation needs to be carefully monitored to ensure that children are able to access the second language so that they will be prepared for formal school instruction in the second language. For some children, additional tutoring or other services may be required to increase exposure to the nonnative language.

As noted in Chapter 1, a multitude of factors, some well understood and others not, have been shown to affect the development of children with hearing loss. Clearly, the family characteristics mentioned here are complex and likely interact and combine with other factors to affect families' abilities to engage in health intervention programs.

Parent Information, Education, and Support

Hearing-Specific Information

In the early months of diagnosis, information about the child's hearing loss and thus potential for auditory learning is often incomplete. During this period, there is an emphasis in audiology and therapy on determining the precise degree of hearing loss in each ear, fitting hearing aids, and establishing exactly what the child hears (Bagatto, Scollie, Hyde, & Seewald, 2010). For children identified with auditory neuropathy spectrum disorder (ANSD), rather than relying on auditory brainstem response (ABR) testing alone, parents are often urged to investigate behavioral testing and observation before proceeding with amplification (Bagatto et al, 2010; Rance, 2005). Decisions about hearing aid prescriptions for children who are "borderline," such as those with mild bilateral or unilateral hearing loss, may be delayed for some time (Fitzpatrick, Durieux-Smith, & Whittingham, 2010; McKay, Gravel, & Tharpe, 2008). Determining whether the use of hearing aids, cochlear implants, or no amplification is the most appropriate for the degree of hearing loss and optimizing the hearing aid fitting can involve several visits to the audiology clinic. As discussed in Chapter 3, not only are objective methods for hearing aid verification required, but observations in intervention sessions, parent questionnaires (Bagatto, Moodie, Seewald, Bartlett, & Scollie, 2011), and discussions with the family can also contribute to hearing aid management decisions (Bagatto et al, 2010; King, 2010).

Throughout these technical areas of management, an important goal is to help parents become familiar with hearing loss and with hearing aids and their characteristics, and to guide them in achieving full-time use of the instruments. Achieving consistent hearing aid use in young children, especially in diverse situations outside the home, remains a challenge for some parents (Bagatto et al, 2011; Moeller, Hoover, Peterson, & Stelmachowicz, 2009). The quality fitting of hearing instruments and education in their full-time use is viewed as the first critical step in audiologic rehabilitation. Providing the infant or young child with optimal access to hearing requires expertise in pediatric audiology and ongoing communication between parents, audiologists, and clinicians/teachers.

As noted in Chapter 3, unlike adults, young children cannot provide feedback to assist with fine tuning of amplification. Therefore, parents, audiologists, and clinicians/teachers work together to evaluate the quality of the sound the child is receiving. Parents can be taught what auditory responses to look for in the home and other settings. These include reactions to sound, such as increased vocalizations, stillness, and searching, as well as vocal variety in the child's babbling. Parents are also coached to report any adverse reactions to sound. With young children, audiologists are concerned with over-amplification as well as with under-amplification, both of which, in the absence of direct feedback from the child, need to be monitored carefully so that appropriate adjustments can be made.

As parents learn about the hearing loss, specific hearing-related information can help them understand the consequences of their child's hearing loss for speech development and the need for full-time use of amplification. Parents specifically underscore the importance of hearing-related information and report that they want ongoing information about the latest technology throughout their child's care (Fitzpatrick et al, 2008). Various materials have been developed to help parents understand audiograms and the specific effects of hearing loss on access to speech and environmental sounds. One very useful tool is a speech sounds audiogram. This commonly used tool helps to translate the child's audiogram through pictures and speech sounds into a format that is meaningful for parents. Various versions of this audiogram exist (see www.audiology.org for an example). Use of such practical tools can help parents understand how hearing loss interferes with acoustic information and how appropriately fitted amplification can enhance their child's access to sound. In addition, simple demonstrations of speech frequency sounds presented at different intensity levels and in different acoustic environments that simulate real-world listening (for example, in quiet and at different signal-to-noise ratios) can be useful for parents, especially those who are having difficulty accepting the full-time use of hearing technology.

Parents' Needs in the Early Stages

Since the implementation of newborn hearing screening, considerable attention has been directed to understanding how best to assist parents in the early months and years of learning about their child's hearing loss (Bernstein & Eriks-Brophy, 2010; Fitzpatrick et al, 2008; McCracken et al, 2008; Tattersall & Young, 2006; Young & Tattersall, 2007). From reports in the literature, supported by parent interviews (Fitzpatrick et al, 2008), we can conclude that, generally, parents

- Place great value on interactions and communication with professionals and find reassurance in knowing that a cohesive team is working with them
- Value coordinated services where there is communication between professionals
- Want information about their child's prognosis for spoken language
- Want clear and specific guidance on how to develop language
- Value contact with other families, especially in the early stages of learning about hearing loss

Luterman and Kurtzer-White (1999) found that parents identified meeting other parents as their most important need at the time of diagnosis of hearing loss. Several years later, Fitzpatrick et al (2008) found that many parents rated this need so high that they recommended it be included as an optional component of early intervention programs to ensure that it is not overlooked by practitioners. In this study, parents also talked about the usefulness of meeting older children with similar hearing loss who had developed language so that they could put hearing loss in perspective and have some sense of the prognosis for their child. From this research we can conclude that in this early period, parents also need help with their feelings as they adjust to parenting a child with hearing loss and that they want to act by getting started with intervention. It is also apparent that the need for this type of support is independent of the severity of hearing loss and that parents of children with mild bilateral and unilateral hearing loss also need support, particularly when the hearing loss is first identified. As expressed by one audiologist (Fitzpatrick, 2011b) in focus group interviews about the impact of learning about hearing loss on parents of children with milder forms of impairment:

The old standard [applies] . . . a hearing loss is a hearing loss, is a hearing loss to the parent.

Research indicates that one of the most important aspects of care in the early stages is equipping parents with ongoing knowledge and information from the time of screening. In a United Kingdom study investigating maternal anxiety during the various stages of the screening and identification processes, knowledge and understanding were found to be protective (Crockett, Baker, Uus, Bamford, & Marteau, 2005). In other research, parents indicated that knowledge was critical to being able to make decisions and feel in control. As stated by one parent, "Knowledge is power" (Fitzpatrick et al, 2008). This includes specific information related to hearing loss and hearing technology, as well as clear directions about the next steps in the process.

Despite the investment in early intervention services and the growing awareness of best practices and the importance of parent support, parents have identified lack of communication between professionals and lack of coordinated services as one of the greatest barriers in working with health and education services (Fitzpatrick et al, 2008). When parents were asked to weigh the key ingredients of early intervention programs, coordination of services was one of the four critical components identified (Fitzpatrick et al, 2007). For example, parents stressed the need for ongoing communication between audiologists and clinicians/teachers. The following quote exemplifies the importance that parents attribute to team communication:

Because we get to see the therapist most often, they know us, they can see the progress or problems. I think the therapist is a window to see what's going on for other people in the team. So I think the therapist needs to talk more to their co-workers, audiologists mostly. (Fitzpatrick, 2007)

Recommendations

These studies, combined with our clinical experience, allow us to summarize the following general guidelines for working with parents in the early months and years when they are adapting to parenting a child with hearing loss:

- Parents have different needs at different times, and they reach stages of adjustment to hearing loss at different times.
- Parents may need some time to deal with the hearing loss before they can begin "intervention" with the child. Early intervention does not have to look like "therapy." It is useful to think about intervention as coaching parents as they interact with their young child as naturally as possible.
- Many parents want opportunities to meet other parents of children with hearing loss and to meet with children or young adults who have hearing loss.
- Parents want information about all of the technology-related options. Practitioners generally try to judge when parents are ready to receive more details, but our work with parents suggests that it seems beneficial to always offer parents information rather than assume that they are not ready for it.
- Professionals with expertise in family counseling in domains such as social work and psychology should be consulted when the family needs additional support.
- Some parents require assistance in finding appropriate resources for their child, such as child care services and nursery schools.
- Parents should be encouraged and provided with strategies to become advocates for their child from the beginning.
- Parents generally benefit from ongoing direct contact with a professional; this helps build trust and confidence in a relationship with the professional.
- When a parent needs to discuss a very specific issue, for example, cochlear implantation, it can be useful to make advance arrangements to have a family member or other individual take care of the child during important discussion meetings.
- Many parents want to be given actionable steps to know what to do next. Therapists frequently find that using a notebook with parents during each session can help keep parents on track (i.e., parents can be assigned specific homework).
- Practitioners should be prepared to discuss the child's prognosis with parents. Parents' concerns about reasonable expectations may be indirectly expressed in questions such as, "Will my child be able to go to a regular school? Will my child be able to attend university?"
- Parents want up-to-date information. Given the availability of Internet resources, clinical programs are no longer the only source or even the primary source for this, but parents want professionals to provide the best available information.

In summary, as noted by Luterman (2006), coping with loss of any type involves a complex process with different decision-making situations and different trigger points generating new or old emotions, such as guilt, stress, inadequacy, and confusion. A thorough discussion of these aspects of counseling is beyond the scope of this text and the reader is referred to readings such as Luterman (2006), Bernstein and Eriks-Brophy (2010), and McGinnis (2010) for further information on supporting families.

■ Creating an Optimal Listening and Learning Environment

Creating a Favorable Listening Environment

The first step in creating an optimal learning environment for the child is to establish consistent hearing aid or cochlear implant use. The situation may be easier for infants who have not yet "found their ears," while for slightly older children, the situation can be a trying one for parents. Therefore, parents may need considerable encouragement and practical tips to help secure hearing aids, such as the use of a bonnet or hearing aid huggie device. Others may need ongoing education and reminders of the importance of ensuring that their child is receiving the very best acoustic information. In particular, the use of hearing aids in children with milder hearing loss seems to be inadequate. In a longitudinal study of seven infants who received amplification early, only two achieved full-time hearing aid use across multiple contexts (Moeller et al, 2009). Less controlled situations, such as driving in a car and outdoor play, were more challenging situations for parents.

Some parents naturally create enriched learning environments, while others need considerable guidance in the form of practical suggestions and learning activities to help them organize the home environment. At this stage, it is not the specific content of the therapy session that is important (i.e., the vocabulary, the type of language); rather, intervention involves helping parents become aware of listening and language learning opportunities in everyday environments. Rehabilitation with young children is essentially about teaching and encouraging parents to provide enriched learning environments. There is good evidence from the general literature that learning in the early years is experiential and contextual (Hart & Risley, 1999). Intervention goals are therefore primarily focused on providing parents with techniques that permit them to offer enriched learning experiences throughout the child's daily activities. In other words, therapy in these very early years is based on natural language models of natural experiences and interactions with people in one's environment. To achieve these goals, parents need to learn how to create the best learning environment possible so that their child has the best possible acoustic access to the auditory centers of the brain.

Historically, with late identification, children with hearing loss entered intervention programs already experiencing a language delay, and clinicians/teachers, while cognizant of the importance of the natural learning environment, were faced with a remedial model of care to address the gap between the child's development and that of hearing peers at the outset. Given early identification, many more children are likely to benefit from a developmental model of spoken language acquisition. Therefore, "therapy" sessions are about providing models for parents that include play situations designed to teach parents how to stimulate audition and language. It should be stressed that the formal sessions are at least partly about coaching parents how to provide stimulating experiences through everyday interactions that extend well beyond the one-hour therapy session.

Equipped with some knowledge about the acoustic properties of speech sounds and how impaired hearing affects audibility (as presented in Chapter 2), parents can be taught specific strategies to optimize the listening environment. Practical strategies include ensuring that: the child is using well-functioning hearing technology during all waking hours, that there is a quiet learning environment in the early stages, and that speech is delivered within the child's earshot (appropriate distance between speaker and listener). In essence, these are necessary strategies or environmental modifications to help compensate for sound that is less rich in quality. The primary concern is ensuring acoustic accessibility of sound to the child's brain to the greatest extent possible through current technologies. In working with parents, strategies aimed at highlighting acoustic salient information are integrated into all of the interventions, as described in subsequent sections of this chapter. Throughout each session, parents are shown and reminded how to provide an optimal listening environment. In particular, intervention sessions conducted in the home can be useful in highlighting to parents how to set up an enriched learning environment. Equally important is the quality and quantity of acoustic information delivered to the child, and making the signal accessible through speech. The application of various intervention techniques is the focus of the next section.

Guiding Parents in Developing Listening and Spoken Language

Our conception of rehabilitation in this book is based on the notion that children with hearing loss require "intervention" to acquire language because of reduced access to sounds in their environment, a situation that interferes with the natural development of speech and language.

In other words, as presented in Chapter 1, the child's brain is wired or programmed to learn language in the same way as peers with normal hearing. Furthermore, as seen in Chapters 3 and 4, most children with hearing loss gain access to the speech spectrum through hearing aids or cochlear implants. Therefore, the goal of auditory or audiologic rehabilitation is to equip the child with the best listening skills possible to facilitate spoken language development in as natural a way as possible. In other words, the premise of this book and the focus of our discussions on intervention is that these children have a hearing problem rather than a language problem.

Auditory-based intervention services have evolved under different funding structures and care models, resulting in some variation from one program to another with regard to frequency and place of service delivery: for example, clinic, community center, or home. Program delivery models seem to have evolved based on regional practices, costs, and clinicians' preferences, and while there is no evidence supporting a preferred model, there are several characteristics common to most services. (See Chapter 12 for a brief description of several programs throughout the world.) These generally include individualized therapy goals, based on an overall assessment process, including audiologic results and so-called diagnostic assessment of the child's abilities through interaction; parent-specific guidance and participation of parents in all sessions; and (auditory-based) therapy through play aimed at teaching listening skills to facilitate spoken language development through hearing. Common elements of most programs include some form of planned therapy that varies in structure and specific activities depending on the child's age and clinician/teacher style and preference.

Prior to the availability of cochlear implant technology, there was a tendency to apply more structured and very specific teaching methods, but many such approaches have transitioned to much less structured interventions that may look more like play sessions with children with normal hearing. It is common practice to apply certain techniques that facilitate listening and learning in children with hearing loss. These specialized techniques may be thought of as ways of embellishing language to make it more accessible for children with hearing loss and are generally applied as a function of the degree of hearing loss or rate of progress of the child.

The notion of patient-centeredness is widely accepted in health care, and a family-centered approach to pediatric hearing programs is widely advocated. See Rhoades and Duncan (2010) for an in-depth treatment of this subject. What parental involvement looks like in actual practice varies depending on the characteristics of the program. The importance of investing in parental engagement has been underscored in several studies on children with hearing loss. In a 20-year longitudinal study of 40 children and families, Schlessinger (1992) found self-esteem of the mother to be the most important predictor of academic success, superseding severity of hearing loss, socioeconomic status, and intervention method. Audiologic rehabilitation described in this book involves intervention sessions that are planned with the overall objective of teaching parents how to develop spoken language through maximizing audition. Consequently, the goals targeted in a specific organized therapy session become part of listening and language learning outside the session at home and elsewhere. To achieve this, clinicians/teachers typically integrate audition, speech, language, and cognition objectives in demonstration-type therapy sessions, which for young children consist of a variety of play activities, book reading, music, and rhymes. Intervention focused on spoken language development for children affected with hearing loss differs from other speech-language interventions in that the clinician/teacher takes into account the auditory functioning of the child throughout the therapy session. In this sense, audiologic rehabilitation refers to the ensemble of events that take place to develop "hearing" so that language acquisition occurs as naturally as possible. In this model, parents view the clinician/teacher with whom they develop a long-term relationship as a key player and the professional primarily accountable for the child's intervention program (Fitzpatrick et al, 2008).

The nature of auditory rehabilitation of hearing is such that it requires expertise related to several domains, notably audiology, speech-language pathology, and education. Accordingly, professionals from these different disciplines have assumed responsibility for managing the ongoing intervention for children with hearing loss and work in concert with other professionals, particularly audiologists, to facilitate listening and spoken language. Increasingly, there is recognition of the need for a specialization in listening and spoken language for children with hearing loss. Efforts to ensure that professionals trained in various disciplines have the required competencies have led to the development of training programs (see the 2010 special issue of *Volta Review*) and an international certification offered by the AG Bell Academy for Listening and Spoken Language Specialists (LSLS) (www.agbell.org). Frequently, care models are team based and include specialists from other disciplines, such as occupational therapy, psychology, social work, and developmental pediatrics. Otolaryngologists are also involved, particularly in the early stages of establishing the diagnosis of a permanent hearing loss. They continue to be involved past the early stages as required to manage middle ear disorders and to provide surgical intervention, including cochlear implantation when appropriate.

Beginning Intervention with Babies

Assessment

One of the first steps in rehabilitation services in any domain generally involves a comprehensive assessment to determine the nature and magnitude of the problem and to plan treatment. For young children who begin intervention after early identification of hearing loss, a focal part of the assessment process is related to the audiologic evaluation, which is aimed at determining the type of hearing disorder and degree of hearing loss. Once hearing loss is confirmed, the rehabilitation process generally starts with the fitting of technology for the majority of children.

Assessment in communication disorders serves several purposes: (1) to compare functioning with that of peers with normal hearing, (2) to monitor progress, and (3) to set treatment goals (McCauley, 2001). In the early months of infancy, the child with hearing loss will have little or no spoken language skills, and therefore most formal speech and language measures are not generally useful. Such a situation may also apply to young children when hearing loss has been identified late (beyond the first year). However, there is a growing recognition of the contribution of preverbal language (Paul & Norbury, 2012), and clinicians/teachers will be keenly interested in determining whether appropriate preverbal language behaviors are in place.

In Chapter 3 it was noted that auditory-specific questionnaires, such as the Parents' Evaluation of Aural/Oral Performance of Children (PEACH) Rating Scale, can help provide information about the child's early auditory behaviors. The PEACH, which is available either in parent diary form or in a shortened version as a rating scale, is a caregiver report designed to provide information about functional auditory behavior in quiet and noisy situations in real-world listening environments (Ching & Hill, 2007). Recent data from a large longitudinal study in Australia suggest that PEACH scores at 6 months of age can predict auditory and spoken language development scores at age 3 years (Ching, 2012). Other caregiver report questionnaires, such as the Infant-Toddler Meaningful Auditory Integration Scale (Zimmerman-Phillips, Robbins, & Osberger, 2000) and the LittlEARS questionnaire (Tsiakpini et al, 2004; Weichbold, Tsiakpini, Coninx, & D'Haese, 2005), have become widely used functional auditory measures in both hearing aid and cochlear implant validation. They are particularly useful with young children who cannot reliably participate in more objective methods, such as speech recognition testing. Bagatto et al (2011) provide a useful critical review of functional auditory questionnaires that can be applied with preschool-age children.

Clinicians/teachers often refer to "diagnostic" assessment (Estabrooks, 2006), meaning that an evaluation of the child's ability to process information and acquire language through hearing is integral throughout the entire intervention process. In practical terms, each time that the clinician/teacher provides services to the family, questions are asked about whether changes are required to optimize the child's intervention. Each session involves observations of the strengths and challenges of the child through the learning process. This ongoing assessment approach assists in planning subsequent interventions.

As the child starts to acquire words and spoken language, assessments can be conducted. The cases described later in this chapter and in Chapter 6 provide examples of some of the current commonly used tools to assess children's communication development. Refer to Paul and Norbury (2012) for lists and descriptions of additional assessment measures.

An assessment of the child's overall developmental status through skilled observations and various tools is of considerable importance. Current literature suggests that 60 to 70% of children with hearing loss have typical development, leaving a high percentage of children with hearing loss who have complex medical and developmental disabilities. Some of these disabilities are not apparent at birth and, in some cases (e.g., autism), may not be diagnosed for several years. Essentially, the clinician/teacher's role extends beyond just listening and language to include consideration of the child's global development so that appropriate referrals to developmental specialists can be made. Because of the close interaction with the child and family, the clinician/teacher may be the first to suspect additional difficulties, and this can facilitate the involvement of and interaction with a team of specialists to obtain more comprehensive assessment. See Chapter 7 for discussion of children with hearing loss and additional developmental disabilities.

When the child's native language (home language) is different from that of the clinician/educator or when the child is exposed to more than one language, interpretation of the assessments must take this information into account. Some of the available assessments will not be useful with respect to children with cultural and linguistic differences. Fortunately, some assessment tools for young children, such as the Communication Development Inventory (Ireton, 1992), as well as auditory questionnaires (e.g., PEACH, LittlEARS), are available in multiple languages. However, caution must be exercised in using and interpreting the results from tools that have been simply translated but not standardized for the population of interest (Langdon & Wiig, 2009). Psychometric properties of assessments should be examined to ensure adherence to normative samples, validity, and accuracy (McCauley & Swisher, 1984). In some cases, support from a native speaker of the language can help the clinician in conducting and interpreting the assessment. Suggestions for modifying standardized tests for assessment of children with linguistic differences and further discussion of assessment practices can be found in Paul and Norbury (2012).

Auditory Learning

Auditory learning for children with hearing loss is often conceptualized in terms of stages of auditory development (Estabrooks, 2006; Ling & Ling, 1978; Pollack, Goldberg, & Caleffe-Schenck, 1997). Erber (1982) presented a framework for auditory teaching that involves four levels of auditory processing: detection, discrimination, identification, and comprehension of speech. It is clear that sound detection is a necessary prerequisite to auditory learning. In other words, hearing technology must provide the child with sufficient access so that speech sounds are audible. However, detection after hearing aid fitting for a young child may not be immediately obvious, particularly with severe to profound hearing loss, and considerable auditory practice may be required before there is consistent sound detection.

Detection refers simply to knowledge of the presence or absence of a sound. Some authors refer to the subsequent stage of learning as auditory awareness. In other words, the child not only is able to detect a sound, such as in an audiometric sound suite, but also shows awareness of sound through searching, stilling, smiling, head turning, vocalizing, or other response. It is frequently in these very early stages of establishing consistent detection and attention, that is, before clear and reliable awareness of sound is demonstrated, that parents require so much support and encouragement. For example, for children with profound hearing loss, during the preimplant stage, detection and awareness can be fairly inconsistent, and parents need support to continue intensive auditory stimulation when there is little feedback from the child. In the case of severe or profound hearing loss, lack of sound awareness, if not demonstrated reliably through behavioral responses, can be an indication to proceed with consideration of cochlear implants. Consistent sound detection and awareness provide early convincing evidence that auditory learning can occur. Very early in intervention, children are introduced and taught to respond to the Ling-6 sound test, a commonly used test comprising the phonemes [m, u, a, i, ʃ, s] that cover the spectrum of speech sounds in English (Ling, 2002). Consistent responses to these six sounds suggest that the child's hearing technology is providing audibility across the speech frequency range.

Once awareness of sound is established, it can be expected that the child will start associating meaning to sounds around him; for example, when Mother says, "up, up, up," the child learns to associate the sound pattern with being held, or "mmm" with being fed. Essentially, in doing this, the child has learned to "discriminate" that sounds are different, to identify words or patterns, and to comprehend (associate meaning to) sounds and words. Children with normal hearing and typical development reach these stages so rapidly and effortlessly that rarely is there reflection about a hierarchy of auditory stages. In other words, these auditory skills emerge very early as part of the typical course of language development.

Depending on hearing loss severity and auditory experience, the auditory development trajectory may be longer for children with hearing disorders. More attention is accorded to stages and discrete auditory skills for these children because of their impaired hearing and the consequent need for specific "training" of hearing. In the next section, we present activities and practical aspects of developing auditory learning in children with hearing loss.

Once detection, awareness, and associating meaning to sound are established, most children with hearing loss are well on their way to learning language through audition. As discussed in Chapters 3 and 4 and earlier in this chapter, through feedback from parents and clinicians/educators, validation of the fitting is achieved, and adjustments or alternative technology (e.g., more powerful hearing aids or cochlear implants) ensure that sound is audible, allowing the auditory experience necessary for language learning to continue.

Listening and Language Facilitation Techniques

One of the most common language facilitation techniques applied in typical adult-child interaction is infant-directed talk (motherese). Infant-directed talk, which includes techniques like variation in pitch, intensity, and duration, has been widely adopted and even expanded in work with children with hearing loss. In auditory-based therapy, the use of acoustic enhancements is incorporated into a strategy often referred to as *acoustic highlighting,* which essentially means slightly changing the typical speech pattern to make the information more audible for the child with hearing loss (Estabrooks, 2006; Simser, 1999). Making speech more acoustically salient is achieved through a variety of techniques that involve some form of exaggeration, such as emphasis (for example, placing a word at the end of a phrase), elongation of vowels, changing the intonation pattern, and repetition. As the child becomes more acoustically competent, the amount of additional acoustic information is reduced and more typical speech patterns are used (Simser, 1999).

Another common strategy in auditory teaching is the use of animal sounds or other interesting sound words (e.g., pop-pop-pop), often referred to as sound–word associations,

meaning that a sound can be associated with a meaningful word or event. While these types of sound are used in play with children with normal hearing, one of the key differences in auditory-based therapy is the frequency and the specific intent or meaning attributed to them. These sounds or short words are intended to be acoustically salient and are selected to help the young child with hearing loss detect and attend to sound in an interactive play environment. These sound-words or beginning words also lend themselves to easy repetition along with the accompanying movement of a toy or other event. For example, "walk-walk-walk" can be repeated as the child walks toward something or as a movable toy moves across a table. Similarly, "ba-ba-ba" can be repeated for an extended period of time as a child plays with a toy boat bobbing in a container of water, or "hop-hop-hop" as a frog hops through the water. Examples of words and expressions that permit acoustic enhancements are provided in "learning to listen" word lists (Estabrooks, 1998; Simser, 1993). Common characteristics of many lists are the use of onomatopoeic words, as discussed above (e.g., "meow"). Some beginning lists also include familiar expressions such as

"Shhh—baby's sleeping," "Brrr, it's cold," and "Don't touch!" because they provide similar opportunities for redundancy and repetition to occur regularly in everyday settings. **Table 5.1** provides examples of some of the "learning to listen" words, including our favorite suggestions for helping parents get started with acoustically salient material. Effectively, any words or short phrases that lend themselves to repetition in multiple situations in a child's life are appropriate. In summary, these specific techniques permit the clinician/teacher to provide the parent with practical strategies to use at home in the early stages. **Table 5.2** provides an example of one clincan/teacher's favorite activities for stimulating auditory and language development with babies. In **Table 5.3**, another clinician/teacher shares how she integrates multiple teaching goals (e.g., audition, speech, language, cognition, and motor) with the use of some of her favorite toys for babies.

Unlike parents of children with normal hearing, parents of children with hearing loss may spend considerable time stimulating the child to detect and attend to sound while receiving little clear reinforcement in the form of language comprehension and expression. Clinicians/teachers working in concert with audiologists need to provide parents with the assurance that auditory stimulation of the brain will facilitate the child's ability to develop spoken communication in the most natural way possible. Other important activities to be encouraged at this stage are singing, reading books, and engaging in any other oral language activity that allows for extensive repetition, rhythm, and redundancy. See Chapter 10 for further discussion of how these activities contribute to emergent literacy.

Even before children use their first words, important language learning is taking place. Parents need coaching to understand the rich contribution not only of auditory stimulation before there is evidence that their child is understanding language, parents need coaching to grasp the contribution not only of auditory stimulation, but also of preverbal language, a contribution to spoken language development that should not be underestimated. In cochlear implant research, preimplant communicative behaviors have been shown to be a good predictor of auditory and language outcomes in children at a later age (Tait, De Raeve, & Nikolopoulos, 2007; Tait,

Table 5.1 Example of "learning to listen" sounds

"Learning to listen" sounds	Example of toy
Aaaaaaaaaaaah!	Airplane
Shhhhhhhh!	Baby or animal sleeping
Up up up up weeeeeeee!	Slide
babababababa	Boat
choo choo oooo	Train
Vrooom vrooom beep beep	Car
Hop hop hop	Rabbit or frog
Walk walk walk	Shoes/person
Uffuffuffuffuff	Butterfly
Sssssssssssssss!	Snake
Round and round and round	Spinning top/helicopter
Quack quack quack	Duck
Mmmmm!	Ice cream/other food
Ha ha ha!	Clown
Hee hee hee hee!	Witch
Ho ho ho ho!	Santa Claus
Ding dong ding dong!	Bells

Table 5.2   An example of a clinician/teacher's favorite activities for stimulating auditory and language development with babies

Favorite activities for babies
Audition To develop on/off perception, I ask parents to dance around with their child when the music is on, and freeze when the music stops. As the child gets older, she begins to imitate by swaying to the music, and vocalizing when it stops
Speech To develop a baby's speech sound repertoire, I like to use mirror play time. Some kids can be very vocal when they see themselves and their caregivers in the mirror. I encourage the parent to imitate the child's vocalization and continue turn taking with their child.
Language To develop the child's receptive understanding of his parents' names, we play a game of hide and seek. One parent walks the baby around the house while calling for the other parent (e.g., "Mommy"). The child then listens for other's response (target: localization) and moves slowly to that parent's hiding spot. The parent is called over and over in order to give the child multiple opportunities to hear the word. Then, when the child finds "mommy," we have a big party "There's mommy; you found her!" Most young kids really love water play. To encourage a child to vocalize for a request, we use a water jug to slowly fill up a tub. We take turns looking and telling the pitcher to "POUR!" Eventually, after a lot of modeling, I hold the pitcher as if I am ready to pour and then we wait. We wait for the child to make a sound to reward her with the water. Once the bucket is full, we bring some "learning to listen" sound objects (e.g., duck, frog, boat).
Communication At all ages, I really enjoy using books in therapy. Early on, books are a great way to help parents learn the strategies involved in "parentese" and acoustic highlighting. We forget about the words on the page and focus on using short, repetitive, acoustically interesting phrases and sounds. We pass the book around the table and each adult gets a chance to practice. At the end, I always give the child the chance to manipulate the book and even turn to his favorite page. The parent is then taught to follow the child's lead and talk about what the child is interested in. For very young children, I like flap books because they allow for an element of surprise. We can also practice action imitation (knock, knock, knock).
Contribution from Erin McSweeney, Children's Hospital of Eastern Ontario, Ottawa, Canada.

Lutman, & Robinson, 2000). Therefore, parents are taught not only to "bathe their children in sound" but also to encourage and recognize preverbal behaviors, such as joint gesturing, joint attention, and turn taking. Research has shown that children with hearing loss can have difficulty because so much of this normal interaction depends simply on the child's awareness of being spoken to and the ability to engage in communication even on a preverbal level.

Early Intervention: Moving On

Clinicians/teachers play an important role in helping parents understand their child's current listening and language levels and helping them learn what to expect and when to move to more advanced listening and language skills. For example, once the child demonstrates understanding of sound patterns (e.g., that "hop, hop, hop" is associated with a frog), parents need to advance to the next stage of word and phrase development. Parents will benefit from ongoing coaching on the expectations for typically developing children and learn to adjust the amount of acoustic information (acoustic cues) provided to the child in order to promote positive audi-

Table 5.3 A clinician/teacher shares how she integrates multiple teaching goals (e.g., audition, speech, language, cognition, and motor activities) while using some of her favorite toys for babies

Integration of teaching goals using favorite toys for babies
Pop-up farm
This is a toy that requires the children to push a button, pull or twist a lever, or turn a wheel, and when they do an animal pops up.
Auditory: stimulation. Every time an animal pops up we say its name and make the correct LTL sound. Also, when the farmer pops up, we sing "Old McDonald."
Language: We say, "Hi cow," "Bye pig," "Where's the chick?"
Speech: encourage child to say LTLs
Fine motor: work on various ways to use fingers
Cognition: problem solving
Pull toy dog
The dog is on a string; his ears can spin around and his tail is a ball on the end of a spring.
Auditory: LTL "woof woof" (have child listen to LTL several times prior to seeing the toy). Emphasize to parents that while talking, they should stress critical words, put pauses around them, be animated, and use lots of intonation.
Language: stimulation ("pull the dog," "look at his tail," "his ears go round and round")
Cognition: cause/effect
Bubbles
Auditory: LTL "up up up" "blow the bubble" "pop"
Language: "all gone" "Where'd it go?" "more bubbles"
Speech: /p/, blowing
Mirror
Use a large, unbreakable mirror with a cloth covering it.
Auditory: "Where's _____?" "Peekaboo"
Language: "Hi _____." "Bye _____."

Abbreviation: LTL, learning to listen.
Contribution from Kelly Rabjohn, Children's Hospital of Eastern Ontario, Ottawa, Canada.

tory experiences. In essence, clinicians/teachers allow the child to follow normal developmental sequences while making embellishments and modifications to enhance the acoustic quality and make the information more accessible. Effectively, teaching of new language forms is occurring in synchrony with the development of more complex auditory skills.

As noted, for children with normal hearing, there seems to be no evidence of specific or discrete stages of auditory development, after the child has started attaching meaning to sound patterns (e.g., animal sounds) and words. That is, it is not clear that young children compartmentalize their auditory learning into sound–word associations, then words, and then multiple words, short phrases, and longer chunks of information. However, children with hearing loss have more restricted auditory access in terms of both quantity and quality of information. Clinicians have therefore generally proposed that some organization of acoustic input into a kind of "auditory hierarchy" of skills is useful in developing children's capacity to acquire spoken language primarily through hearing (Estabrooks, 2006; Simser, 1993; Sindrey, 1998). These hierarchies seemed to have evolved because, in general, children with hearing loss, particularly severe to profound loss, need more practice to process speech information through the auditory channel. Presenting the auditory information in acoustically salient "chunks" has been adopted in early audition-based intervention.

Although there is a general tendency to refrain from using the term "auditory training" in an effort to dispel the notion that developing language through audition is an isolated activity, the goal of these hierarchies is to train or fine-tune the child's hearing, a tuning exercise that does not seem to be required for children with normal hearing. This process has often been referred to as organizing auditory input to help children maximize use of residual hearing (or electrically stimulated hearing through cochlear implants) (Estabrooks, 2006; Ling, 2002).

The development of auditory-specific skills for the purpose of equipping the child with the auditory experience is an important characteristic of audition-based intervention. Although auditory skill teaching is not separated from experiential language learning and speech development, many clinicians/teachers guide the parents through a series of auditory goals and activities. Several practitioners have developed checklists or criterion-referenced tools to guide intervention. Some of these are also used as informal assessment tools to assist clinicians/teachers in monitoring progress. These checklists vary in the number of discrete skills, but common is the notion of moving from simple to complex auditory skills. Examples are described by Simser (1993) and Pollack, Goldberg, and Caleffe-Schenck (1997). Pollack et al describe nine stages of auditory development, ranging from awareness of sound to understanding of speech, and provide numerous suggestions for materials, activities, and parent guidance for each stage. As noted above, Erber (1982) proposed a hierarchy of four auditory response levels as a way to conceptualize and organize auditory skills development: detection, discrimination, identification, and comprehension. Other clinicians have used these categories and have identified types of specific auditory skills falling in each one (Estabrooks, 2006). It is important to note that prior to the availability of cochlear implantation, many of the early auditory skills hierarchies involved very discrete auditory development because of children's limited access to sound. Some of these specific plans for skill building may be very useful for children who are progressing slowly in auditory skills or who do not have access to optimal hearing—for example, when cochlear implants are not available.

It is essential to understand that working with babies and families in the first two years after early identification of hearing loss is about facilitating access to sound, rich auditory stimulation, and providing an embellished language environment so that learning occurs as naturally as possible. Therapy is about guiding and encouraging parents and involves constantly monitoring the child's auditory and language abilities so that action can be taken to ensure optimal hearing with the best available technology. **Tables 5.4** and **5.5** provide examples of expectations for typical children in the 19- to 24-month and 25- to 30-month ranges.

Tables 5.6 and **5.7** provide a clinician/teacher's sample lesson plans for a young child (case described below) identified following newborn hearing screening. These lesson plans at hearing aid fitting and 1 year later illustrate how therapy goals change to focus on more advanced auditory, language, and cognitive skills as the child progresses over the 1-year period. The clinician/teacher's notes related to parents also demonstrate the importance of parental input in audition-based learning.

Jordan is an 8-year-old boy with bilateral sensorineural hearing loss who was born at 28 weeks' gestation. He spent two days in the neonatal intensive care unit, where his hearing was first screened and hearing loss was confirmed at 3 months' corrected age. Auditory brainstem results showed a mild to severe hearing loss in the right ear and moderate to severe hearing loss in the left ear. He was fitted with binaural hearing aids at 5 months' corrected age, and he and his family were immediately enrolled in weekly auditory-verbal therapy sessions at their local hospital. No other developmental concerns were identified. He currently attends a grade 2 class in a French immersion program in his neighborhood school.

The appendix to this chapter provides a detailed example of a typically developing child with hearing loss identified before 6 months of age. This example provides the results of a comprehensive assessment undertaken by his clinician/teacher, her interpretation of the results, and a lesson plan for the child at 1 year, 5 months. The same type of information is also summarized for the child 1 year later. The summary provides an overview of the sequential assessments and intervention for young children as well as a good example of expectations for auditory and language growth for typically developing children with hearing loss.

Table 5.4   Typical stages for 19- to 24-month-old children

Listening (audition)

- Auditory memory of two items
- Discriminates songs
- Comprehends a variety of phrases
- Discriminates descriptive phrases

- Follows a two-step direction, e.g., Get your ball and throw it.
- Identifies by category

Receptive language

- Completes two requests with one object
- Chooses two familiar objects
- Comprehends action phrases
- Points to a range of body parts, e.g., elbow, cheek

- Begins to understand personal pronouns— "my," "mine," "you"
- Recognizes new words daily
- Increases comprehension—decodes simple syntax
- By 24 months understands 250–300 words

Expressive language

- Occasionally imitates two- or three-word phrases
- Uses new words regularly
- Increases expressive vocabulary to 30 words or more
- Attempts "stories"—longer utterances in jargon to get message across

- Begins to use own name when talking about self
- Uses possessive pronouns ("mine")
- May ask "where" questions ("Where car?")
- By 24 months may use two- or three-word phrases with nouns, some verbs and some adjectives

Speech

- Approximates words
- Substitutes /w/ for /r/
- Uses suprasegmental features
- Most vowels and diphthongs present
- Consonants [k, g, t, ng] emerging

- Consonants [p, b, m, h, n, d] established—used in initial position in words
- Consonants often omitted in medial and final positions

Cognition

- Imitates symbolic play, e.g., household activities
- Uses one object as a symbol for another
- Places triangle, circle, square in shape board
- Imitates vertical strokes
- Threads three beads
- Begins to tear paper

- Imitates ordering of nesting cups
- Begins to categorize objects in play
- Uses two toys together
- Stacks blocks/builds tower
- Completes simple pull-out puzzle
- Activates mechanical toy

Social communication

- Begins to develop more self-confidence and is happy to be with other people
- Initiates pretend play
- Responds to requests from adults

- Practices adult-like conversation about familiar themes
- Uses words to interact
- Requests information, e.g., "What is this?"
- Develops turn taking in conversation

Source: Reprinted with permission from Cochlear Limited. (2005). *Listen, learn, and talk* (2nd ed.). Alexandria, Australia: SOS Printing Group.

Table 5.5 Typical stages for 25- to 30-month-old children

Listening (audition)	
• Auditory memory of two items in different linguistic contexts • Listens to familiar songs on tape	• Comprehends longer utterances • Listens from a distance

Receptive language	
• Begins to understand complex language • Comprehends more complex action phrases • Understands functions, e.g., "What do we use for drinking?"—points to cup • Begins to understand size differences, e.g., big/little	• Begins to understand prepositions, e.g., "in," "on," "under" • Receptive vocabulary increases • Begins to understand concept of quantity, e.g., "one," "all" • Understands pronouns, e.g., "he," "she," "they," "we"

Expressive language	
• Uses two- and three-word phrases more consistently • Uses some personal pronouns, e.g., "me," "you" • Asks for help using two or more words, e.g., "wash hands" • Begins to name primary colors • Refers to self by pronoun "me"	• Repeats two numbers counting • Answers "wh" questions, e.g., "What's that?," "What's . . . doing?," "Who?" • Recites nursery rhymes and favorite songs • Understands and answers "Can you . . . ?" • Uses negation, e.g., "don't," "no"

Speech	
• Loves experimenting with prosodic features • Begins to use stress correctly • Repeats words and phrases • Consonants [f, y] emerging • Consonants, e.g., [m, p, b] used in final position	• Word/phrases shortened; medial consonants often omitted • Tends to overpronounce words • Different pronunciation of the same word common • Whispers

Cognition	
• Continues symbolic play, e.g., talking on the phone • Completes actions, e.g., hand claps and high fives • Uses toys appropriately • Performs related activities at play • Turns one page at a time	• Imitates vertical, horizontal lines and circle • Matches identical picture to picture and shape to shape • Puts two parts of a whole together • Understands number concepts of one and two

Social communication	
• Enjoys talking, e.g., pretends to have a conversation on the phone • Completes actions, e.g., "Give me five" • Begins to develop parallel play with other children	• Talks more in play • Shares toys • Asks for help using two or more words • Uses longer utterances

Source: Reprinted with permission from Cochlear Limited. (2005). *Listen, learn, and talk* (2nd ed.). Alexandria, Australia: SOS Printing Group.

Table 5.6 First lesson plan for a young child at hearing aid fitting (age is 8 months, corrected age is 5 months)

Child	Audition (1 day after hearing aid fitting)	Speech/language	Cognition
	(1) Detection (2) [a]—airplane (3) Water play—duck, fish, boat	(1) Baby toy (2) Book—Hallowe'en (3) Hallowe'en wind-ups	(1) Swipe at toy (2) Pull toy
Parent report	Likes: monkey, frog (hop), bath, ducks Turns from tummy to back and back to tummy, pushes up from tummy, stiffness in hips Songs: "ABCD," "Wheels on the Bus"		
Suggestions for parents	Beginning vocabulary list, rhyming sheet		

Contribution from: Deirdre Neuss, Children's Hospital of Eastern Ontario, Ottawa, Canada.

Table 5.7 Lesson plan for a young child 1 year after hearing aid fitting (age is 1 year, 8 months, corrected age is 1 year, 5 months)

Child	Audition	Speech/language	Cognition
	(1) Detect and try identification of six sounds (2) Select two words—"night night," "sit down," "baby," "dog" (therapist note: yes–1x)	(1) Where's the spider? —under hat, shoe (2) Verbs—weebles (therapist note: DND) (3) Hot—with stove (4) Book—Hallowe'en (5) Bubbles (4) Vehicles (therapist note: DND)	(1) Match picture to picture
Therapist notes	Imitations: bye bye, woof woof, banf, sit down, night night, spider, walk walk, fall down, __ + bye bye, hot, pu/pumpkin, wagon, all done, round & round, witch sound, m-m- / some juice		
	Spontaneous: yeah, sound for boo, uh oh, tu/truck, tried itsy bitsy spider		
Assessment	Administered the Integrated Scales of Development—Feb./05; J's C.A.= 12 months (corrected age = 9 months); J was able to do many items in the 7–9-month range in the areas of audition, receptive language, expressive language, speech, cognition, and social communication.		
	Administered the Rossetti—March/05; J's C.A.= 13 months (corrected age = 10 months)		
	Jordan was able to do many items in the 9–12-month range in the areas of Interaction-attachment, pragmatics, gesture, play, language comprehension, language expression		
	Based on the List of Suggestions for Beginning Vocabulary, J. was able to understand 30 words and say 21 words in October/05 when he was 1 year, 8 months C.A. and 1 year, 5 months corrected age. (1 year hearing age.) Progress is good.		

Abbreviations: C.A., chronological age; DND, did not do.
Contribution from Deirdre Neuss, Children's Hospital of Eastern Ontario, Ottawa, Canada.

Learning beyond the Home

For many children, the learning environment extends well beyond the home. This means that much of the listening and language exposure is in not only noisy but busy environments. Chapter 8 will address in detail the use of additional technology to enhance the signal-to-noise ratio in difficult listening environments, such as preschool and classrooms. In addition to optimizing the environment through the use of special technology, such as remote microphone systems, child care workers can be coached and encouraged to be part of the team helping the child maximize listening and spoken language. Whenever possible, it is recommended that the clinician/teacher visit the child care or early education facility to observe the learning environment and make recommendations to improve sound quality and develop strategies for facilitating listening and spoken language development. Just as considerable time is spent in engaging parents, it is important to engage all those who are involved in interacting with the child, so that the auditory and language experience is enriched to the extent possible in interactive group environments. Strategies include sharing the child's listening and language goals with child care providers. It is helpful if child care workers can observe a session with parent and child in the clinic or home; if this is not possible, a session can be conducted at the child care facility. Given the number of hours some children spend learning in child care facilities, learning language from other children and adult models who are not parents, this investment seems very worthwhile.

Other children may receive care in various other environments, including home day care and with other family members. Similarly, individuals can attend sessions to learn techniques and understand the intervention goals. It is highly recommended that clinicians/teachers and all others responsible for the child's audiologic rehabilitation become aware, through site visits, of all of the child's learning environments and encourage the inclusion of others in therapy sessions. These practices can help ensure that acoustic modifications are implemented where feasible and that all providers and caregivers have some minimal level of knowledge about hearing loss and are equipped with practical suggestions to facilitate listening and spoken language development. As indicated by teachers of school-age children, one of the greatest challenges is engaging parents and others involved in the child's care when there is a long distance to the therapy center. Geographical distance to a cochlear implant center and intervention in the early years have emerged as important barriers affecting the development of children with cochlear implants at school age (Fitzpatrick & Olds, submitted manuscript; Hyde, Punch, & Grimbeek, 2011).

Expectations for Early Language Acquisition

What can we expect for the "average" 2- to 3-year-old identified with hearing loss in the first few months of life? In an era of evidence-based practice in health care, the notion of outcomes permeates policy and practice decisions. There has been an increasing interest in the outcomes of children with hearing loss more generally (Moeller, Tomblin, Yoshinaga-Itano, Connor, & Jerger, 2007), perhaps partially motivated by extensive research in pediatric cochlear implantation and the need to document the effectiveness of universal newborn hearing screening. Certainly, as a starting point, newborn screening has considerably changed the age at which children with congenital deafness start to access hearing, with the average age of identification lowered from an average of 2.5 years to 3 to 6 months of age (Nelson, Bougatsos, & Nygren, 2008; Thompson et al, 2001). In children with severe to profound deafness, early cochlear implantation before 1 year of age has become common practice in several regions. A summary of studies of children who received cochlear implants before age 12 months suggests favorable outcomes (Vlastarakos et al, 2010).

An analysis of clinical data for 43 children identified since the implementation of a newborn screening program at an average age of

13.4 months (with a standard deviation [SD] of 11.6) who were followed in a listening and spoken language program showed that, on average, children at 3 years of age obtained scores comparable to their hearing peers on receptive vocabulary, receptive and expressive language, and speech production as measured by standardized tests (Fitzpatrick, 2011a). However, population-based data from a large Australian study that included auditory and language measures for more than three hundred 3-year-old children showed that on average they were functioning below their peers with normal hearing. Like other studies, there was considerable individual variability in children's spoken language abilities. It seems reasonable to conclude that in the first 2 to 3 years, a substantial number of children can be well on their way to acquiring spoken language through hearing and can be expected to use spoken language forms that are comparable to or closely aligned with those of their peers with normal hearing. However, it also seems that some children will continue to require substantial specific teaching well beyond these early years.

Mild Bilateral and Unilateral Hearing Loss

In recent years, a new population of children have appeared on clinical caseloads—children with mild bilateral and unilateral hearing loss. Until the implementation of UNHS initiatives, these children were identified on average at 4 to 5 years of age and therefore were not commonly enrolled in early intervention programs (Durieux-Smith, Fitzpatrick, & Whittingham, 2008; Fitzpatrick, et al, 2010). Newborn screening programs vary with respect to the severity of hearing loss targeted (Hyde, 2011). Some services do not specifically target the early identification of mild bilateral hearing loss, having set the target disorder at 40 dB hearing level (HL) or greater. The Joint Committee on Infant Hearing (2007) identified the need to address even very mild hearing loss. Regardless of the defined target disorder, it can be expected that at least those children with unilateral hearing loss of moderate or worse degree are being identified early through screening initiatives.

Follow-up studies from UNHS programs show that estimates of prevalence of mild bilateral and unilateral hearing loss vary widely due to the differences in definition of the target disorder (Canadian Working Group on Childhood Hearing, 2005; National Workshop on Mild and Unilateral Hearing Loss, 2005). Current screening technologies allow accurate identification of hearing losses of 30 dB HL in the neonatal period (Canadian Working Group on Childhood Hearing, 2005). For example, prevalence rates of 0.83/1,000 have been reported for unilateral hearing loss of 40 dB HL (Prieve & Stevens, 2000) and greater, while Johnson et al (2005) estimated an overall prevalence rate of 0.55/1,000 for both mild and unilateral hearing loss in the neonatal population. Watkin & Baldwin (2011), in a follow-up of a screening cohort of 35,668 children at school age, found that 2.4/1,000 children had mild bilateral (1.2/1,000) or unilateral hearing loss (0.81/1,000), representing 58% of 130 children identified with hearing loss in the cohort. In our clinical program, where children with hearing loss of all degrees of severity are identified and managed, mild bilateral and unilateral hearing loss accounts for more than 40% of the clinical pediatric audiology population (Fitzpatrick, 2011b; Fitzpatrick et al, 2010).

One of the reasons provided as a justification for targeting children with mild/UHL in screening programs is the risk of progressive hearing loss, including deterioration in audiometric levels or progression from one ear to both ears. In a recent review of 337 children confirmed with mild bilateral or unilateral loss since the implementation of UNHS, 74 (22%) experienced some deterioration in hearing, and 50 of these children showed deterioration of at least 20 dB in pure-tone average (500, 1,000, 2,000 Hz) in one or both ears (Fitzpatrick & Whittingham, submitted paper). These data, now beginning to emerge from newborn screening follow-up studies, suggest that careful monitoring of hearing loss of any degree, including mild and unilateral hearing loss, is critical to ensure that children are provided with optimal access to hearing throughout their development.

There is considerable uncertainty around best practices in the management of children with mild bilateral or unilateral hearing loss (Fitzpatrick et al, 2010). Most of the outcome data come from studies of children who were identified late prior to screening, and suggest that about one-third experienced difficulties in speech understanding in noise, as well as difficulties in language, academic, and psychosocial development. A recent study that examined 74 school-age children with unilateral hearing loss found that they had poorer language skills than their siblings (Lieu, Tye-Murray, Karzon, & Piccirillo, 2010). Information about the impact of early-identified unilateral and mild bilateral hearing loss on development is limited, but some research suggests that roughly 30% of children experience some delays relative to their peers with normal hearing. Taken together, these studies suggest that children are at risk for learning difficulties and should at a minimum be carefully monitored from the time of identification.

It is also important to recall that parents of children with hearing loss are affected by the diagnosis of a hearing disorder, regardless of the severity of the impairment. Audiologists also point to the fact that "a big hearing loss is hard to see" and "small losses even more so"; therefore, parents need to understand how even a so-called minimal degree of hearing loss can affect the child's learning. Current literature suggests that if our assessments reveal that direct intervention is not considered necessary on a regular basis for these young children, at the very least parents need some support and these young children should be carefully monitored by audiologists and clinicians/teachers for both changes in hearing severity and negative effects on auditory and spoken language skills. As practitioners, our interest is in making hearing accessible for *all* children, regardless of audiometric hearing levels. Although, language stimulation techniques are not substantively different for these children, it is reasonable to expect that the rate of progress will be faster in children with milder hearing loss relative to their peers with more severe hearing loss.

Summary

There is considerable emphasis on supporting parents in the beginning stages of audiologic rehabilitation as they learn to adapt to parenting a child with hearing loss. Parents are taught specifically how to create a listening and learning environment and are shown techniques considered effective in making sounds more accessible to young children with hearing disorders. Given the limited feedback from the child in the early stages, it is very important to monitor the child's overall auditory and linguistic development to ensure that optimal hearing is achieved through hearing aids and/or cochlear implants. Children with hearing loss identified in infancy, whose development is otherwise typical, can be expected to be well on their way to developing spoken language as they enter the toddler years and to have developed skills closely aligned with those of their peers with normal hearing. Parents will continue to need ongoing support and guidance to continue therapy sessions throughout the preschool years.

Acknowledgments

We are grateful to all of the listening and spoken language specialists, Erin McSweeney, Deirdre Neuss, Kelly Rabjohn, Rosemary Somerville, and Pamela Steacie, from the Audiology program at the Children's Hospital of Eastern Ontario for their many contributions to this chapter.

Appendix

This is an example of assessment and intervention plans for a child with hearing loss. Intervention plans at 1 year, 5 months and at 2 years, 5 months are described. (Contribution from Erin McSweeney, Children's Hospital of Eastern Ontario, Ottawa, Canada.)

▪ Assessment and Intervention

Background

Ben is 1 year, 5 months of age. He was diagnosed with a moderate/severe to severe sensorineural hearing loss at birth (he failed his otoacoustic emissions [OAE] screening at birth, and the loss was confirmed with an auditory brainstem response [ABR] 1 month later). He was subsequently fit with binaural hearing aids (Phonak [Zurich, Switzerland] Certena SP) at age 2 months. He started attending weekly auditory-verbal therapy (AVT) sessions at the age of 4 months. He also attends a weekly music therapy session at the center. Ben is cared for at home by his mother. English is the only language spoken in the home. There are no developmental concerns for this child.

Assessment Results

Language

When Ben was 11 months of age, the Preschool Language Scale—Fourth Edition (PLS-4) was administered to assess Ben's language skills. This test targets receptive and expressive language skills in the areas of attention, play, gesture, vocal development, social communication, vocabulary, concepts, language structure, integrative language skills, and phonological awareness (sound awareness). Results were obtained both through parent report and through direct elicitation. **Table 5.8** shows Ben's results

Ben's scores on the PLS-4 were all within the normal range, indicating that both his receptive and expressive language skills are developing as expected compared with his hearing peers. Auditorily, Ben demonstrated an understanding of simple words and phrases (e.g., "come with me," "no," "mommy," "daddy"). In play routines of up to 1 to 2 minutes, he was able to use more than one object at a time. Expressively, Ben was able to produce a variety of consonants and could combine these sounds with vowels to form reduplicative syllables (e.g., "mama," "dada").

Table 5.8

Composites	Standard scores normal range: 85–115	Percentile normal range: 16–84
Auditory comprehension: understanding of language	97	42
Expressive communication: spoken language skills	112	79
Total language score	105	63

Vocabulary

The MacArthur Communicative Development Inventory: Words and Gestures was completed by Ben's mother. This is a vocabulary checklist that records the words the child understands and says from set categories, such as animal names, toys, food, people, action words, descriptive words, and pronouns. Ben's results according to his mom are presented in **Table 5.9**.

Ben's receptive and expressive vocabulary both fall within the normal range for his age.

His vocabulary includes a variety of nouns and action words, as well as a few pronouns and prepositions. He has a good understanding and expression of family names ("mommy," "daddy," "ginger"). He also recognizes and can request familiar toys and foods (e.g., "ball," "duck," "cheerios," "banana"). Recently, Ben has been able to identify some body parts and articles of clothing, including ears, eyes, hat, and shoes.

Table 5.9

Chronological age	Words understood (number/percentile)	Words understood *and* said (number/percentile)
17 months	157/27th	51/49th

Speech

Ben's speech production skills have grown significantly over this term. His consonant and vowel inventory are age appropriate. Ben is able to combine sounds to form syllables and words beginning with a consonant and ending with a vowel (e.g., "bee," "ha," "no"). Ben is now just beginning to combine sounds to form words ending with a consonant sound (e.g., "down," "up," "pop," "ball"). Finally, in terms of Ben's speech imitation skills, he is often spontaneously imitating sounds, syllables, and some words. He can also accurately imitate the pitch, length, and loudness of utterances.

Global Development

The Child Development Inventory Profile (CDI), a parent questionnaire, was administered when Ben was 1 year, 5 months of age to assess his development in the following developmental domains: social, self-help, gross motor, fine motor, expressive language, language comprehension, letters, and numbers. Ben's scores were all within the normal range for his age group, and he did not present as being at risk for developmental concerns.

Therapy Plan: Age 1 year, 5 months

Audition:
- Hearing equipment check
- Gain independence in play audiometry (stimulus-response task): We played with bean bags, and tossed them into the bucket when we heard one of the Ling-6 sounds. We worked on Ben's being able to wait for the sound (eliminated false positives).
- Auditory selection of one item (by name) from a closed set: put the bear's clothing away, one item at a time at clean-up time.
- Inputting for recognition of musical instruments by sound: played with the instruments (piano, drums, bells, and cymbals). Eventual goal is for Ben to recognize and identify the correct instrument by sound.

Speech:
- Imitation of "new" two-word phrases: While introducing body parts vocabulary with a book (Karen Katz's *Where Is Baby's Belly Button?*) we took turns saying two-word phrases (e.g., "mommy's nose," "daddy's nose," "Ben's eyes"). We bombarded Ben with these two-word phrases, and used the hand cue sparingly to have Ben imitate the phrase.

Language:
- Receptively, follows instructions with two related commands: We reviewed familiar articles of clothing while dressing up bear. Ben was told to "Get the socks/shoes/hat/shirt, and put them on the bear."
- Vocabulary: learning to identify body parts.
- Parent goal to develop Ben's expressive language: to expand on his utterances. When Ben uses one word, parent should expand utterance to two words (e.g., Ben: "ball"; Mom: "a big ball").

Cognition:
- Matching similar objects: After reading our book, we completed a Mr. Potato Head (Hasbro, Pawtucket, RI, USA). Ben was able to match all of the parts of the face to his own face.

■ Assessment and Intervention 1 Year Later

Background

Ben is now 2 years, 6 months of age. He continues to wear his hearing aids during all waking hours. There has been no change to his hearing status. Ben is still attending weekly AVT sessions. In the fall he will begin attending a local preschool group two mornings per week.

Assessment Results

Language

At 2 years and 5 months of age, the Preschool Language Scale—Fourth Edition (PLS-4) was administered to assess Ben's language skills. This test targets receptive and expressive language skills in the areas of attention, play, gesture, vocal development, social communication, vocabulary, concepts, language structure, integrative language skills, and phonological awareness (sound awareness). Ben's results were above average compared with children his age with typical hearing. His results are shown in **Tables 5.10** and **5.11**.

Table 5.10

Composites	Standard scores normal range: 85–115	Percentile normal range: 13–84
Auditory comprehension: understanding of language	126	96
Expressive communication: spoken language skills	124	95
Total language score	128	97

Table 5.11

Auditory comprehension	
Strengths	*Areas for development*
• Identifies colors • Understand the quantity concepts "one" and "all" • Follows two-step related commands • Understands the descriptive concepts "big," "wet," "little"	• Understanding the use of objects (e.g., "What do you use to drink water?") • Understanding the pronouns "he," "she," "him," "her" • Making inferences (e.g., "Annie scraped her knee. How did she get hurt?") • Identifying categories of objects (e.g., "Show Ma all the things we eat.")
Expressive communication	
Strengths	*Areas for development*
• Uses words that describe physical states (e.g., "sleepy," "cold") • Uses quantity concepts: one, two, three • Uses a variety of nouns, verbs, modifiers, and pronouns in spontaneous utterances • Answers *what* and *where* questions	• Using plurals • Consistently using verb + *ing* (e.g., "eating," "sleeping") • Naming a variety of pictures, objects • Telling how an object is used (e.g., "Tell me what you do with a spoon.")

Vocabulary

The MacArthur Communicative Development Inventory: Words & Sentences was completed by Ben's mother. This is a vocabulary checklist that records the words the child understands and says from set categories, such as animal names, toys, food, people, action words, descriptive words, and pronouns. Ben's results according to his mom are given in **Table 5.12**.

Ben's expressive vocabulary is within normal limits. Ben is able to form two- and three-word utterances. Based on a language sample collected at the age of 2 years and 6 months, Ben's mean length of utterance (MLU) is 3.2.

Table 5.12

Chronological age	Words produced (number/percentile)
30 months	576/70th

Speech

Ben's speech production skills are following typical development. Informally, his voice quality, intonation, pitch, intensity, and rate are all judged to be within normal limits. Upon visual assessment at rest and in speech production, Ben's oral motor structures (lips, tongue, teeth, jaw, palate) are unremarkable.

Global Development

At the age of 2 years, 4 months, the Child Development Inventory Profile (CDI) was completed to assess Ben's global development in the areas of social skills, self-help, gross motor, fine motor, expressive language, language comprehension, letters, numbers, and general development. All scores were within normal limits. Results from this assessment indicate that, over all, Ben's development is progressing as expected compared with his age-matched hearing peers.

Therapy Plan: Age 2 years, 5 months

Audition:
- Hearing equipment check
- Introduction to auditory memory for three items (in a closed set). Upon entering the therapy room, we noticed a very big mess. The toys were everywhere! Ben had to clean up the toys (by threes), sorting them into buckets labeled with the numbers 1, 2, 3. As this was one of Ben's first attempts at this task, mom repeated the three items once, and then helped him as needed.

Speech:
- Bombardment of final /s/ in possessives. Parent goal: acoustically highlight the /s/ sound by getting close to Ben, stretching the "s" sound, and using a more quiet voice to highlight the target.

Language:
- Expressively, Ben will use "I" instead of "Ben" in first-person requests (e.g., "I want . . ."). When completing our painting activity, Ben had to ask for the paint color he wanted using "I want the [*color*] paint."
- Expressive: input for use of possessive "'s." After completing our flower paintings, we toured the center and showed our artwork to various staff members. As we went through each person's painting, the staff member or mom highlighted "this is Ben**'s** flower," "this is Erin**'s** flower," "this is mommy**'s** flower," etc.

- Receptively, Ben will comprehend and begin to answer "who" questions. We went through Ben's experience book and looked at the new entries (pictures and words) mom had added. We prompted Ben with questions (e.g., "Who made the birthday cake?" "Who's hiding behind the tree?"). Also, during our turn-taking activities, we prompted with "Whose turn is it?"
- Receptively, with assistance, Ben will follow three-step commands. We reviewed a sequence story about a girl planting a seed and growing flowers in her garden. We took turns planting various seeds (put the big seed in the dirt, cover it up, and give it some water).
- Receptive vocabulary: introduce new vocabulary related to planting (e.g., "seed," "soil," "pot," "watering can").

Cognition:
- What's missing? Before completing our flower paintings, Ben was asked to find the two missing parts from each sheet (e.g., stem, leaves, petals, sun, clouds).
- Turn-taking skills: During our painting, we set the expectation that each person at the table would have a chance to use the paintbrush (there was only one). Ben is working on being patient and waiting for his turn.

References

Bagatto, M., Scollie, S. D., Hyde, M., & Seewald, R. (2010). Protocol for the provision of amplification within the Ontario Infant Hearing Program. *International Journal of Audiology, 49*(Suppl. 1), S70–S79. 10.3109/14992020903080751.

Bagatto, M. P., Moodie, S. T., Malandrino, A. C., Richert, F. M., Clench, D. A., & Scollie, S. D. (2011). The University of Western Ontario Pediatric Audiological Monitoring Protocol (UWO PedAMP). *Trends in Amplification, 15*(1), 57–76.

Bagatto, M. P., Moodie, S. T., Seewald, R. C., Bartlett, D. J., & Scollie, S. D. (2011). A critical review of audiological outcome measures for infants and children. *Trends in Amplification, 15*(1), 57–76. 10.1177/1084713811420304.

Bernstein, A., & Eriks-Brophy, A. (2010). Supporting families. In E. A. Rhoades & J. Duncan (Eds.), *Auditory-verbal practice: Toward a family-centered approach* (pp. 225–257). Springfield, IL: Charles C Thomas.

Burger, T., Spahn, C., Richter, B., Eissele, S., Löhle, E., & Bengel, J. (2005). Parental distress: The initial phase of hearing aid and cochlear implant fitting. *American Annals of the Deaf, 150*(1), 5–10.

Canadian Working Group on Childhood Hearing. (2005). *Early hearing and communication development: Canadian Working Group on Childhood Hearing (CWGCH) resource document.* Ottawa.

Ching, T. Y. C. (2012). *Predicting developmental outcomes of early- and late-identified children with hearing impairment, including those with special needs: Findings from a population study.* Paper presented at the Newborn Hearing Screening 2012, Cernobbio, Italy.

Ching, T. Y. C., & Hill, M. (2007). The Parents' Evaluation of Aural/Oral Performance of Children (PEACH) Scale: Normative data. *Journal of the American Academy of Audiology, 18*(3), 220–235.

Crockett, R., Baker, H., Uus, K., Bamford, J., & Marteau, T. M. (2005). Maternal anxiety and satisfaction following infant hearing screening: A comparison of the health visitor distraction test and newborn hearing screening. *Journal of Medical Screening, 12*(2), 78–82.

Durieux-Smith, A., Fitzpatrick, E., & Whittingham, J. (2008). Universal newborn hearing screening: A question of evidence. *International Journal of Audiology, 47*(1), 1–10.

Erber, N. (1982). *Auditory training.* Washington, DC: A.G. Bell Association.

Estabrooks, W. (Ed.). (1998). *Cochlear implants for kids.* Washington, DC: Alexander Graham Bell Association for the Deaf.

Estabrooks, W. (Ed.). (2006). *Auditory-verbal therapy and practice.* Washington, DC: Alexander Graham Bell Association for the Deaf and Hard of Hearing.

Fitzpatrick, E. (2007). Population infant hearing screening to intervention: Determinants of outcome from the parents' perspective. Doctoral thesis, University of Ottawa, Ottawa.

Fitzpatrick, E., Angus, D., Durieux-Smith, A., Graham, I. D., & Coyle, D. (2008). Parents' needs following identification of childhood hearing loss. *American Journal of Audiology, 17*(1), 38–49.

Fitzpatrick, E., Coyle, D. E., Durieux-Smith, A., Graham, I. D., Angus, D. E., & Gaboury, I. (2007). Parents' preferences for services for children with hearing loss: A conjoint analysis study. *Ear and Hearing, 28*(6), 842–849.

Fitzpatrick, E., Durieux-Smith, A., Eriks-Brophy, A., Olds, J., & Gaines, R. (2007). The impact of newborn hearing screening on communication development. *Journal of Medical Screening, 14*(3), 123–131.

Fitzpatrick, E., Graham, I. D., Durieux-Smith, A., Angus, D., & Coyle, D. (2007). Parents' perspectives on the impact of the early diagnosis of childhood hearing loss. *International Journal of Audiology, 46*(2), 97–106.

Fitzpatrick, E. M. (2011a). *Defining typical development for children with hearing loss.* Paper presented at Australasian Newborn Hearing Screening Conference 2011, Perth, Australia.

Fitzpatrick, E. M. (2011b). *New challenges from newborn hearing screening: Children with mild bilateral and unilateral hearing loss.* Paper presented at the Australasian Newborn Hearing Screening Conference 2011, Perth, Australia.

Fitzpatrick, E. M. (2011c). *Newborn hearing screening: Making it work.* Paper presented at the Canadian Association of Speech-Language Pathology and Audiology Conference 2011, Montreal, Canada.

Fitzpatrick, E. M., Durieux-Smith, A., & Whittingham, J. (2010). Clinical practice for children with mild bilateral and unilateral hearing loss. *Ear and Hearing, 31*(3), 392–400.

Fitzpatrick, E. M., & Olds, J. (submitted manuscript). Beyond hearing: Perspectives from teachers on school functioning of children with cochlear implants.

Fitzpatrick, E. M., Whittingham, J., & Durieux-Smith, A. (submitted manuscript). Mild bilateral and unilateral hearing loss in children: A 20-year view of characteristics and practices.

Hart, B., & Risley, T. R. (1999). *The social world of children learning to talk.* Baltimore, MD: Paul H. Brookes Publishing Co.

Hyde, M. (2011). Principles and methods of population screening in EDHI. In R. Seewald & A.-M. Tharpe (Eds.), *Comprehensive handbook of pediatric audiology* (pp. 283–337). San Diego, CA: Plural Publishing, Inc.

Hyde, M., Punch, R., & Grimbeek, P. (2011). Factors predicting functional outcomes of cochlear implants in children. *Cochlear Implants International, 12*(2), 94–104.

Ireton, H. (1992). *Child development inventories*. Minneapolis, MN: Behavior Science Systems, Inc.

Johnson, J. L., White, K. R., Widen, J. E., Gravel, J. S., James, M., Kennalley, T., . . . Holstrum, J. (2005). A multicenter evaluation of how many infants with permanent hearing loss pass a two-stage otoacoustic emissions/automated auditory brainstem response newborn hearing screening protocol. *Pediatrics, 116*(3), 663–672.

Joint Committee on Infant Hearing. (2007). *Year 2007 position statement: Principles and guidelines for early hearing detection and intervention.* Retrieved from www.asha.org/policy.

King, A. M. (2010). The national protocol for paediatric amplification in Australia. *International Journal of Audiology, 49*(Suppl. 1), S64–S69.

Langdon, H. W., & Wiig, E. H. (2009). Multicultural issues in test interpretation. *Seminars in Speech and Language, 30*(4), 261–278.

Lieu, J. E. C., Tye-Murray, N., Karzon, R. K., & Piccirillo, J. F. (2010). Unilateral hearing loss is associated with worse speech-language scores in children. *Pediatrics, 125*(6), e1348–e1355.

Ling, D. (2002). *Speech and the hearing-impaired child: Theory and practice* (2nd ed.). Washington, DC: Alexander Graham Bell Assoication for the Deaf.

Ling, D., & Ling, A. H. (1978). *Aural habilitation: The foundations of verbal learning in hearing-impaired children*. Washington, DC: Alexander Graham Bell Association of the Deaf, Inc.

Lü, J., Huang, Z., Yang, T., Li, Y., Mei, L., Xiang, M., . . . Wu, H. (2011). Screening for delayed-onset hearing loss in preschool children who previously passed the newborn hearing screening. *International Journal of Pediatric Otorhinolaryngology, 75*(8), 1045–1049 10.1016/j.ijporl.2011.05.022.

Luterman, D. (2006). The emotional impact of hearing loss. In D. Luterman (Ed.), *Children with hearing loss: A family guide* (pp. 9–35). Sedona, AZ: Auricle Ink Publishers.

Luterman, D., & Kurtzer-White, E. (1999). Identifying hearing loss: Parent's needs. *American Journal of Audiology, 8*, 8–13.

Marmot, M., & Wilkinson, R. (Eds.). (2006). *Social determinants of health* (2nd ed.). Oxford: Oxford University Press.

McCauley, R. J. (2001). *Assessment of language disorders in children*. Mahwah, NJ: Lawrence Erlbaum Associates, Inc.

McCauley, R. J., & Swisher, L. (1984). Use and misuse of norm-referenced tests in clinical assessment: A hypothetical case. *Journal of Speech and Hearing Disorders, 49*(4), 338–348.

McCracken, W., Young, A., & Tattersall, H. (2008). Universal newborn hearing screening: Parental reflections on very early audiological management. *Ear and Hearing, 29*(1), 54–64.

McGinnis, M. D. (2010). A support provider's goals. In E. A. Rhoades & J. Duncan (Eds.), *Auditory-verbal practice: Toward a family-centered approach* (pp. 349–377). Springfield, IL: Charles C Thomas Publisher, Ltd.

McKay, S., Gravel, J. S., & Tharpe, A. M. (2008). Amplification considerations for children with minimal or mild bilateral hearing loss and unilateral hearing loss. *Trends in Amplification, 12*(1), 43–54.

Meinzen-Derr, J., Lim, L. H. Y., Choo, D. I., Buyniski, S., & Wiley, S. (2008). Pediatric hearing impairment caregiver experience: Impact of duration of hearing loss on parental stress. *International Journal of Pediatric Otorhinolaryngology, 72*(11), 1693–1703.

Moeller, M. P., Hoover, B., Peterson, B., & Stelmachowicz, P. (2009). Consistency of hearing aid use in infants with early-identified hearing loss. *American Journal of Audiology, 18*(1), 14–23.

Moeller, M. P., Tomblin, J. B., Yoshinaga-Itano, C., Connor, C. M., & Jerger, S. (2007). Current state of knowledge: Language and literacy of children with hearing impairment. *Ear and Hearing, 28*(6), 740–753.

National Workshop on Mild and Unilateral Hearing Loss. (2005). Workshop proceedings. Breckenridge, CO: Centers for Disease Control and Prevention.

Nelson, H. D., Bougatsos, C., & Nygren, P.; 2001 US Preventive Services Task Force. (2008). Universal newborn hearing screening: Systematic review to update the 2001 US Preventive Services Task Force Recommendation. *Pediatrics, 122*(1), e266–e276 10.1542/peds.2007-1422.

Niparko, J. K., Tobey, E. A., Thal, D. J., Eisenberg, L. S., Wang, N. Y., Quittner, A. L., & Fink, N. E.; CDaCI Investigative Team. (2010). Spoken language development in children following cochlear implantation. *Journal of the American Medical Association, 303*(15), 1498–1506.

Paradis, J., Crago, M., Genesee, F., & Rice, M. (2003). French-English bilingual children with SLI: How do they compare with their monolingual peers? *Journal of Speech, Language, and Hearing Research, 46*(1), 113–127.

Paul, R., & Norbury, C. F. (2012). *Language disorders from infancy through adolescence: Listening, speaking, reading, writing, and communicating* (4th ed.). St. Louis, MO: Elsevier Inc.

Pipp-Siegel, S., Sedey, A. L., & Yoshinaga-Itano, C. (2002). Predictors of parental stress in mothers of young children with hearing loss. *Journal of Deaf Studies and Deaf Education, 7*(1), 1–17 10.1093/deafed/7.1.1.

Pollack, D., Goldberg, D., & Caleffe-Schenck, N. (1997). *Educational audiology for the limited-hearing infant and preschooler: An auditory-verbal program* (3rd ed.). Springfield, IL: Charles C Thomas.

Prieve, B. A., & Stevens, F. (2000). The New York State universal newborn hearing screening demonstration project: Introduction and overview. *Ear and Hearing, 21*(2), 85–91.

Rance, G. (2005). Auditory neuropathy/dyssynchrony and its perceptual consequences. *Trends in Amplification, 9*(1), 1–43 10.1177/108471380500900102.

Rhoades, E. A. (2008). Working with multicultural and multilingual families of young children with hearing loss. In J. R. Madell & C. Flexer (Eds.), *Pediatric audiology: Diagnosis, technology and management* (pp. 262–268). New York: Thieme Medical Publishers.

Rhoades, E. A. (2010a). Core constructs of family therapy. In E. A. Rhoades & J. Duncan (Eds.), *Auditory-verbal practice: Toward a family-centered approach* (pp. 137–163). Springfield, IL: Charles C Thomas.

Rhoades, E. A. (2010b). Enablement and environment. In E. A. Rhoades & J. Duncan (Eds.), *Auditory-verbal practice: Toward a family-centered approach* (pp. 81–96). Springfield, IL: Charles C Thomas.

Rhoades, E. A., & Duncan, J. (Eds.). (2010). *Auditory-verbal practice: Toward a family-centered approach*. Springfield, IL: Charles C Thomas.

Rhoades, E. A., Price, F., & Perigoe, C. B. (2004). The changing American family & ethnically diverse children with hearing loss and multiple needs. *Volta Review, 104*, 285–305.

Schlessinger, H. (1992). The elusive X factor: Parental contributions to literacy. In M. Walworth, D. Moores, & T. O'Rourke (Eds.), *A free hand*. Silver Springs, MD: TJ Publishers.

Shulman, S., Besculides, M., Saltzman, A., Ireys, H., White, K. R., & Forsman, I. (2010). Evaluation of the universal newborn hearing screening and intervention program. *Pediatrics, 126*(Suppl. 1), S19–S27.

Simser, J. (1993). Auditory-verbal intervention: Infants and toddlers. *Volta Review, 95*(3), 217–229.

Simser, J. (1999). Parents: The essential partners in the habilitation of children with hearing impairment. *Australian Journal of Education of the Deaf, 5*, 55–62.

Sindrey, D. (1998). *Cochlear implant auditory training guidebook*. Washington, DC: Alexander Graham Bell Association for the Deaf.

Sininger, Y. S., Grimes, A., & Christensen, E. (2010). Auditory development in early amplified children: Factors influencing auditory-based communication outcomes in children with hearing loss. *Ear and Hearing, 31*(2), 166–185.

Tait, M., De Raeve, L., & Nikolopoulos, T. P. (2007). Deaf children with cochlear implants before the age of 1 year: Comparison of preverbal communication with normally hearing children. *International Journal of Pediatric Otorhinolaryngology, 71*(10), 1605–1611.

Tait, M., Lutman, M. E., & Robinson, K. (2000). Preimplant measures of preverbal communicative behavior as predictors of cochlear implant outcomes in children. *Ear and Hearing, 21*(1), 18–24.

Tattersall, H., & Young, A. (2006). Deaf children identified through newborn hearing screening: Parents' experiences of the diagnostic process. *Child: Care, Health and Development, 32*(1), 33–45.

Thompson, D. C., McPhillips, H., Davis, R. L., Lieu, T. L., Homer, C. J., & Helfand, M. (2001). Universal newborn hearing screening: Summary of evidence. *JAMA, 286*(16), 2000–2010.

Tsiakpini, L., Weichbold, V., Kuehn-Inacker, H., Coninx, F., D'Haese, P., & Almandin, S. (2004). *LittlEARS Auditory Questionnaire*. Innsbruck, Austria: MED-EL.

Vlastarakos, P. V., Proikas, K., Papacharalampous, G., Exadaktylou, I., Mochloulis, G., & Nikolopoulos, T. P. (2010). Cochlear implantation under the first year of age—the outcomes: A critical systematic review and meta-analysis. *International Journal of Pediatric Otorhinolaryngology, 74*(2), 127–132.

Watkin, P. M., & Baldwin, M. (2011). Identifying deafness in early childhood: Requirements after the newborn hearing screen. *Archives of Disorders in Childhood, 96*, 62–66.

Weichbold, V., Tsiakpini, L., Coninx, F., & D'Haese, P. (2005). Development of a parent questionnaire for assessment of auditory behavior of infants up to two years of age. *Laryngo-Rhino-Otologie, 84*(5), 328–334 10.1055/s-2004-825232.

Young, A., & Tattersall, H. (2005). Parents' of deaf children evaluative accounts of the process and practice of universal newborn hearing screening. *Journal of Deaf Studies and Deaf Education, 10*(2), 134–145.

Young, A., & Tattersall, H. (2007). Universal newborn hearing screening and early identification of deafness: Parents' responses to knowing early and their expectations of child communication development. *Journal of Deaf Studies and Deaf Education, 12*(2), 209–220.

Zimmerman-Phillips, S., Robbins, A. M., & Osberger, M. J. (2000). Assessing cochlear implant benefit in very young children. *Annals of Otology, Rhinology, and Laryngology, 185*(Suppl.), 42–43.

6 Continuing Listening and Learning in Early Childhood

This chapter describes audiologic rehabilitation for children from approximately 2½ years of age. Children who benefited from early intervention can generally be expected to build on the early foundations of listening and continue to advance their listening and spoken language skills. This chapter also addresses intervention for children who were identified after the first year of life. Assessment of children in the preschool years and various intervention techniques are described. Stages of auditory development are discussed and typical intervention sessions are provided to illustrate the important components of intervention. Parents continue to be the focal point of the intervention program during the preschool period.

■ Parent Guidance

As discussed in the previous chapter, in the early years of hearing loss management, the rehabilitation program is centered on parent guidance and is aimed at teaching parents about hearing loss, its impact on child development, and how to create optimal learning environments. Parent stressors change over time after the diagnostic period, but parents continue to require ongoing support (Meinzen-Derr, Lim, Choo, Buyniski, & Wiley, 2008). Although information needs may evolve as parents acquire more experience with hearing loss, ensuring that parents are well informed and supported throughout their child's early development is fundamental to the intervention process. Once the child is demonstrating the potential to develop spoken language, parents generally continue to require considerable guidance to optimize the child's communication skills. In contrast to the very early stages, many parents have acquired skills in creating an optimal listening and language learning environment at this later stage. Parents will, however, often need specific guidance in developing listening, language, and communication skills in their child. Accordingly, while parents continue to participate actively in therapy, sessions frequently involve more child-focused activities aimed at demonstrating the teaching of specific auditory and language targets.

Guiding Parents in Auditory and Language Stimulation

During the toddler years, our work with parents varies somewhat depending on their previous experience with auditory-based intervention. Parents fall into two broad categories: (1) those whose children have received early intervention in the first year of life, which is the general expectation when children have congenital deafness and access to universal newborn hearing screening (UNHS); and (2) those whose children start late intervention. In the first section of this chapter, we describe intervention when parents have been enrolled in early family-centered services and have received coaching from the early months of their child's life, as described in Chapter 5. The subsequent section addresses situations where parents come to intervention much later due to identification of hearing loss beyond the first year of life.

Continuing the Intervention Program

Children with typical development who receive early intervention can be expected to develop auditory skills and spoken language in the first 2 years. However, because of their hearing disorder, children with hearing loss can have delayed language and literacy skills despite early intervention and good hearing technology. Even when children's spoken language is equivalent to that of their peers with normal hearing, intervention is generally continued (although frequency may be modified) to equip the child as much as possible with high-level auditory skills. The rationale for continuing intervention is that these children are at risk for developing delays in spoken language and related areas, especially as they enter school, and working with them to develop more advanced listening and language skills, as well as early literacy skills, is generally advocated (Fitzpatrick & Doucet, in press).

Furthermore, research suggests that parents prefer to continue active participation in an intervention program where they receive specific guidance about appropriate auditory and language goals to target at different stages. Parents also indicate that they appreciate receiving specific ideas on how to stimulate language outside planned therapy sessions (Fitzpatrick, Angus, Durieux-Smith, Graham, & Coyle, 2008). In this research, when asked to describe their needs after identification of hearing loss, many parents indicated that the most important need

after hearing aids was specific guidance, which they articulated as "knowing what to do next," "what to teach my child" and "how to develop my child's language." One parent described these benefits from the therapy experience:

> I guess [what helped] was mostly just working with the therapist, . . . and just realizing, that really, it's just still just a child developing along the normal stages, and as long as I was inputting and reinforcing and doing all the things you do with any other child, that he was learning. They really showed me techniques to work with him to maximize his hearing. (Fitzpatrick, 2007)

Intervention sessions generally continue throughout the preschool years, and typically involve goals in audition, speech, language, and cognition. The activities conducted in sessions with young children should generally target the integration of these goals in a seamless manner. To create an individualized intervention plan, the clinician/teacher requires a good understanding of the child's functioning, which is generally undertaken through a comprehensive assessment of the child's abilities.

Assessment

Ongoing assessment of the child's communication is a hallmark of the rehabilitation program. In other words, assessment is integrated into therapy and is not conducted as a specific event to determine the need for or type of intervention, as it might be more generally for children with speech-language disorders. Like other developmental areas, communication development changes rapidly in the early childhood years. In addition, children with hearing loss are at risk for fluctuations and permanent declines in hearing that affect access to spoken language. Regular evaluation of the child's hearing levels and validation that the hearing instruments are appropriate are central to audiologic rehabilitation.

Comprehensive assessment has several goals: to measure progress for an individual child, to compare the child's development against his peers with normal hearing, and to identify gaps in the various language domains. Although some children who have received a strong early foundation in language stimulation can follow typical developmental trajectories, it is well documented that a large number of children will lag somewhat behind their peers and need specific instruction to develop certain language skills (Fitzpatrick, 2011a; Nicholas & Geers, 2006). As noted in Chapter 5, information gleaned from the ongoing assessments informs future therapy goals.

Assessment Protocols

As described in Chapters 3 and 5, several parent report questionnaires have been developed specifically to permit a functional evaluation of the child's hearing abilities. In recent years, with an increased number of tools and a

growing recognition of the need to document outcomes, there seems to be a trend toward greater inclusion of these tools in audiologic protocols. These tools can provide the care team with important information related to the child's overall auditory awareness and development, particularly when hearing instruments or cochlear implants are first fit. Increasingly, these tools are systematically developed and validated for broader clinical evaluation of functional outcomes in pediatric audiology and rehabilitation. See Bagatto, Moodie, Seewald, Bartlett, and Scollie (2011) for a review.

Beyond auditory skills, overall communication assessment with young children generally involves a combination of standardized measures and other, less structured tools. For children enrolled in a regular intervention program (e.g., weekly intervention sessions), assessment is generally incorporated into the sessions and, for young children, is completed during several therapy encounters. Concurrently, parent guidance and auditory and language stimulation are taking place and, in fact, form part of the assessment of the child's needs.

Standardized (Norm-Referenced) Assessments

Since the goal of audiologic rehabilitation is to develop spoken language skills that are aligned with the skills of peers with normal hearing, standardized measures typically make up one pillar of the assessment. A set of norm-referenced measures (for children with normal hearing) that tap different domains is commonly administered. Examples of typical assessment measures are provided in case examples throughout this chapter. These measures help to situate the child's language development in relation to his peers with normal hearing and can assist in identifying particular areas of strengths and weaknesses, such as vocabulary or syntactic structures. For extensive descriptions of commonly used speech and language assessment tools, see Paul and Norbury (2012).

Other Assessment Tools

In addition to standardized tests, language sample analysis is commonly conducted to provide detailed information about a child's spontaneous language abilities. Clinicians/teachers may choose to use the samples more informally to examine, for example, whether certain morphological markers are in place or whether the child is using a variety of vocabulary and elaborate sentence structures, and to calculate the mean length of utterance (MLU). At other times, highly systematic procedures using language analyses techniques or specialized analysis software may be undertaken (see Chapter 9). **Table 6.1** provides a brief sample of 20 sequential utterances from a child with moderate to severe hearing loss, extracted from a 100-utterance language sample at 2 years, 6 months of age. Based on a total of 100 utterances collected, a MLU of 3.2 was calculated for the child.

At the time of this writing, a new tool has emerged to assess children's spoken language development. The Language Environment Analysis (LENA) program is designed to capture child and caregiver interaction in naturalistic environments. The information, which is collected via a recording device worn by the child, is used in the home or other child play setting and permits an assessment of the child's language environment. The analysis provides details on specific aspects of interest, such as number of vocalizations, turn taking, and the acoustic quality of the environment (for information on the technical aspects of the device, see www.lenafoundation.org).

Tools and scales are frequently used to monitor progress and development of auditory and language skills. Some of these are criterion-referenced tools that clinicians/teachers use to informally document progress on an ongoing basis. As described in Chapter 5, based on their clinical experience and expectations at different stages of auditory, speech, and language development, clinicians have developed numerous "checklists" specifically for children with hearing loss. These checklists, many of which are unpublished, are frequently shared among colleagues and several published examples are available also (Estabrooks, 2006; Simser & Steacie, 1993). A survey conducted with clinicians/teachers working in auditory-based intervention programs indicated that these types of tools are widely used and have been found to be helpful with young children for counseling parents, monitoring progress, and setting goals (Neuss et al, in press). Some tools focus specifically on auditory skill development, and others, such as the St. Gabriel's Curriculum (Truohy, Brown, Mercer-Moseley, & Walsh, 2005), serve as a guide for planning intervention in multiple domains, including audition, language, early communication, speech, and cognition.

Table 6.1   Brief sample of 20 sequential utterances from a child with moderate to severe hearing loss, extracted from a 100-utterance language sample at 2 years, 6 months of age

Utterance	Morphemes per utterance
1. I want dry	3
2. This hand	2
3. Go the garbage	3
4. I want this	3
5. I put garbage	3
6. It's George	3
7. I have a bath too	5
8. Look Erin look	3
9. No I is bunny	4
10. Bunny treat	2
11. He bring special treat	4
12. Tractor	1
13. I got book	3
14. I want play to a bubbles	7
15. I need George	3
16. Sit down George sit down	5
17. Farmer and car and truck and turtle	7
18. Here's the pen and chair right there	8
19. Sit down right there	4
20. Tanis red paper	3

Contribution from Erin McSweeney, Children's Hospital of Eastern Ontario, Ottawa, Canada.

Various clinical protocols have evolved, and in recent years there has been an increasing interest in documenting progress in real-life settings. One extensive assessment protocol has "packaged" several tools that measure progress in everyday environments and targets the domains of audition, communication (including spoken language), and speech (Archbold, Phil, & O'Donoghue, 2009; Nikolopoulos, Archbold, & Gregory, 2005). The Nottingham Early Assessment Package (NEAP), described in the pediatric cochlear implant literature, includes a range of measures that monitor progress from infancy to adulthood. A protocol developed more specifically to monitor clinical processes related to hearing aid fitting and functional auditory outcomes, the UWOPedAMP protocol, has been described by Bagatto et al (2011).

Evidently, one of the challenges in working with young children is reaching an appropriate balance between assessment and intervention so that sessions are not invested simply in conducting assessments, especially when children are seen once weekly, as is common practice in many preschool programs. Assessments should be selected judiciously at various points of care to monitor progress and ensure that optimal technology and intervention plans are in place so that adjustments can be made when required.

Intervention

As discussed in Chapter 5, from the time of hearing loss identification, listening is developed or "trained" to help the child process spoken language patterns as naturally as possible. An understanding of what constitutes age-appropriate language for young children is important for planning specific intervention goals. A comprehensive description of typical language development is beyond the scope of this text, and useful information about typical language development is available in various resources, such as speech-language pathology and early childhood education textbooks. **Tables 6.2**, **6.3**, and **6.4** provide a snapshot of expectations for typically developing children at ages 2½ to 3, 3 to 3½, and 3½ to 4. Applying knowledge about typical language development, the clinician/teacher works with the child and family to develop language through listening.

Over all, clinicians determine through their combined assessments whether an individual child is meeting expected targets following normal developmental sequences and decide which language structures should be emphasized next through play and daily living activities. Clinicians/teachers often talk about being "one step ahead of the child," and this is one of the strategies they transmit to parents in their demonstration therapy sessions. Clinicians/teachers refer to the need to move from simple to complex targets when working with children, that is, always building on what is known, whether teaching new speech or new language targets. Such a course would seem to be appropriate for children with hearing loss given what is known about typical language development.

Stimulating Meaningful Language

Since most language learning occurs outside planned therapy sessions, an essential part of the clinician/teacher's work is helping parents to capitalize on everyday situations that make language more naturally meaningful to their child. Examples include getting dressed and undressed, preparing snacks and meals, getting ready to go outside, or any other experiences that occur several times throughout a child's day. These daily experiences naturally create an opportunity to solidify emerging language forms and provide exposure to new vocabulary and language structures. Reflecting on a situation where a young child has just acquired new shoes, considerable new vocabulary can be introduced, for example, *size, tan, sole, heel, leather, slip-on, squeaky, open-toe, buckle, scuff, stylish,* and *elegant, as* well as phrases like *fit to a tee, go with your dress, squeeze into it,* and *worth waiting for.*

As noted in Chapter 5, as the child acquires auditory experience and progresses in auditory skill and language development, the amount of acoustic highlighting is reduced. Similar to other areas of development, as children's auditory abilities mature, they learn to become more and more confident and to take risks (**Fig. 6.1**). Frequently, parents need specific coaching to remind them that the child no longer requires repetition and should be expected to process information the

first time it is delivered. In other words, while considerable emphasis was placed on acoustic enhancements during early auditory stimulation, a deliberate effort is now made to deemphasize elements of speech to "fine-tune" the child's hearing abilities. For example, "The *boy* is going for a ride in the wagon," first presented in listening exercises with much emphasis on *boy* versus *girl,* is later deemphasized and presented without additional emphasis on the nouns. Specific exercises and games using rhyming words may be presented to sharpen auditory skills and teach the child that minor acoustic differences can result in new words. Through play, games, and books, sentences containing longer and longer chunks of information are presented to help develop auditory memory skills. Similarly, parents need to be coached to expose the child to more and more complex language structures.

As mentioned in Chapter 5, when intervention sessions are provided in clinical or similar settings, occasional home visits can be very useful and help provide families with practical tips and examples for integrating language targets in the home environment. An ongoing goal is to transfer targets from clinical teaching situations to everyday experiences. Many early childhood resources provide excellent ideas for auditory and language activities (see examples

Table 6.2   Age 31 to 36 months: typical stages of development in listening, receptive language, expressive language, speech, cognition, and social communication

Listening (audition)	
• Continues to expand auditory memory—three-item auditory memory with different linguistic features	• Sequences two pieces of information in order • Listens to stories on tape • Follows two to three directions

Receptive language	
• Understands most common verbs • Understands and responds to more complex language and commands • Carries out two to three verbal commands in one sentence • Understands several prepositions, e.g., "in," "on," "under"	• Expands concept development • Identifies parts of an object • Understands time concept, e.g., "today," "yesterday," "tomorrow" • Understands "What is missing?"/"Which one does not belong?"

Expressive language	
• Knows gender vocabulary • Talks about what has drawn • Gives both first and last names when asked • Relates recent experiences • Converses in three- to four-word simple sentences • Begins using more complex language • Uses questions, e.g., "who," "what," "where," "why"	• Uses pronouns, e.g., "he," "she," "they," "we," "you," "me" • Uses some plurals • Uses possessives • Uses more negatives, e.g., "not," "none," "nobody" • Begins to use "and"/"because" • Names three or more colors

Speech	
• Makes some substitutions—[f] for [th], [w] for [r] • Medial consonants still inconsistent • Final consonants inserted more regularly • Consonants [l, r, sh, s, z, ch] emerging	• Vowels and diphthongs established • Omits some unstressed parts of speech • Pronunciation becomes more correct • Whispers frequently

Cognition	
• Shares toys and takes turns more appropriately • Develops parallel play • Begins to develop interest in writing and drawing • Begins fantasy play • Matches six color cards • Sorts and categorizes, e.g., blocks and pegs	• Names object when part of it is shown in a picture • Adds two missing body parts to a drawing • Shows interest in how and why things work • Completes two or three interlocking puzzle pieces • Imitates drawing a cross

Social communication (pragmatics)	
• Takes turns and shares • Recites rhymes • Acts out songs; sometimes changes endings • Engages in make-believe activities • Begins to ask permission of others	• Expresses feeling • Initiates conversation • Uses questions for a variety of reasons, e.g., to obtain information, to request

Source: Reprinted with permission from Cochlear Limited. (2005). *Listen, learn, and talk* (2nd ed.). Alexandria, Australia: SOS Printing Group.

Table 6.3   Age 37 to 42 months: typical stages of development in listening, receptive language, expressive language, speech, cognition, and social communication

Listening (audition)

- Auditory memory increases to five items
- Sequences three or more pieces of information in order
- Retells a short story
- Follows three directions
- Processes complex sentence structures
- Tracks a six-word sentence

Receptive language

- Can listen to a 10–15 minute story
- Comprehends an increasing level of complex language
- Understands more difficult concepts, e.g., quality, texture, quantity
- Understands concept of day/night, e.g., distinguishes day from night activities
- Follows directions using concepts of empty/full, same/different
- Understands locational prepositions, e.g., "next to"
- Begins to understand comparatives, e.g., "I am taller than you"
- Understands ~ 900 words

Expressive language

- Holds conversations using many correct grammatical structures (plurals, possession, pronouns, prepositions, adjectives)
- Uses "when" and "how many" questions
- Uses "so"/"because"
- Relays a message
- Describes what objects can be used for
- Starts to answer "what if?" questions
- Answers "What is missing?"
- Identifies which one does not belong and answers "Why?"
- Attempts to answer problem-solving questions, e.g., "What if?"
- Uses ~ 500 intelligible words

Speech

- Uses some blends, e.g., [mp, pt, br, dr, gr, sm]
- Consonants [j, v, th] emerging
- Some substitutions still made, e.g., [gw] for [gr] in blends
- Pronunciations of words more stable from one production to the next

Cognition

- Begins one-to-one correspondence
- Follows directions using concepts, e.g., "empty," "full," "same," "different"
- Develops more difficult concepts, e.g., quality, quantity, texture
- Compares objects
- Begins simple problem solving
- Develops imagination

Social communication (pragmatics)

- Takes turns
- Plays with other children more appropriately
- Shows understanding of others' feelings/needs
- Interacts through simple conversation
- Initiates conversation
- Enjoys role plays

Source: Reprinted with permission from Cochlear Limited. (2005). *Listen, learn, and talk* (2nd ed.). Alexandria, Australia: SOS Printing Group.

Table 6.4 Age 43 to 48 months: typical stages of development in listening, receptive language, expressive language, speech, cognition, and social communication

Listening (audition)

- Processes longer and more complex language structures, e.g., "Can you find something that lives in a tree, has feathers and a yellow crest?"
- Follows directions with more difficult concepts, e.g., "Put the thick blue square behind the empty jug"
- Retells longer stories in detail—five or more sentences
- Tracks an eight-word sentence

Receptive language

- Continues to expand vocabulary comprehension
- Understands singular/plural
- Understands difference between past/ present/future
- Answers final word analogies
- Identifies objects missing from scene
- Understands day/morning/ afternoon/night
- Makes comparisons of speed/weight
- Understands 1,500–2,000 words

Expressive language

- Uses "his"/"her"/"their"
- More consistent use of plurals—irregular and regular
- Talks about pictures and storybooks
- Uses more sophisticated imaginative play
- Uses negatives and some modals, e.g., "shouldn't"/"won't"/"can't"
- Uses comparisons
- Makes inferences
- Develops colloquial expressions
- Uses How much? How? questions
- Uses 800–1,500 words
- Uses more complex language structures
- Spontaneous utterances are mostly grammatically correct

Speech

- Reduces omissions and substitutions
- Most consonants established
- More blends emerging in initial and final positions
- Rate and rhythm normal
- Uses appropriate loudness level
- Uses appropriate intonation
- [For accompanying chart, see *Sounds of Speech* p. 43]

Cognition

- Draws simple objects
- Understands time concepts, e.g., "today/ "tomorrow"/"yesterday"/"morning"/ "afternoon"/"night"
- Tells how many fingers and toes
- Associates an object with an occupation, e.g., thermometer/doctor
- Continues to develop imagination
- Concentration increases
- Copies simple picture line drawings
- Matches patterns
- Makes inferences

Social communication (pragmatics)

- Increases confidence and self-esteem
- Requests made from others, e.g., shop/retail assistant
- Uses intonation appropriately
- Initiates conversation
- Adapts to changes of topic
- Uses language for different communicative intent, e.g., obtaining information, giving information, expressing needs/feelings, bargaining

Source: Reprinted with permission from Cochlear Limited. (2005). *Listen, learn, and talk* (2nd ed.). Alexandria, Australia: SOS Printing Group.

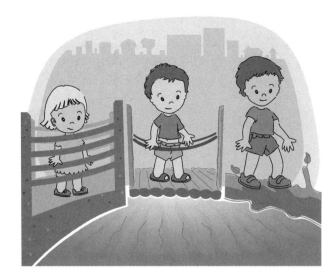

Fig. 6.1 Building confidence in auditory skills can be compared with developing motor skills to cross a bridge. A young child needs substantial support in the beginning stages, but less and less support as her auditory abilities improve and she becomes more confident.

of resources at the end of this chapter). **Table 6.5** provides an example of how constructing a simple large wall calendar at home can capitalize on daily experiences and expand a child's learning through enriching auditory, language, and literacy skills. For this activity, a new large calendar with plenty of writing space is hung on the wall each month. During the month, there is considerable opportunity for repetition and reinforcement of receptive and expressive language. Concepts of time, such as "yesterday," "today, and "tomorrow,"

Table 6.5   Using a wall calendar to stimulate audition, language, and early literacy

- Daily news: When the child is very young, parents write a simple sentence about an event in the child's life (e.g., a visit to grandparents or to the zoo, buying new shoes) and either paste on a picture of the event or add a drawing. If the child is a little older, she can help decide on the news item of the day and even produce the sentence that the parent writes to accompany the picture or drawing. These entries can be read regularly and are good starting points for conversations. Since the child's and family members' names appear frequently, the child will start to recognize some of these familiar words in a meaningful context.

- Emergent literacy (reading, writing, and phonological awareness): With the young child, parents can direct attention to letters and words that come up frequently. As the child ages, she can start recognizing the days of the week and the month. Basic phonological awareness activities can be done using the calendar—e.g., rhyming, counting words in sentences, recognizing letters, playing with words and sounds.

- Linguistics concepts: Calendars can be used to place emphasis on different language goals (e.g., conjunctions, pronouns, prepositions, verb tense). Calendars can reinforce the understanding of verb tense (e.g., "Yesterday, we went to visit grandma," "Next week will be Jeffrey's birthday!").

- Concepts of time: Date/time vocabulary (e.g., yesterday, next week), the days of the week, the months, the year.

- Weather: Weather vocabulary (e.g., "It's snowing, "The wind blows hard"), clothing related to the weather changes.

- Numeracy: Counting the days until the child's birthday, locating a certain date on the calendar.

- Anniversaries and special events: Writing birthdays, special holidays, and vocabulary related to these events (e.g., words, idiomatic expressions, sentences).

are not mastered by a young child before age 3 to 4 years; and more complex concepts of time, such as "next week" or "last year," may not be acquired before the child is 5 years old. A calendar will help promote early literacy skills while making these concepts of time more concrete for the child as well as facilitating learning of numerous other concepts. Each day's calendar space can be filled with information through writing and pictures. At the end of the month, the squares for the different days can be cut out and stapled together to form a book. These books can be used over and over to work on conversations skills, to review specific vocabulary, or simply to read the daily news written for that month.

Advancing the Child's Auditory and Language Skills

Given the reduced access to hearing, children with hearing loss are at risk for phonological processing difficulties, and good oral language skills are associated with literacy abilities in school (National Institute for Literacy, 2008). In early language learning more generally, there is a growing interest in promoting early literacy development through a focus on spoken language, which involves teaching of vocabulary, phonemic awareness, and letter–sound relationships. Therefore, it seems logical that rehabilitation programs with a focus on auditory and spoken language development contribute to literacy success in children. Exposing children to diverse forms of language through different types of oral and written material appears to enhance literacy skills. Emergent literacy and literacy at school age are the subject of Chapter 10. The point here is that strong auditory skills not only favor spoken language but also provide an important foundation for other skills. Competent auditory and advanced language learning are also critical for the development of theory of mind, that is, understanding the perspectives of others and awareness that others can have different feelings, thoughts, and emotions about an experience. Because of reduced hearing and particularly due to limitations in overhearing different types of conversation, children with hearing loss are at risk for not developing an age-appropriate theory of mind.

By the time, the child enters school at around 5 years of age, auditory skills should be well developed. **Table 6.6** provides examples of expected auditory abilities of typical 5-year-old children.

Listening beyond the Clinic and Home

During the preschool years, it is common for children to attend child care, nursery school, or playgroup programs at least on a part-time basis. Crucial to developing spoken language is interaction with peers with normal hearing. Parents are therefore generally encouraged to expose children to typical speech and language patterns and social interaction through programs with children with normal hearing when possible. As the child ages, it is evident that listening and language acquisition extend well beyond the home environment. Parents can enlist the support of child care services and inform them about the child's intervention targets. Direct contact between the child care environment and the clinician/teacher is highly desirable so that the clinician can observe the child in the learning environment, evaluate the acoustic conditions, inform child care workers about hearing loss and hearing instruments, and provide input about auditory and language stimulation. Also of importance, the child care program can inform the clinician/teacher about the child's interactions with peers and highlight any issues related to social or other areas of development. In some cases, communication exchange through e-mail or a communication book can be established so that the clinician/teacher can update the early childhood educators and the educators can provide input about the child's real-world functioning. These strategies can help prevent or at the very least minimize difficulties for the young child in a preschool setting.

As shown in several studies, degradation of the auditory signal is one of the greatest barriers to receiving auditory input. A considerable body of research has documented the challenges in classroom-type environments (Crandell & Smaldino, 2000). Therefore, for example, consideration should be given to the use of remote microphone technology, and a determination must be made of the most appropriate technology in view of the child's age and the pace

Table 6.6   Auditory abilities of a typical 5-year-old child

- Differentiate between all phonemes, including those with similar acoustic characteristics, such as p vs. t vs. k.

- Carry out phonological processing skills, such as: "If we replace *h* in hat with *m*, what is the new word? What words rhyme with *hot*?"

- Identify 90–100% of recorded words in a list of 25 words, e.g., PBK.

- Identify 90–100% of phrases using recorded material, e.g., HINT.

- Auditory memory for five or more critical items. Examples include following a direction, such as "Put the frog and the cat in the sandbox, and put the puppy in the pool with the baby"; "On my trip, I would like to take a tie, scarf, shampoo, sweater, and a cap."

- Repeat sentences 10 or more words in length.

- Follow multiple directions, e.g., "Put your bottle in the recycle bin, then get your raincoat and stand beside the window."

- Understand a short story and answer several questions.

- Understand complex question forms, such as "How would we decide whether we should wear boots?" "What might occur if we put too many people in the canoe?" "If you were a polar bear, what would be your favorite food?"

Abbreviations: PBK, Phonetically Balanced Kindergarten Test; HINT, Hearing in Noise Test.

and variety of learning settings occurring in a given environment (Flexer, 2004). For example, children sit in a group for storytelling and other activities for short periods of the day, but much of the interaction occurs in one-to-one and small group interaction with peers and adults. Chapter 8 provides detailed information about the advantages and considerations involved in selecting and using optimal technology to enhance learning in various environments.

The child's everyday listening life also extends to other situations, including time spent with grandparents, other family members, and friends, much of which may take place in other individuals' homes and in other listening environments. Thinking about how to achieve the best possible access to sound beyond the clinic and home is therefore important and also involves, where possible, the provision of education and information to all individuals involved in interaction with the child. Parents and clinicians/teachers can partner to transfer clinic-based teaching to everyday settings.

From Preschool to School

Over their child's development, parents pass through several stages and events that may trigger stress and concern. One such event is the transition into school. In their questionnaire with 162 parents of children at different times since diagnosis, Meinzen-Derr et al (2008) found that parents whose children had been diagnosed for more than 60 months had higher stress levels than those of children with shorter times since diagnosis. The time before school entry can be a period where parents need additional attention and time to talk about their apprehension and concerns about this next phase in their child's learning. Therefore, the preparation of parents for school can become an important aspect of the rehabilitation process in the intervention years prior to school entry. As discussed in the next chapter, as children transition to school, in addition to ongoing parent support and education, specific practical strategies can be applied in the final year prior to school entry to introduce the child and family to school and to make the school system aware of the child's needs.

Children Who Experience Late Intervention

Late Identified/Late Intervention

Despite vast improvements in early identification, some children are late identified for various reasons, including the lack of availability of newborn screening, onset of hearing loss at some point postscreening (i.e., child passed the screening test), or lack of follow-up from screening due to parental or systemic factors (Watkin & Baldwin, 2011). Children identified with mild bilateral hearing loss often enter the system later, as they are not always targeted through universal screening initiatives. These children and others who are late identified due to delayed onset of hearing loss may enter the habilitation process with various levels of previous auditory experience and language. Finally, some children will be identified in infancy but experience progressive hearing loss (Fitzpatrick, 2011b; Fitzpatrick, Durieux-Smith, & Whittingham, 2010; Watkin & Baldwin, 2011).

Parents of children who did not benefit from early identification sometimes start intervention with a sense of guilt and urgency (Fitzpatrick, Graham, Durieux-Smith, Angus, & Coyle, 2007). As reported by one mother of a child whose profound hearing loss was confirmed at 18 months of age:

> She could have had a better start to language. . . . So because we started behind the 8 ball, we always felt like we were trying to catch up. . . . I would say that was our biggest issue—we were always feeling behind.

Depending on the severity of hearing loss, the child may enter the intervention program with some language, although in most cases it is delayed relative to typical hearing peers. At any age or stage, a comprehensive assessment is undertaken using standardized speech-language measures, if appropriate for the child's level, and careful evaluation of the child's auditory and language capacities is performed through the intervention sessions. As noted, spoken language acquisition is based on typical language trajectories. If a child with impaired hearing has little or no language, it is impera-

tive to take him or her through the early stages of listening that have been previously described.

A common starting point for a child who starts late without language or auditory function is with "learning to listen" words—that is, acoustic material that permits considerable repetition and strong intonation patterns—when amplification is introduced. However, it is important to ensure that these beginning activities be presented using materials appropriate to the child's overall developmental level. For example, for a 2-year-old child with no previous sound exposure, the repeated [ba-ba-ba] sound associated with a boat might be introduced by having the child sort boats, airplanes, and cars, or work on a puzzle with different colors of airplanes—activities that would not be selected for stimulating a 5-month-old baby with the same sound–word association. Such activities are performed extensively to attempt to establish natural patterns of sound because the child has missed out on a period of auditory stimulation. Most parents will require considerable guidance and encouragement to carry on this important work in the early period.

For young children, the validation of the fitting of acoustic aids or cochlear implants is a crucial component of the intervention program. The audiologic assessment can provide useful information to the audiologist about the amount of amplified hearing, the maximum output of the hearing aid(s), and the frequency range of the hearing instrument(s). However, this information helps verify the fitting and does not provide information about the child's functioning with the technology. Behavioral audiometric information will generally be available by age 2 years, and hearing aid adjustments are frequently required over a period of time to achieve an optimal fitting. Through auditory based intervention, the clinician/teacher can provide valuable information based on the child's functioning using formal or informal (experiential) benchmarks established for other children with hearing loss with similar listening experience.

Delayed-Onset and Progressive Hearing Loss

Evidence about delayed-onset and progressive hearing loss is continuing to accumulate in postnewborn screening studies. Prior to UNHS,

it was difficult to discern the true onset of hearing loss, and in the absence of known etiology, many children were presumed to have congenital loss. Data emerging from UNHS programs suggest that more children than anticipated are at risk for delayed-onset or progressive hearing loss. For example, in an examination of data from a newborn screening program, Fitzpatrick and Whittingham (submitted manuscript) found that 27% of 75 children with mild bilateral or unilateral hearing loss had passed screening but later presented with hearing loss. Of a clinical population of 337 children with milder forms of hearing loss, 22% experienced deterioration in audiometric hearing levels. These findings have implications for audiologic rehabilitation in that they underscore the importance of a constant follow-up in audiology to ensure that the child has optimal hearing technology for his or her hearing loss. Any suspicion of deterioration of hearing warrants follow-up evaluations in audiology.

Not surprisingly, parents can be seriously affected when they observe or learn through assessment that the child's hearing has deteriorated. In some cases, the situation can be exacerbated when it involves new decision making about cochlear implantation and parents had previously thought that their child would be able to hear without surgical intervention. For other parents, the gradual loss of hearing that becomes evident over a series of audiologic test sessions can be particularly stressful.

Since the introduction of meningitis vaccines, the incidence of acquired hearing loss due to exogenous causes has decreased in developed countries. However, in our multicultural societies, children from other countries may present with acquired hearing loss. Children undergoing ototoxic treatments are also at risk for hearing loss.

For children with late entry to audiologic rehabilitation, our key message is that it is critical to realize that parents are starting at the beginning and may need intensive guidance to adjust to the diagnosis of hearing loss. Parents are moving through the process of learning about and coping with the hearing loss at different stages, sometimes having themselves observed the deterioration in auditory function or the delay in language that is characteristic of unidentified and perhaps later-onset or progressive hearing loss. Likewise, for the child with no auditory experience, it is important to begin at the beginning and to take the child through the auditory learning stages while considering age and developmental status.

Auditory Neuropathy Spectrum Disorder

As discussed in Chapter 4, both audiometric and speech recognition results for children with auditory neuropathy spectrum disorder (ANSD) have been reported as highly variable (Rance, 2005; Rance, Barker, Sarant, & Ching, 2007). Furthermore, ANSD may not be identified in children in the neonatal period, particularly if there are no risk factors for hearing loss. ANSD is more frequently identified in infancy in the course of newborn screening programs, in infants who are at risk and who are screened using automated auditory brainstem response screening techniques (Bagatto, Scollie, Hyde, & Seewald, 2010). In addition, because of the complications in sorting out effective hearing abilities in children with ANSD, given the variability in the child's functioning, decision making regarding the most appropriate technology options for these children can take some time. In general, a diagnostic process is advocated to determine whether the child can benefit from conventional hearing aids and auditory stimulation. Given the fluctuating hearing levels and the lack of correlation between apparent audiometric levels and auditory abilities, more time may be needed to tease out the best options in comparison with children with sensorineural hearing loss of cochlear origin. In listening and spoken language intervention, clinical practices are similar to those for children with sensorineural hearing loss, and many children can develop auditorially based on similar expectations.

Case Examples of Children Identified after 12 Months of Age

Child with Late-Identified Hearing Loss

Sammy was referred to the audiology program at 16 months of age because of concerns raised by his early childhood providers shortly after they moved to Canada. He was identified with a bilateral severe hearing loss and was fitted with bilateral hearing aids within a month. Over a 16-month period, he developed beginning auditory skills and some two-word combinations. However, his therapist judged that his progress, given the excellent family input, was not comparable to that of typical 2-year-olds in the early intervention program. The use of cochlear implants was discussed with the parents over a period of several months as Sammy, with a pure-tone average of 91 and 93 dB HL in the left and right ears, was considered within the "borderline" category of candidacy. He eventually received a unilateral cochlear implant at age 2.8 years. After the initial fitting of his cochlear implant, he continued to work with the clinician/teacher, who noted that he was not able to detect "s" with his cochlear implant alone. This information was discussed with the audiologist, and further fine tuning of the cochlear implant map was performed while Sammy was at the clinic for his therapy

session. A new program was created, but the old program, which was clearly comfortable for Sammy, was retained in his speech processor in case the parents observed adverse reactions to the new program. Subsequent to the reprogramming of his speech processor, during play activities in the therapy session, Sammy demonstrated the ability to respond to all sounds of the Ling Six-Sound Test, suggesting that he now had access to all sounds of the speech spectrum in English. Therapy and more fine tuning of the speech processor program continued over the next 6 months as Sammy learned to respond to and process the new sounds through his speech processor. Sammy has been using his cochlear implant combined with a hearing aid in the contralateral ear and is now considered to be receiving optimal acoustic information.

Child with Delayed-Onset Hearing Loss

(Contribution from Kelly Rabjohn, Children's Hospital of Eastern Ontario, Ottawa, Canada.)

Katie passed newborn hearing screening but returned to the audiology clinic at 18 months of age due to parental concern about her language. She was identified with bilateral moderate to severe hearing loss, was fitted with binaural hearing aids within 2 weeks, and began attending weekly auditory-verbal therapy sessions. There were no other developmental concerns. A language assessment at 18 months, when intervention began using the Preschool Language Scale (PLS-4), showed that Katie's language was already significantly delayed. She was functioning at the 4th per-

centile. Katie progressed well in therapy, and by 3 years of age was able to close the gap. **Table 6.7** presents a summary of the first lesson plan prepared by her clinician/teacher. As shown, the clinician/teacher starts with the beginning stages of auditory development, as discussed above. That is, to begin stimulating Katie's auditory learning, the clinician/teacher introduces the parents to several different sounds and words that permit considerable repetition and redundancy in the acoustic information presented. She then provides the parents with a list of "learning to listen" words to help them get started with auditory stimulation at home.

Child with Progressive Hearing Loss

(Contribution from Rosemary Somerville, Children's Hospital of Eastern Ontario, Ottawa, Canada.)

Jenny was born prematurely at 29 weeks' gestation and presented with a history of anoxia. At 5½ months of age, a bilateral moderate hearing loss was confirmed through auditory brainstem response testing, and she was fitted with binaural hearing aids within a couple of months. By age 2½ years, her hearing loss had progressed to severe to profound levels. The initial audiogram and the audiogram prior to implantation are shown in **Fig. 6.2a,b**. With well-fitted hearing aids, sound field detection levels were in the 30 to 35 dB range. Her clinician/teacher was very concerned that although she was detecting all the sounds of

the speech spectrum, she was struggling with listening and her progress was slower than expected, particularly in capturing high-frequency information, such as the "s" marker for plurals, or in differentiating rhyming words. There were also concerns that she was becoming frustrated and more withdrawn. The clinician/teacher advocated for a cochlear implant, but there was still some hesitation due to her borderline hearing levels. She received a unilateral cochlear implant shortly after her fourth birthday. Jenny was very unhappy during the activation of the implant, but with support, her mother was able to encourage her to adapt to the new sounds. Within weeks, her personality changed and she was described by her family

Table 6.7   Summary of a clinician/teacher's first intervention session with a child identified at 18 months of age

Introduced Ling Six Sounds test.

LTLs ("moo," "neigh neigh," "oink oink oink") with puzzle and later with barn (stressed talking in short phrases, use LTLs, use lots of expression and intonation, pick sounds with different patterns).

"Up up up boom" with clown. Emphasize: Starting with toy out of sight first, talk about it, then show it. Make activity exciting and fun ("boom").

Baby play ("brush your hair," "have a drink," "wash wash wash your toes," etc. Emphasize: Talking all day during "normal" daily activities, and that bath time is a time when she can't hear; therefore, play doll routines around bath so that she hears the language in some context).

Penguins on slide: "up up up wee." Emphasize: Talk before show, talk during "outdoor" activities, talk about toy and demo before allowing child access to toy—so she keeps listening.

Discussed aids (reviewed care, listening check, retention issues).

Chose five LTLs to practice for the week.

Abbreviation: LTLs, "learning to listen" words.
Contributed by Kelly Rabjohn, Children's Hospital of Eastern Ontario.

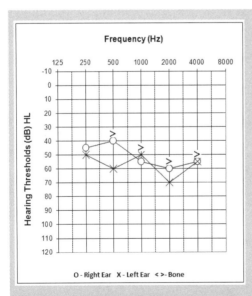 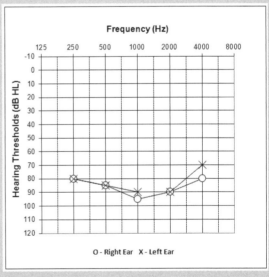

Fig. 6.2a,b   **(a)** Audiogram showing hearing loss prior to deterioration of thresholds. **(b)** Audiogram showing severe to profound hearing loss prior to cochlear implantation.

as more perky and talkative. **Table 6.8** displays preimplant as well as postimplant speech recognition and language scores after 1 year of implant use. At age 8½ years, she received a second implant, underwent a short period of intensive therapy to develop auditory skills through the new device, and soon adapted to the new input. Her speech recognition scores while she was wearing the second implant only are also shown in **Table 6.8**.

Table 6.8 Speech recognition scores obtained with unilateral cochlear implant and with second implant

			Post-CI				
		Pre-CI	3 Mths	6 Mths	1 Year	4 Year	Second CI (left ear alone)
PBK recorded	Words	0%	12%	52%	56%	76%	72%
	Phonemes	23%	53%	83%	86%	90%	85%
MLNT recorded	Words	21%	50%	67%	88%	92%	83%
	Phonemes	48%	81%	88%	91%	96%	93%
	HINT in quiet	DNT	–	65%	79%	96%	93%
	HINT +10 S/N	–	–	–	–	–	78%
GFTA		87	–	–	99	–	–
PPVT		87	–	–	80	–	–
PLS AC		98	–	–	104	–	–
EC		83	–	–	89	–	–

Abbreviations: CI, cochlear implant; PBK, Phonetically Balanced Kindergarten Test; MLNT, Multisyllabic Neighborhood Test; HINT, Hearing in Noise Test; S/N, signal-to-noise ratio; GFTA, Goldman-Fristoe Test of Articulation; PPVT, Peabody Picture Vocabulary Test; PLS, Preschool Language Scale; AC, auditory comprehension; EC, expressive communication.
Note: Speech-language tests are normed on children with normal hearing, where 100 represents the mean standard score (standard deviation of 15).
Contribution from Rosemary Somerville, Children's Hospital of Eastern Ontario, Ottawa, Canada.

◼ Summary

Children with hearing loss typically continue to benefit from intervention during the preschool years, and parents continue to require specific guidance in helping their children develop listening and spoken language skills. Assessment of the child's abilities is important for measuring progress, situating the child relative to peers, and planning intervention goals. Regardless of the starting point, which can vary with age of identification or due to interruptions in early intervention, parents can be guided to follow a developmental sequence in stimulating their child's acquisition of spoken language. Children who come to intervention at later ages will need intensive support to "catch up" to peers with normal hearing and may lag behind for some time. There is good evidence that the majority of children who have access to early intervention and receive optimal auditory and language stimulation can develop spoken language skills commensurate with age-matched peers, enabling them to attend regular education programs.

◼ Acknowledgments

We are grateful to the listening and spoken language specialists, Erin McSweeney, Deirdre Neuss, Kelly Rabjohn, Rosemary Somerville, and Pamela Steacie, from the Audiology Program at the Children Hospital of Eastern Ontario for their contributions to this chapter.

References

Archbold, S., Phil, M., & O'Donoghue, G. M. (2009). Education and childhood deafness: Changing choices and new challenges. In J. K. Niparko (Ed.), *Cochlear implants: Principles and practices* (2nd ed., pp. 313–321). Philadelphia, PA: Lippincott Williams & Wilkins.

Bagatto, M., Scollie, S. D., Hyde, M., & Seewald, R. (2010). Protocol for the provision of amplification within the Ontario infant hearing program. *International Journal of Audiology, 49*(Suppl. 1), S70–S79. 10.3109/14992020903080751.

Bagatto, M. P., Moodie, S. T., Malandrino, A. C., Richert, F. M., Clench, D. A., & Scollie, S. D. (2011). The University of Western Ontario Pediatric Audiological Monitoring Protocol (UWO PedAMP). *Trends in Amplification, 15*(1), 57–76.

Bagatto, M. P., Moodie, S. T., Seewald, R. C., Bartlett, D. J., & Scollie, S. D. (2011). A critical review of audiological outcome measures for infants and children. *Trends in Amplification, 15*(1), 57–76. 10.1177/1084713811420304.

Crandell, C. C., & Smaldino, J. J. (2000). Classroom acoustics for children with normal hearing and with hearing impairment. *Language, Speech, and Hearing Services in Schools, 31,* 362–370.

Estabrooks, W. (Ed.). (2006). *Auditory-verbal therapy and practice.* Washington, DC: Alexander Graham Bell Association for the Deaf and Hard of Hearing.

Fitzpatrick, E. (2007). Population infant hearing screening to intervention: Determinants of outcome from the parents' perspective. Doctoral thesis, University of Ottawa, Ottawa.

Fitzpatrick, E., Angus, D., Durieux-Smith, A., Graham, I. D., & Coyle, D. (2008). Parents' needs following identification of childhood hearing loss. *American Journal of Audiology, 17*(1), 38–49.

Fitzpatrick, E., Graham, I. D., Durieux-Smith, A., Angus, D., & Coyle, D. (2007). Parents' perspectives on the impact of the early diagnosis of childhood hearing loss. *International Journal of Audiology, 46*(2), 97–106.

Fitzpatrick, E. M. (2011a). Defining typical development for children with hearing loss. Presented at the Australasian Newborn Hearing Screening Conference 2011, Perth, Australia.

Fitzpatrick, E. M. (2011b). New challenges from newborn hearing screening: Children with mild bilateral and unilateral hearing loss. Paper presented at the Australasian Newborn Hearing Screening Conference 2011, Perth, Australia.

Fitzpatrick, E. M., & Doucet, S. P. (In press). When should children be discharged from an auditory-verbal program? In W. Estabrooks (Ed.), *101 FAQs about auditory-verbal practice.* Washington, DC: AG Bell Association.

Fitzpatrick, E. M., Durieux-Smith, A., & Whittingham, J. (2010). Clinical practice for children with mild bilateral and unilateral hearing loss. *Ear and Hearing, 31*(3), 392–400.

Fitzpatrick, E. M., & Whittingham, J. (Submitted manuscript). Mild bilateral and unilateral hearing loss in children: A 20-year view of characteristics and practices.

Flexer, C. (2004). Classroom amplification systems. In R. J. Roeser & M. P. Downs (Eds.), *Auditory disorders in school children* (pp. 284–305). New York: Thieme Medical Publishers.

Meinzen-Derr, J., Lim, L. H. Y., Choo, D. I., Buyniski, S., & Wiley, S. (2008). Pediatric hearing impairment caregiver experience: Impact of duration of hearing loss on parental stress. *International Journal of Pediatric Otorhinolaryngology, 72*(11), 1693–1703.

National Institute for Literacy. (2008). *Developing early literacy: Report of the National Early Literacy Panel.* Retrieved from http://www.pathstoliteracy.org/sites/default/files/uploaded-files/NELPReport09.pdf

Neuss, D., Fitzpatrick, E. M., Durieux-Smith, A., Olds, J., Moreau, K., Ufholz, L.-A., & Schramm, D. (In press.). A survey of assessment tools used by certified auditory-verbal therapists for children from birth to 3 years.

Nicholas, J. G., & Geers, A. E. (2006). Effects of early auditory experience on the spoken language of deaf children at 3 years of age. *Ear and Hearing, 27*(3), 286–298.

Nikolopoulos, T. P., Archbold, S. M., & Gregory, S. (2005). Young deaf children with hearing aids or cochlear implants: Early assessment package for monitoring progress. *International Journal of Pediatric Otorhinolaryngology, 69*(2), 175–186.

Paul, R., & Norbury, C. F. (2012). *Language disorders from infancy through adolescence: Listening, speaking, reading, writing, and communicating* (4th ed.). St. Louis, MO: Elsevier, Inc.

Rance, G. (2005). Auditory neuropathy/dys-synchrony and its perceptual consequences. *Trends in Amplification, 9*(1), 1–43. 10.1177/108471380500900102.

Rance, G., Barker, E. J., Sarant, J. Z., & Ching, T. Y. C. (2007). Receptive language and speech production in children with auditory neuropathy/dyssynchrony type hearing loss. *Ear and Hearing, 28*(5), 694–702.

Simser, J., & Steacie, P. (1993). A hospital clinic early intervention program. *Volta Review, 95*(5), 65–74.

Truohy, J., Brown, J., Mercer-Moseley, C., & Walsh, L. (2005). *St. Gabriel's curriculum: A guide for professionals working with children who are hearing impaired (birth to six years).* St Gabriel's School for Hearing Impaired Children, Sydney, Australia.

Watkin, P. M., & Baldwin, M. (2011). Identifying deafness in ealy childhood: Requirements after the newborn hearing screen. *Achives of Disorders in Childhood, 96,* 62–66.

7 Adapting Intervention for Children with Hearing Loss and Other Special Needs

In Chapters 5 and 6, we described audiologic rehabilitation for children with hearing loss of varying degrees who otherwise have typical development. It is estimated that 60 to 70% of children fall in this category, while the other 30 to 40% of children with hearing loss have one or more other disabilities (Gallaudet Research Institute, 2009; Picard, 2004). While there is a tendency to discuss children with additional developmental disabilities as a group, it is important to recognize that they represent a highly heterogeneous subset of children, and that there are many categories and sub-categories of additional disabilities. In this chapter, we are primarily concerned with children whose cognitive or other sensory or language impairments limit or preclude the typical development of spoken language. Our discussion is primarily focused on children with hearing loss who would experience difficulties developing spoken communication, even in the absence of a hearing disorder.

▦ Effects of Additional Disabilities on Listening and Spoken Language

There appears to be a growing trend for more children with hearing loss and additional disabilities to access intervention services focused on listening and spoken language development. This may be due to an apparent growth in the number of children with hearing loss and additional disabilities (Gallaudet Research Institute, 2009; Guardino, 2008). It may also be partly due to an increase in the actual prevalence of additional disabilities in the general population (e.g., survival of more babies from neonatal intensive care units) (Boyle et al, 2011). The rise in the number of children frequenting services may also be related to more refined and elaborate assessment techniques that permit differential diagnoses. There is also likely a heightened awareness of the range of disabilities, resulting in more children placed in a "special needs" category.

Over the last two to three decades, the shift in practice to include all children with special needs in regular early education programs has also likely contributed to the increase in children who receive hearing technology and access auditory rehabilitation. For example, in the early years of cochlear implantation, the presence of additional disabilities was often an exclusion criterion for candidacy, whereas more children with additional disabilities have received cochlear implants in the last decade (Edwards, Frost, & Witham, 2006; Fitzpatrick & Brewster, 2008; Meinzen-Derr, Wiley, Grether, & Choo, 2011). Consequently, there is a growing interest in providing optimal auditory rehabilitation services to these children and in helping them make use of auditory input.

The following section is intended to provide a brief introduction to some of the most common disabilities that interfere with typical development in children with hearing loss. For a more comprehensive review, a special monograph edited by Rhoades, Price, and Perigoe (2004) provides considerable information on the subject. Descriptions of clinical features of numerous syndromes can be found in Northern and Downs (2002) and in the online Mendelian Inheritance in Man database (www.ncbi.nlm.nih.gov/omim).

Classification of children according to type of disability is problematic with respect to communication development because there is generally a spectrum of cognitive and global development across syndromes and disorders. A recent review of clinical data for 363 children identified with hearing loss in a 10-year period showed that 23% (82) presented with at least one developmental disability (see **Table 7.1** for types of disabilities). As shown in **Table 7.1**, of the 82 children, 26 had hearing loss and developmental disabilities associated with a syndrome. Our main interest in this chapter is the effect of other disabilities on the child's ability

Table 7.1   Clinical profile of 82 children identified with hearing loss and developmental delays

Nonsyndromic n = 56 (68%)		Syndromic n = 26 (32%)	
Learning disability	2 (3.6%)	Goldenhar	2 (7.7%)
ADHD	2 (3.6%)	Di George	2 (7.7%)
Cognitive disability	4 (7.1%)	Down syndrome	5 (19.2%)
Autism	4 (7.1%)	CHARGE	6 (23.1%)
Communication	6 (10.8%)	Other:	11 (42.3%)
Motor disability	19 (33.9%)	Pfeiffer, Noonan, San Filippo, Smith Magenis, Treacher Collins, oculocutaneous albinism, Moebius, partial 11q and 18q	
Other	19 (33.9%)		

to process auditory information and develop functional oral communication. Essentially, for this purpose, we view children with additional disabilities as falling into two broad categories: (1) children who have the potential for spoken language acquisition, although progress may be slower or different compared with other peers with hearing loss, and (2) children who show limited or no ability to acquire spoken language as their primary mode of communication. In other words, depending on the severity of the additional disorders, some children are not expected to develop spoken language through listening despite access to usable hearing. In our experience, it is primarily this type of classification, rather than one based on medical diagnosis, that guides our discussion of expectations for listening and spoken language development with parents, and ultimately guides our intervention objectives. In the future, the integration of genetic testing and counseling with audiology and rehabilitation services may also provide guidance in clinical care.

Parent Guidance

One of the main differences in working with families of children with additional disabilities is that the family is adapting to and coping with the knowledge that their child has multiple developmental and learning challenges. Sometimes, the hearing loss is secondary, in that other disabilities have greater consequences for the child's overall development. In other cases, the child's immediate health may be the primary concern rather than the effects of the hearing loss.

A second difference is that an interdisciplinary team of specialists is necessarily involved in providing care for children with multiple disabilities and their families. This differs from other children with hearing loss, where the primary and ongoing contacts for the parent are usually the professionals involved in managing the hearing loss (e.g., audiologist and clinician/teacher). Therefore, the emphasis placed on audiologic rehabilitation, one of many services, and the timing of care may differ for these children. In particular, in the early months and years, parents are interacting with many more professionals, are required to constantly adjust their expectations, and will possibly learn about their child's limitations from different perspectives. One of the consequences is that parents can often feel quite overwhelmed with all of the information and need more time to adjust to addressing hearing-specific issues. For some parents, adjusting to caring for a child with disabilities involves a long process (Luterman, 2006). Therefore, although the information provided to parents about hearing loss and its effects is not different from typical care, the "dose" and timing of information may need to be adjusted according to the professionals' judgment of parent readiness.

Audiologic Care

Confirmation of hearing loss may take longer for children with complex medical issues and developmental needs (Madell & Flexer, 2008). Although objective techniques, including auditory brainstem response (ABR) audiometry, otoacoustic emissions, and immittance measures, provide valuable information, interpretation can be complicated for children with certain neurological difficulties. In addition, the child's health status or other medical appointments that place extra demands on the family may take precedence over audiologic testing. For older children, in whom behavioral audiometry would generally be sufficient to identify hearing loss, objective techniques may need to be employed, and confirmation with behavioral measures may be slower or behavioral testing may result in more limited information for some children. For more in-depth information about behavioral evaluation for children with multiple disabilities, consult resources such as Madell and Flexer (2008).

Due to the complexity of identifying and confirming hearing loss, subsequent audiologic decisions can be more challenging for children with special needs. For example, for both practitioners and parents, decision making related to hearing aid and cochlear implant recommendations may be more difficult. This may be partly due to more limited information about the child's hearing loss, as well as indecision on the part of parents in light of other health priorities. Adding to the complexity of sorting out the degree and type of hearing impairment is that some children with developmental issues, such as Down syndrome, have structural abnormalities that are also associated with middle ear disease and conductive hearing loss (Northern & Downs, 2002). Research related to clinical management confirms that time from identification to hearing aid fitting is generally longer and that the fitting can be delayed for children with additional disabilities (Durieux-Smith, Fitzpatrick, & Whittingham, 2008; Spivak, Sokol, Auerbach, & Gershkovich, 2009). The number of visits involved in confirming hearing loss and fitting amplification can increase the burden for families.

As discussed in Chapter 3, validation of hearing aids or cochlear implants through audiologic evaluations, such as speech recognition testing or more informal therapy observations, is an important part of the process in achieving optimal amplification. Validation of the child's responses to sound can be much more challenging and take longer for children with additional developmental disabilities.

Similarly, cochlear implant research suggests that the presence of additional disabilities can result in late implantation because the child's medical and developmental conditions can complicate decision making (Fitzpatrick, Johnson, & Durieux-Smith, 2011). In this clinical study, additional time was required for children to be classified as cochlear implant candidates, and the wait time to surgery of up to 21 months suggested that there was considerable uncertainty regarding implantation. For some children, other factors can interact with developmental issues to slow the decision-making process, including middle ear disorders and uncertainty of audiologic responses due to inconsistent test results. Similar results were reported in a recent study in the United Kingdom that interviewed parents of children with complex needs about access to cochlear implants (McCracken & Turner, 2012). Stacey, Fortnum, Barton, and Summerfield (2006) reported that children who had received cochlear implants in the United Kingdom were more likely to have fewer disabilities than those with profound hearing loss who did not receive implants. All of these factors affect the "starting point" for access to hearing for these children. Therefore, many children begin intervention already experiencing an important delay in hearing in addition to their other non-hearing-related difficulties.

The magnitude of the decision related to cochlear implant surgery may account for an increasing number of studies related to children with additional developmental disabilities who receive cochlear implants. In a systematic review, Schramm, Fitzpatrick, Olds, and Sampson (2007) reported on 19 observational studies that included comparison groups and that specifically addressed outcomes in children with cochlear implants and other disabilities. An additional 38 observational, case series, or case studies without comparison groups were excluded from the review. Children who had motor or sensory disabilities without neurological disabilities generally performed at comparable levels to typically developing peers. Based on seven studies that examined outcomes in a total of

103 children grouped under the category of neurological disabilities in the review (e.g., children described as having cognitive delay, autism, communication disorders, and global developmental delay), the authors concluded that children experienced some gains in speech perception, but at a slower rate than children without disabilities. Four other studies that included children with neurological impairments (e.g., global developmental delay), as well as children with other disabilities (e.g., motor disabilities, learning disabilities), led to a similar conclusion that, over all, these children showed less gain in auditory skills on speech perception testing than their peers with typical development. Since the review, other studies have consistently shown that auditory skills development progresses at a slower rate in children with developmental delays and cochlear implants (Meinzen-Derr, Wiley, Grether, & Choo, 2010; Meinzen-Derr et al, 2011; Wiley, Meinzen-Derr, & Choo, 2008).

▪ Adjusting Intervention

Audiologic rehabilitation for children with additional disabilities has the overall goal of supporting families in their decision to use hearing technology and of developing spoken language through listening when possible. As seen in previous chapters, this process starts by providing the child with audiologic rehabilitation, which includes the best technology and auditory-focused, family-centered intervention. The primary difference in the approach is that *expectations and service delivery need to be adjusted.* For example, developing spoken language with a cochlear implant may not be realistic for a child with severe cognitive delay, however, spoken language may be within reach for a child with mild cognitive delay. As noted above, studies of children with mild cognitive/developmental delays who received cochlear implants have shown that they make gains in auditory and communication skills, but their rate of progress is slower than that of children without cognitive delays (Edwards et al, 2006; Holt & Kirk, 2005).

An important part of the clinician/teacher's role is to help families understand their children's potential and set appropriate expectations for their children. Research with parents suggests that they want to provide their children with every opportunity to hear even when spoken language is not a realistic expectation (Olds, Fitzpatrick, Steacie, McLean, & Schramm, 2007), as indicated by two parents when discussing decision making:

My child has other handicaps but we wanted to give him the maximum possible.

I'd always be wondering, if we didn't get it, you'd have that wonder in the back of your mind—if we had gotten it, where would he have gotten to?

It is important to note that for some children, the presence of additional disabilities will be identified prior to audiologic assessment, while others will be referred to diagnostic audiology through screening programs and other routes without suspicion of other issues that might interfere with communication. Examples of the latter include children without syndromic features, such as those with autism spectrum disorder (ASD) and other developmental involvement. A Canadian report showed that ASD is frequently not reliably identified until an average age of 2 to 3 years (Ouelette-Kuntz et al, 2009). Furthermore, some researchers have reported that children with hearing loss and ASD are likely to be identified later than other children (Donaldson, Heavner, & Zwolan, 2004; Steinberg, 2008). The diagnosis of ASD in the presence of hearing loss may be complicated due to characteristics of ASD and hearing loss that may look similar, such as impairment in social communication and language delays.

Assessment

As described previously, the assessment process takes place on an ongoing basis. Many children may not be able to complete typical speech-language assessments because of motor, speech, language, or cognitive difficulties. Audiologic assessment is often limited to primarily objective test methods. For children with additional disabilities, clinicians/teachers may rely more on observations through intervention and parent input than on standardized (formal) assessment tools. A tool, such as the Focus on the Outcomes of Communication Under Six (FOCUS), may be useful in documenting communication development in this population of children. The FOCUS is a tool to be completed by clinicians that has recently been developed to capture communication outcomes across a spectrum of disabilities (Thomas-Stonell, Oddson, Robertson, & Rosenbaum, 2010). Assessment tools specific to hearing that employ parent questionnaires to document functional hearing outcomes have been proposed to attempt to document the benefits of access to hearing for young children, and may also be very useful in working with children who have other disabilities (Bagatto et al, 2011; Bagatto, Moodie, Seewald, Bartlett, & Scollie, 2011). For children with cochlear implants, there has been an interest in examining caregivers' perceptions of benefits that may be difficult to quantify through typical quantitative speech recognition or language testing (Olds et al, 2007; Wiley, Jahnke, Meinzen-Derr, & Choo, 2005; Wiley et al, 2008). These studies document quality-of-life–type benefits that are not hearing specific, but that may be related to the fact that a child is more connected to the environment through some access to hearing.

An interdisciplinary team is typically involved in the assessment and treatment of children with complex medical and developmental disabilities. The assessments of other team members provide important information when planning audiologic rehabilitation goals and guiding parents about expectations. Working with specialists, such as a developmental pediatrician, neurologist, occupational therapist, psychologist, and other specialists as required, the clinician/teacher, with the parent, defines the child's treatment goals in alignment with the parent's values and hopes. In some cases, depending on the age of identification and the severity of the child's difficulties, the clinician/teacher may be the first person to recognize the presence of an additional disability and may actually trigger the referral to other specialists, for example, in children with dysphasia, oral-motor difficulties, or mild global developmental delay.

Working with the team, the clinican/teacher can better define the child's treatment goals. Just as therapy is individualized for all children depending on their stage of development and progress in various language domains, this notion is even more critical for children with additional needs. When spoken language is not the primary goal, the objective of the assessment is different and the tools selected are adapted accordingly. One way of proceeding is to develop common treatment goals based on the child's global (broader) needs. Teams can work together, even offering joint therapy sessions to integrate goals for the child within the respective areas of development. For example, an occupational therapist and rehabilitation specialist may offer a joint session to work on feeding and listening awareness at the same time. Early intervention workers are often included in rehabilitation sessions to assist with carry-over of the therapy goals in their stimulation activities with children and parents. The underlying issue is that these children can be expected to develop at a different rhythm, and typically take longer to reach treatment goals.

Intervention

There has been little specific research on optimal interventions for children with hearing loss and additional disabilities. Drawing from case studies, commentaries, and clinical discussions, some of the adjustments required in serving children with additional disabilities are summarized below:

- The involvement of other interventionists, such as early interventions (e.g., infant development workers, communication disorders assistants), may change how intervention is delivered. In addition to guiding parents, training is provided to the professionals who are closely involved in the child's care. Such a situation occurs, for example, when a child in a preschool setting is accompanied by a developmental worker because of physical disabilities and cognitive delay.

- Early interventionists, such as child development workers, frequently have an important role in providing auditory stimulation, ensuring that hearing technology is functioning, and presenting oral language as part of the overall communication goals in a way that is accessible for the child. In many cases, not unlike parents, these individuals participate in intervention sessions to learn specific auditory techniques.

- Children with cognitive delays can be expected to take more time to acquire language and concepts, and they may require more concrete experiences to grasp new

information. For example, in learning new vocabulary, children with typical development may glean more information from books and pictures, whereas children with delays may need activities that permit them to manipulate actual objects.

Case Examples

Reflecting on our clinical work, particularly related to cochlear implantation in children with additional disabilities, several examples of children *commonly* encountered in clinical practice are presented below to illustrate how decision making and intervention were adjusted for children with additional disabilities. Throughout these examples, we highlight parents' decisions and intervention modifications aimed

at helping children to develop auditory skills through hearing technology. The case examples have been contributed by clinicians/teachers who work with children with hearing loss and additional disabilities across a spectrum of disorders and highlight a range of children, some of whom demonstrated the potential to develop auditory skills and spoken language, and others who did not.

Children with Disabilities and Mild or No Cognitive Delay that Affect Spoken Language Development

Child with Down Syndrome and Developmental Delay

(Case example contributed by Pamela Steacie, Children's Hospital of Eastern Ontario, Ottawa.)

Karine was born with Down syndrome, and at 2 years of age was diagnosed with a mild cognitive disability, as well as an attention disorder a few years later. She passed newborn hearing screening, but was referred at age 2 due to speech and language concerns. Audiologic testing was difficult and involved ABR testing, with results consistent with a moderately severe loss. Karine attended weekly auditory-verbal therapy sessions, but progress was slow. By age 4, hearing levels had progressed to a profound sensorineural hearing loss in the left ear and a severe loss in the right ear. She received a cochlear implant in the left ear at 4½ years of age, and with further deterioration of thresholds to a profound loss in the right ear, a

second implant at 5½ years. Although auditory and spoken language skills showed a faster rate of progress after cochlear implantation, overall progress was slower than that expected for children with typical development. At age 5, Karine obtained a standard score of 65 on the Peabody Picture Vocabulary Test (receptive vocabulary), placing her well behind the average standard score of 100 for children with normal hearing. Due to Karine's oral language skills at school entry, a decision was made for Karine to spend half-time in a special class where she received intensive support for spoken language, and half-time in a regular kindergarten class. Her oral language skills continued to improve, and within 2 years she was able to attend a regular classroom with full-time support from an educational assistant.

Child with a Syndrome and Global Developmental Delay

(Case example contributed by Rosemary Somerville, Children's Hospital of Eastern Ontario, Ottawa.)

Brittany was born with a syndrome accompanied by craniofacial anomalies, and was diagnosed shortly after birth with global developmental delay. At 10 months of age, ABR testing was consistent with a bilateral mild to moder-

ate conductive hearing loss. She was fitted with a bone conduction hearing aid. The craniofacial anomalies severely affected oral motor skills, and she was introduced to sign language and her parents were encouraged to continue developing her auditory skills. Following reconstructive craniofacial surgery a few months before her fourth birthday, audiologic tests showed primarily a conductive hearing loss, and she began using conventional postauricular hearing aids and intervention with a focus on oral language devel-opment was resumed. Despite the late start in oral language development, oral language skills at almost 5 years of age were, with the exception of speech, at age-appropriate levels.

Child with CHARGE Syndrome who Developed Age-Appropriate Auditory and Language Skills

(Case example contributed by Deirdre Neuss, Children's Hospital of Eastern Ontario, Ottawa.)
Keenan was born with CHARGE syndrome, and was diagnosed at 3 months of age with a moderate to severe hearing loss in the right ear and a severe loss in the left ear. He was fitted with binaural hearing aids at 4 months of age and attended weekly therapy sessions. There was no evidence of cognitive delay. Keenan adapted well to his hearing aids and followed a developmental trajectory in auditory and spoken language development that was consis-tent with children without disabilities. Speech production was, however, more problematic compared with other children with similar degree of hearing loss, and his speech was characterized as hypernasal; therefore, a spe-cific emphasis was placed on improving speech intelligibility. An assessment of Keenan's lan-guage at 5 years of age revealed age-appropri-ate scores on the Peabody Picture Vocabulary Test (receptive vocabulary) and the Clinical Evaluation of Language Fundamentals (various language subtests).

Children with Disabilities and Severe Cognitive Delay that Impact Spoken Language Development

Alternative modes of communication, including sign language or augmentative communication, may be the primary mode of communication for children with additional disabilities for whom spoken language is not achievable. Furthermore, for some children, hearing loss may be secondary to other disorders. A recent examination of long-term clinical results for 13 children with severe cognitive delay who had been recipients of cochlear implants for 10 years or more showed that 5 of 13 had discon-tinued use of their implant a few years post-implant. The remaining 8 children reportedly used their implants, but did not achieve open-set speech recognition. However, they showed some auditory improvement on the Infant Toddler Meaningful Auditory Integration Scale (IT-MAIS). Interviews with families of children with severe delays indicate that many parents value the additional auditory information that the child receives (Olds et al, 2007).

The following examples illustrate auditory-based intervention for children whose devel-opmental profile suggests that limited or no spoken language skills can be expected to emerge.

Child with CHARGE Syndrome, Global Developmental Delay, and Limited Progress in Auditory Development

(Case example contributed by Kelly Rabjohn, Children's Hospital of Eastern Ontario, Ottawa.)
Janine was born with CHARGE syndrome, spent the first 6 months of her life in hospital, and continued to be admitted to hospital sev-eral times during the first year of her life. At that time, she was fed through a gastrostomy tube and had a tracheotomy, but complications prevented the use of the speaking valve. At 3 months of age, a bilateral sensorineural severe to profound hearing loss was diagnosed, and she was fitted with binaural hearing aids at 6 months. She attended weekly auditory-verbal therapy sessions. Although she was somewhat delayed in gross motor skills, preverbal com-munication was developing well, for example, she was noted to wave bye-bye and blow kisses at 12 months. Due to limited auditory progress with hearing aids, sign language was introduced around 12 months, and she underwent cochlear implant surgery at 17 months. The delay to cochlear implantation was due to health con-cerns and some indecision on the part of her parents. A "sandwich" approach to intervention was used, which involved saying the word or phrase, signing it, and then presenting it orally,

again. By 4 months postimplant, Janine was turning to sounds and had a small corpus of ~ 30 signs. By 1 year postimplant, she could select one object (e.g., ball) from a set of three familiar objects through audition alone. Her listening ability seemed to vary from day to day. By 6 years of age, she could understand several "learning to listen" sound-word associations (e.g., meow for cat) and could sign short phrases. Although detection levels with the cochlear implant were in the 30–35 dB range, Janine's auditory development did not progress beyond a basic level, and she continued to communicate through sign language using short phrases.

Child with Autism Spectrum Disorder

(Case example contributed by Pamela Steacie, Children's Hospital of Eastern Ontario, Ottawa.)

After being referred through newborn hearing screening, Nathalie was identified with a severe loss in the right ear and a profound loss in the left ear at 10 weeks of age. Within 2 weeks, she was fitted with binaural hearing aids and started attending weekly auditory-verbal therapy. Although her parents worked very hard to provide enriched, repetitive language stimulation, her progress with hearing aids was very slow. By 1 year of age, she understood just four sound-word associations, but used no spontaneous language. There were limited vocalizations, but no real babbling of repeated syllables. By 18 months of age, she understood ~ 15 words and imitated 6 words, but there was no spontaneous use of words. She had no consonants in her repertoire. She detected speech sounds across the speech spectrum (all six Ling sounds) and could identify single items in a small set.

Nathalie rarely made eye contact, was not pointing, did not engage in symbolic play, and did not show much interest in the people around her. She was observed to perseverate on some actions, such as rotating certain toys repeatedly for minutes at a time. At this point she was referred for developmental testing. A few signs were introduced experimentally to see if she would be more responsive to sign than word, but consistent with her lack of interest in interacting with people, she showed no interest.

Nathalie underwent cochlear implant surgery at 19 months of age. Her auditory skills improved and she began to produce a few word approximations, though very infrequently, and she showed some progress in learning new words, although at a very slow rate. Within 6 months postimplant, she could hum songs. She began a daycare program with support from an integration advisor who worked closely with the auditory-verbal therapist. Due to limited progress in both spoken and sign language, a picture exchange system was introduced experimentally; she quickly learned to communicate preference for a toy using this communication mode. At age 2½, she was diagnosed with "probable high-functioning autism." She continued to receive services from an auditory-verbal therapist and from a speech-language pathologist specializing in autism. An example of a therapy session plan showing the integration of listening, spoken language, and autism intervention goals is presented in **Table 7.2.**

Assessments of Nathalie's language were challenging due to lack of focus and her inability to point or imitate on demand. Although there was progress, her language functioning at age 3½, as demonstrated on the PLS-4, was at the 1 year 9 month level for auditory comprehension, and at the 1 year 2 month level for expressive language. Speech abilities were very limited; other abilities, such as counting and number and letter recognition, were far beyond her language or social skills.

At age 4½, Nathalie began an intensive behavioral intervention (IBI) program 4 days per week, and attended junior kindergarten 1 day per week. She received specialized services in listening and spoken language through the school program. At age 5, Nathalie received a second cochlear implant, and although the initial adjustment was difficult, she achieved full-time use within a few weeks. She demonstrated good auditory benefit with a second implant. Having access to sound appears to have mitigated the effects of Nathalie's autism, allowing her to develop verbal comprehension and some speech sounds. Overall, hearing has helped her to engage more with the world around her.

Table 7.2 Example of therapy plan for child with ASD and her mother showing integration of auditory goals and autism intervention goals (age 34 months, after 4 months of autism intervention)

Therapy plan for child with autism
To improve compliance with nonpreferred activities, each activity was paired with a large foam puzzle number that was removed from its foam square at the beginning of the activity and replaced in the foam square at the end of the activity. After five activities, Nathalie was permitted to choose a favorite toy and play with it while her mother and the clinican/teacher chatted.
Audition: *AVT goal:* Select picture cards representing six Ling sounds. (She did, and she spontaneously imitated them all—/m/, /u/, /a/, and /i/ were produced correctly; she produced a raspberry for /ç/ and inhaled loudly for /s/.)   *AVT goal:* Select single items from a group of rhyming words. (She did.)
Speech: *Combined autism/AVT goals:* Approximate "my turn" by producing /m/ or /ma/ (speech goal and also expressive language goal) to have a turn playing with a high-interest toy. (She had previously mastered the autism goal of pointing to herself to communicate that she wanted it to be her turn.)
Language: *Combined goals:* Autism goal: Symbolic play with a cat (preferred animal) performing a variety of pretend actions (sleeping, having a drink, going up the stairs, and going in the car). AVT goal: Follow simple instruction.   *Combined goals:* Autism goal: Model and take pictures of a daily activity (preparing and eating a strawberry) involving a sequence/two-to-three-word phrases. (She had great difficulty following a sequence of actions, e.g., coming into the therapy room, taking off her coat, hanging it up, and sitting on her chair.) AVT goal: Comprehension of three-word phrases, and some new vocabulary.   *Activity:* We all washed our hands (because our hands were dirty), washed a strawberry (because it was dirty), cut the top off the strawberry (Don't eat the stem! Don't eat the leaves!), and ate the strawberry (it was juicy and sweet). Because our hands were juicy, we had to wash them again.

Contributed by Pamela Steacie, Children's Hospital of Eastern Ontario, Ottawa.

Other Children with Complex Needs

Children may present with additional disorders that affect specific areas of development but they have intact cognitive function. Although spoken language development may be quite possible, therapy targets may differ or therapy strategies may be adapted. Examples include children with oral motor difficulties, such as those with cleft palate, and children with cerebral palsy but no cognitive delay. In these cases, practitioners, for example who are not speech-language pathologists, will typically ensure that this expertise is added to the audiologic rehabilitation team, as speech skills will be affected by non–hearing-related speech errors that may require specific intervention strategies. Children with severe visual impairment will require adaptations through the use of different materials. Other situations may present themselves with children who are medically fragile, which delays parent decision making, or who, for medical reasons, had a delay in treatments such as cochlear implant surgery.

Despite the improvements in assessment and knowledge, clinical experience shows that a small number of children without a clear diagnosis of additional disabilities do not develop hearing and language like their peers with typical development. Practitioners may describe children in this category using adjectives such as "slow," "different," or "atypical" when compared to their peers with typical development. These children present particularly challenging issues for both professionals and parents, and decision making about optimal interventions is complex and may be delayed. As exemplified below, some children eventually receive a specific diagnosis, but it can take considerable time.

Child with Specific Language Impairment

Andrea is a 17-year-old girl who was born with serious health and motor problems. She received medical care in the hospital as an infant, where she was diagnosed with a severe sensorineural hearing loss. She was fitted with hearing aids at the age of 8 months, and her parents started receiving weekly services in listening and spoken language intervention at home. Andrea showed no reaction to sound, and very little reaction to people or to objects around her until 12 to 15 months. Around that time, there was a drop in her hearing, and further testing revealed a severe to profound hearing loss. She received a cochlear implant at 2 years of age and continued with listening and spoken language intervention services three times weekly. Andrea was very slow in showing reactions with the implant. Her initial reactions were to music, and she appeared to have little interest in language. Progress in oral communication was very slow despite good detection thresholds with the cochlear implant. During the same period, she received services in physiotherapy and occupational therapy, and made substantial progress in fine and gross motor skills. Her parents provided a stimulating environment in listening, spoken language, and overall life experiences.

She started attending regular school at 5 years, and at school entry she presented with a severe language delay, and at her parents' request, she repeated kindergarten. She received specialized spoken language services four times a week. Gradually, Andrea showed some progress in spoken language, with better progress noted in listening skills. At 10 years old, her speech was still almost unintelligible, she was experiencing serious learning problems, and was delayed in reading and writing, but her listening skills and language comprehension had continued to improve. She was evaluated at an institute for children with disabilities to determine her learning potential and was diagnosed with severe specific language impairment. Services from the clinician/teacher were increased to 8 hours a week, and Andrea made regular progress in oral communication. Over the years, her improvement in every field of learning has been impressive. At age 17, she now has intelligible speech, and although she continues to present serious language and learning delays, she is able to express herself using increasingly complex sentences. She has an adapted educational program in school while integrated with her peers with normal hearing all day except for the individualized sessions with the clinician/teacher. She is fully integrated in her community, playing volleyball with peers with normal hearing, learning to play the piano, and attending various youth activities. It is expected that she will attend the local community college, where a special program will be implemented to assist her in transitioning to life as an independent adult.

▪ Summary

Over all, children with disabilities in addition to their hearing loss will require services from interdisciplinary teams to address their multiple challenges. A strong team working together can help align parents' expectations and hopes for their children with realistic developmental outcomes in multiple areas. In this chapter, we emphasize the enormous range of performance in communication development in children with hearing loss who have additional disabilities. The wide spectrum of disabilities, even within one syndrome or type of disability, and the functional consequences for early development of audition and language mean that outcomes and the rehabilitation process will vary considerably from one child to another. Furthermore, for some children, the presence of other disabilities will be identified in synchrony with the diagnosis of their hearing loss, while for others, complex needs will be identified after hearing loss identification and intervention have been initiated. These situations can influence parent guidance and the time at which adjustments to intervention and new decisions are undertaken. The main message of this chapter is that audio- logic rehabilitation, taking into account parents' preferences, will involve necessary and constant adjustment of intervention objectives and tech- niques for these children so that they can attain optimal benefit from hearing technology.

Acknowledgments

We are grateful to Klio Kazinska and Nathalie Wakil for collecting and preparing data pre- sented in this chapter. We are also grateful to the listening and spoken language specialists, Erin McSweeney, Deirdre Neuss, Kelly Rabjohn, Rosemary Somerville, and Pamela Steacie, from the Audiology Program at the Children Hospital of Eastern Ontario for their many con- tributions to this chapter.

References

Bagatto, M. P., Moodie, S. T., Malandrino, A. C., Richert, F. M., Clench, D. A., & Scollie, S. D. (2011). The Uni- versity of Western Ontario Pediatric Audiological Monitoring Protocol (UWO PedAMP). *Trends in Amplification, 15*(1), 57–76.

Bagatto, M. P., Moodie, S. T., Seewald, R. C., Bartlett, D. J., & Scollie, S. D. (2011). A critical review of audiological outcome measures for infants and children. *Trends in Amplification, 15*(1), 23–33.

Boyle, C. A., Boulet, S., Schieve, L. A., Cohen, R. A., Blumberg, S. J., Yeargin-Allsopp, M., . . . Kogan, M. D. (2011). Trends in the prevalence of devel- opmental disabilities in US children, 1997–2008. *Pediatrics, 127*(6), 1034–1042.

Donaldson, A. I., Heavner, K. S., & Zwolan, T. A. (2004). Measuring progress in children with autism spectrum disorder who have cochlear implants. *Archives of Otolaryngology—Head & Neck Surgery, 130*(5), 666–671.

Durieux-Smith, A., Fitzpatrick, E., & Whittingham, J. (2008). Universal newborn hearing screening: A question of evidence. *International Journal of Audiology, 47*(1), 1–10.

Edwards, L. C., Frost, R., & Witham, F. (2006). Develop- mental delay and outcomes in pediatric cochlear implantation: Implications for candidacy. *Inter- national Journal of Pediatric Otorhinolaryngology, 70*(9), 1593–1600.

Fitzpatrick, E., & Brewster, L. (2008). Pediatric cochlear implantation in Canada: Results of a sur- vey. *Canadian Journal of Speech-Language Pathol- ogy and Audiology, 32*(1), 29–35.

Fitzpatrick, E. M., Johnson, E., & Durieux-Smith, A. (2011). Exploring factors that affect the age of cochlear implantation in children. *International Journal of Pediatric Otorhinolaryngology, 75*(9), 1082–1087.

Gallaudet Research Institute. (2009). *Regional and national summary report of data from the 2007– 2008 Annual Survey of Deaf and Hard of Hearing* *Children and Youth*. Washington, DC: Gallaudet University.

Guardino, C. A. (2008). Identification and place- ment for deaf students with multiple disabilities: Choosing the path less followed. *American Annals of the Deaf, 153*(1), 55–64.

Holt, R. F., & Kirk, K. I. (2005). Speech and language development in cognitively delayed children with cochlear implants. *Ear and Hearing, 26*(2), 132–148.

Luterman, D. (2006). The emotional impact of hear- ing loss. In D. Luterman (Ed.), *Children with hear- ing loss: A family guide* (pp. 9–35). Sedona, AZ: Auricle Ink Publishers.

Madell, J. R., & Flexer, C. (Eds.). (2008). *Pediatric audi- ology: Diagnosis, technology and management*. New York: Thieme Medical Publishers.

McCracken, W., & Turner, O. (2012). Deaf children with complex needs: Parental experience of access to cochlear implants and ongoing support. *Deafness & Education International, 14*(1), 22–35.

Meinzen-Derr, J., Wiley, S., Grether, S., & Choo, D. I. (2010). Language performance in children with cochlear implants and additional disabilities. *Laryngoscope, 120*(2), 405–413.

Meinzen-Derr, J., Wiley, S., Grether, S., & Choo, D. I. (2011). Children with cochlear implants and developmental disabilities: A language skills study with developmentally matched hearing peers. *Research in Developmental Disabilities, 32*(2), 757–767.

Northern, J. L., & Downs, M. P. (2002). *Hearing in chil- dren* (5th ed.). Baltimore, MD: Williams & Wilkins.

Olds, J., Fitzpatrick, E. M., Steacie, J., McLean, J., & Schramm, D. (2007). *Parental perspectives of out- come after cochlear implantation in children with complex disabilities*. Paper presented at the 11th International Conference on Cochlear Implants in Children, Charlotte, NC.

Ouelette-Kuntz, H. M. J., Coo, H., Lam, M., Yu, C. T., Bretenbach, M. M., Hennessey, P. E., . . . Crews, L. R. (2009). Age at diagnosis of autism spectrum disorders in four regions of Canada. *Canadian Journal of Public Health, 100*(4), 268–273.

Rhoades, E. A., Price, F., & Perigoe, C. B. (2004). The changing American family and ethnically diverse children with multiple needs [Monograph]. *The Volta Review, 104*(4), 285–305.

Picard, M. (2004). Children with permanent hearing loss and associated disabilities: Revisiting current epidemiological data and causes of deafness. *The Volta Review, 104*(4), 221–236.

Schramm, D., Fitzpatrick, E., Olds, J., & Sampson, M. (2007). *Systematic review of cochlear implants in children with multiple disabilities.* Paper presented at the 11th International Conference on Cochlear Implants in Children, Charlotte, NC.

Spivak, L., Sokol, H., Auerbach, C., & Gershkovich, S. (2009). Newborn hearing screening follow-up: Factors affecting hearing aid fitting by 6 months of age. *American Journal of Audiology, 18*(1), 24–33.

Stacey, P. C., Fortnum, H. M., Barton, G. R., & Summerfield, A. Q. (2006). Hearing-impaired children in the United Kingdom, I: Auditory performance, communication skills, educational achievements, quality of life, and cochlear implantation. *Ear and Hearing, 27*(2), 161–186.

Steinberg, A. G. (2008). Understanding the need for language. *Odyssey: New Directions in Deaf Education, 9*(1), 6–9.

Thomas-Stonell, N. L., Oddson, B., Robertson, B., & Rosenbaum, P. L. (2010). Development of the FOCUS (Focus on the Outcomes of Communication Under Six), a communication outcome measure for preschool children. *Developmental Medicine and Child Neurology, 52*(1), 47–53.

Wiley, S., Jahnke, M., Meinzen-Derr, J., & Choo, D. (2005). Perceived qualitative benefits of cochlear implants in children with multi-handicaps. *International Journal of Pediatric Otorhinolaryngology, 69*(6), 791–798.

Wiley, S., Meinzen-Derr, J., & Choo, D. (2008). Auditory skills development among children with developmental delays and cochlear implants. *The Annals of Otology, Rhinology, and Laryngology, 117*(10), 711–718.

8 Auditory Learning Environments: Ensuring Acoustic Accessibility

Carol Flexer and Jane R. Madell

If the family's desired outcomes for their child include spoken language, literacy, social competencies, and life development consistent with hearing peers, then, beginning in infancy, every encounter, location, and environment must be viewed from an acoustic accessibility perspective. That is, in order for a child's auditory brain centers to grow and develop, the child's brain must be stimulated with sufficient quality and quantity of auditory events.

Every sound has to pass through an environment before it reaches the child's technology, and then on to the child's brain. Therefore, acoustic access must be available to the child in all life settings—home, school and playground, car, and after-school activities. Said another way, the first step in attainable and sustainable listening and spoken language outcomes is acoustic accessibility. The purpose of this chapter is to discuss the concept of acoustic accessibility, including the use and management of environments and remote microphones for infants and children in all of their learning domains.

▪ Why It Is Important to Confirm that a Child Has Acoustic Accessibility

Neurological Implications: Children Have Organic Listening Limitations

To begin with, we "hear" with the brain. The ears are just a way in. The problem with hearing loss and with poor auditory environments is that intact sound is barred from reaching the brain. The purpose of having favorable listening environments and amplification technologies, including FM systems (remote microphone systems), is to enhance acoustic saliency by channeling intelligible words efficiently and effectively to the brain (Cole & Flexer, 2011).

Brain development research shows that sensory stimulation of the auditory centers of the brain is critically important, and indeed, influences the actual organization of auditory brain pathways (Berlin & Weyand, 2003; Boothroyd, 1997; Chermak, Bellis, & Musiek, 2007; Chapter 1 of this book). The fact is, the brain can only organize itself based on the stimuli it receives. When complete acoustic events are received, the brain organizes itself accordingly through the development of neural pathways. Conversely, when hearing loss filters speech sounds and prevents these same sounds from reaching auditory centers within the brain, the brain organizes itself differently. "When we want to remember (or learn) something we have heard, we must hear it clearly because memory can be only as clear as its original signal . . . muddy in, muddy out" (Doidge, 2007,

p. 68). Signal enhancement, such as that provided by personal or sound field technology, is really about brain stimulation with subsequent development of auditory neural pathways.

It is important to recognize that children are not small adults; they are not able to listen like adults listen. Indeed, children bring different listening capabilities to a communicative and learning situation than do adults in two main ways. First, human auditory brain structure is not fully mature until about age 15 years; thus a child does not bring a complete neurological system to a listening situation (Bhatnagar, 2002; Boothroyd, 1997). Second, children do not have the years of language and life experience that enable adults to fill in the gaps of missed or inferred information (such filling in of gaps is called auditory/cognitive closure). Leibold and Neff (2011) found that children require years of listening experience to learn to focus on the most informative aspects of complex speech sounds in the presence of interfering noise. Therefore, because children require more complete, detailed auditory information than adults, all children need a quieter room and a louder signal (Anderson, 2001). The goal is to *develop* the brains of children, unlike adults where sound enters a *developed* brain.

▪ Barriers to Acoustic Accessibility in Home and School Environments

The major factors that affect auditory learning in the classroom include the hearing and attention capabilities of the child and the actual classroom environment. Additional variables include the speech of the teacher and pupils and their relative positions in the room. Because the speech of talkers is filtered through the physical environment of a room and the auditory/attentional system of the listener, these variables are of primary consideration.

Distance

As speech sounds travel away from the talker, they lose 6 dB of amplitude for every doubling of distance. A telling example of the interplay between classroom acoustics, distance from the sound source, and speech was reported by Leavitt and Flexer in 1991. Using the Rapid Speech Transmission Index (RASTI), they demonstrated that 83% of the speech energy delivered in the front of a typical classroom-sized environment was available to a listener in the front row. However, in the back row of the same classroom, only about 50% of the speech energy was available. RASTI is a measure of speech energy as it traverses a room, and is an index of the amount of energy available to be perceived when influenced by signal-to-noise ratio (SNR) and reverberation time (RT), not the amount actually perceived. Even less of the signal would be available if the listener has a hearing loss, or reduced auditory/language processing. These factors would hinder the student's actual perception of the available speech energy. That is, add the impact of the classroom acoustical environment to the distortion imposed by a damaged auditory or linguistic system and it becomes apparent why simply using a hearing aid is not likely to result in satisfactory communication in the classroom.

Signal-to-Noise Ratio (SNR)

Background noise in a room reduces speech recognition by covering up or masking important acoustic/linguistic cues in the message. This masking is especially true for the consonants that carry most of the intelligibility of speech necessary for accurate perception. Background noise in a room tends to mask the weaker consonant phonemes significantly more than the more intense vowel phonemes.

SNR is the relationship between a primary signal, such as the teacher's speech, and background noise. Noise is anything and everything that conflicts with the auditory signal of choice and may include other talkers, heating or cooling systems, classroom or hall noise, playground sounds, computer noise, and wind, among others (Nelson & Blaeser, 2010). The quieter the room and the more favorable the SNR, the clearer the auditory signal will be for the brain. The further the listener is from the desired sound source and the noisier the environment, the poorer the SNR and the more garbled the signal will be for the brain. The dominant source of noise in a room is the children in the room and the number of acoustic events that are co-occurring.

Adults with normal hearing and intact listening skills require a consistent SNR of approximately +6 dB for the reception of intelligible speech (Bess & Humes, 2003). Children need a much more favorable SNR because their neurological immaturity and lack of life and language experiences reduce their ability to perform auditory/cognitive closure. Moreover, all children, and especially children with hearing loss, require the signal to be 10 times louder than competing sounds. Interestingly, children with sensorineural hearing loss have a spatial processing disorder, a particular type of auditory processing disorder that makes them less able to attend to target sounds coming from one direction by suppressing sounds coming from other directions (Ching, van Wanrooy, Dillon, & Carter, 2011). Therefore, children with sensorineural hearing loss require an SNR higher than required by their normal-hearing peers in the classroom if they are to equally understand speech when there is background noise. Due to noise, reverberation, and variations in teacher position, the SNR in a typical classroom is unstable and averages out to only about +4 dB and may be as low as 0 dB; often less than ideal even for adults with normal hearing and normal auditory processing capabilities (Smaldino, 2011).

A key concept regarding the value of enhancing the SNR is acoustic saliency. Tallal (2004) found that children with language impairment make more errors on acoustically nonsalient as compared with acoustically salient grammatical morphemes. To explain, in a sentence context, acoustically nonsalient morphemes are shorter in duration and softer than louder phonemes in adjacent portions of the utterance. Thus, the environmental management of enhancing the SNR of spoken instruction has the added benefit of increasing acoustic saliency of more difficult to hear speech sounds.

Distance Hearing/Incidental Learning

Incidental learning through "overhearing" refers to times when the child listens to speech that is not directly addressed to him or her and learns from it. Akhtar, Jipson, and Callanan (2001) found that typically developing children as young as 2 years of age can acquire new words from overheard speech, showing the active role played by children in acquiring language. Further, Knightly, Jun, Oh, and Au (2003) found that childhood overhearing helped improve speech perception and phonologic production of all languages heard. Unfortunately, children with hearing losses, even minimal ones, have reduced overhearing potential because they cannot receive intelligible speech well over distances. This reduction in distance hearing, also called *earshot*, can pose substantial problems for classroom and life performance because distance hearing is essential for the passive/casual/incidental acquisition and use of spoken communication. Therefore, in school and at home, a child's distance hearing needs to be extended as much as possible through the use of technology to enable him or her to overhear language (Ling, 2002).

Effects of Reverberation Time

Reverberation time (RT) refers to the amount of time it takes for a steady state sound to decrease 60 dB from its peak amplitude. In a reverberant room, speech is reflected from various hard room surfaces so that some of the speech elements are delayed in reaching the ear of the listener. The reflected speech overlaps with the direct speech signal (the signal not reflected before reaching the listener's ear) and covers up or masks certain acoustic speech components. Because vowels are more intense than consonants, a long RT tends to produce a prolongation of the spectral energy of vowels, which then covers up less intense consonant components. A reduction of consonant information can have a significant effect on speech recognition because the vast majority of the acoustic information that is important for speech recognition is provided by consonants (Smaldino, 2011). Speech recognition, therefore, tends to decrease with increases in reverberation time.

▪ Managing the Acoustic Environment

There are some noise sources that can be controlled and others that cannot. It is essential that we control the things we can control to provide children with an appropriate listening and learning environment. For infants, we are primarily concerned about the home environment. For toddlers, we are concerned about the home, the playground, and possibly daycare. As children get older, nursery school, primary school, and after-school activities become concerns.

A discussion of environmental modifications must be preceded by a discussion of "necessary versus sufficient" benefit. There is general agreement that acoustic accessibility is a necessary prerequisite for academic success. However, acoustic accessibility and enhanced signal saliency in the absence of additional accommodations may not be sufficient for children with hearing loss.

An analogy in the visual realm might involve a child who has difficulty drawing geometric figures. A necessary first step in addressing this problem would be ensuring clear lighting that enhances visual saliency of the drawing field. The lighting alone might be insufficient to correct a child's drawing of geometric designs; additional supports may be necessary. One doesn't remove the lights if they did not solve the entire problem. One keeps the lighting as a necessary first step and then adds additional instruction and accommodations. In a similar vein, one does not remove FM systems if they do not solve the entire problem of access to instructional information for a child with hearing loss. One adds other accommodations, such as pretutoring of instructional information for topic redundancy, to achieve sufficiency.

Managing the Acoustic Environment for Infants

Tiny infants are often in a parent's arms, which puts them at the ideal distance to both hear and see the speaker. However, it is still necessary to control the acoustic environment. As much as possible, extraneous noise sources should be turned off. Radio, TV, or background music should not be on when speaking with infants. If the infant is in the kitchen at meal time or during meal preparation, the dishwasher should not be turned on. Whenever possible, infants should be close to the talker. When that is not possible, an FM system will provide a good acoustic signal to the infant, permitting ongoing auditory stimulation to the brain.

Managing the Acoustic Environment for Toddlers

Once infants start to move on their own, they are frequently out of excellent earshot positioning. Once this happens, families will need to work harder to ensure consistent audition. Some of the same principles apply to toddlers as apply to infants. As much as possible, extraneous noise sources should be turned off. Radio, TV, or background music should not be on when speaking with toddlers. The dishwasher should be off during meal time. Carpeting or other absorbent materials should be in as many places as possible to reduce noise from foot traffic and toys. If carpeting cannot be installed in all rooms, it should at least be in noisy places, such as the children's room or play corner where blocks and other noisy toys are likely to be used. If children attend daycare, it would make a significant difference in the child's listening and learning if the daycare center could use absorbent materials in noisy areas, work to keep the classroom quiet, and have the child with hearing loss seated close to the teacher during critical listening activities. If the day care setting has tables and chairs, chair "socks" should be used to reduce the noise of moving furniture; these are commercially available or can easily be made using old tennis balls, cutting an X on the top, and slipping them under table and chair legs.

Managing the Acoustic Environment for School-Aged Children

Classrooms are very noisy places. Unless the school was built recently, classrooms are likely to have high ceilings, large windows, and hard walls. This poor acoustic environment, combined with a larger group of children is, of course, a recipe for acoustic disaster. It is critical that we do as much as possible to control the noise.

ANSI Standards for Classroom Noise and Reverberation

Because undesirable acoustics (noise and reverberation) can be a barrier to listening and learning in the classroom, a working group composed of a wide variety of stakeholders produced the first American standard, which was published in 2002 (ANSI/ASA S12.60-2002), *Acoustical Performance Criteria, Design Requirements, and Guidelines for Schools.* A second review of the standard resulted in some minor modifications and a separate part devoted to issues unique to portable classrooms.

The first part of the revised standard, *American National Standard Acoustical Performance Criteria, Design Requirements, and Guidelines for Schools, Part 1: Permanent Schools* (ANSI/ASA S12.60-2010) is a refined version of the 2002 standard. The primary performance requirement for furnished but unoccupied classrooms is basically unchanged from the 2002 standard. Specifically, the one-hour average A-weighted background noise level (A-weighting is based on the equal loudness contour for human hearing—attenuating low frequencies) cannot exceed 35 dB (55 dB if C-weighting is used—C-weighting does not attenuate low frequencies), and for average size classrooms, the reverberation time (RT60) cannot exceed 0.6 seconds [35/55 dB(A/C) and 0.7 seconds if the volume is greater than 10,000 but less than or equal to 20,000 cubic feet]. Among other changes are improvements of the requirements for exterior walls and roofs in noisy areas, consideration of activities close to classrooms, clarification of the definition of a "core learning space," addition of the limit of 45 dB(A) for sound in hallways, clarification and simplification of measurement procedures, and addition of the requirement that if a classroom audio distribution system (CADS) is believed appropriate, it should provide even coverage and be adjustable so as not to disturb adjacent classes (Smaldino, 2011).

The second part of the revised standard, *American National Standard Acoustical Performance Criteria, Design Requirements, and Guidelines for Schools, Part 2: Relocatable Classroom Factors* (ANSI/ASA S12.60–2010), phases in performance requirements for portable classrooms. The current standard sets a 41 dB(A) limit for background noise in unoccupied classrooms that would be lowered to 38 dB(A) in 2013, and to 35 dB(A) in 2017. Reverberation time (RT60) in unoccupied relocatable classrooms must not exceed 0.5 seconds in classrooms with volumes of 10,000 cubic feet or less, and 0.6 seconds in classrooms with volumes of 10,000–20,000 cubic feet. Both parts of the standard are available without charge from the Acoustical Society of America store (http://asastore.aip.org).

A third part of the standard is currently under development and will focus on control of noise from informational technology in the classroom. At this writing, compliance with the revised standards remains voluntary. Refer to Smaldino and Flexer (2012) for detailed discussions of measurement and management of classroom acoustics.

Smart Phone, Tablet, and Laptop Apps for the Measurement of Classroom Acoustics

A recent online search of basic sound level meter apps available for Apple and Android platforms identified several that could be useful for the measurement of classroom acoustics. Of this small group, a few appeared to have been designed by audio professionals for use by professionals, or could possibly be considered equivalent to stand-alone, Type II sound level meters (SLMs). The others seem to be designed more for estimation purposes only, lacking features such as A-weighting, spectral analysis, and measures of reverbera-

tion time. While the options may be limited, the well-designed apps can be extremely useful (Smaldino, 2011).

Because parents and professionals who work with children with hearing loss are very focused on acoustic accessibility in all of a child's learning domains, we should have SLM apps on our phones to at least obtain a general idea of the noise levels in a room. In addition, there are more sophisticated applications to obtain precise sound and reverberation measurements.

Classroom Noise Accommodations

Open classrooms (where several classes are in one open space with dividers such as bookcases separating groups) are a terrible acoustic environment for any child and make learning extremely difficult. Children with hearing loss are at a significant additional disadvantage since they require an even better listening environment than children with typical hearing. No child with hearing loss or other

auditory function disorders should be placed in an open classroom. The classroom selected should be located away from particularly noisy areas, such as the gym, lunchroom, or bathrooms. Ideally, acoustic floor materials should be installed in classrooms and in hallways to reduce noise. Ensuring that all areas in a preschool program are covered with acoustic flooring may be more difficult because young children have more free time and have activities that allow them to wander about the room. Absorbent materials should at least be placed in noisy areas, like the block corner. Acoustic tiles should be placed on walls and ceilings to reduce reverberation. Tennis balls or "chair socks" should be placed on the feet of all movable chairs and tables to reduce the noise made as chairs scrape on the floor. Windows and doors should be kept closed to reduce extraneous noise. It is important to monitor the noise from the heating, ventilation, and air conditioning systems, which can generate considerable noise if they are not cleaned regularly. Computers can also be noisy and should be monitored.

Strategic Seating

No matter how good the classroom accommodations, if a child is not seated close to the talker, listening will be difficult. An FM system will permit the child to hear words spoken directly into the transmitter, but other listening will continue to be difficult. Seating should be in the front third of the classroom, off to the side, with the better hearing ear facing the classroom. This placement should permit the student to turn and face the group, monitor the activity occurring in the room, and both identify the talker and see the talker's face. The student should have permission to move about the classroom as needed to hear. For example, if math is taught in the front of the room and reading at the back, the student may need to move to hear. For small group work, the student with hearing loss should be assigned to a table that is at the side of the room, and should be permitted to sit with his or her back to the wall to reduce the amount of noise swirling around.

Teaching Accommodations to Improve Listening

Teachers should be advised to try and keep the classroom quiet, encouraging students not to talk among themselves or chatter during desk work time, and not to call out answers. The teacher should be encouraged to use "clear speech," speak at a normal or slightly slower conversational rate with pauses, and speak at a normal pitch to facilitate listening and auditory processing. The teacher should be asked to face the student with hearing loss when speaking to him and to call him by name to be sure that he knows she is speaking to him. It is important that the teacher confirm that the child understands what is being said. Questions like *"Did you hear that?"* or *"Do you understand?"* are not useful because the child will likely answer in the affirmative whether or not she actually hears. By asking specific informational questions, the teacher is more likely to determine what the child does and does not understand. If the child does not understand, teachers should be encouraged to reword rather than simply repeat the statement. Students should be encouraged to ask for clarification when they do not understand and should be made comfortable when they do so. Assignments should be written on the board or in a handout to be certain that the child receives the correct assignment. If possible, the teacher may consider assigning a buddy to the student with hearing loss. The buddy can help the student with hearing loss get assignments and know what page to turn to. As students grow older and note taking becomes more difficult, it may be helpful for the student with hearing loss to receive a copy of class notes from another student who is a good note taker. In high school or beyond, it may be useful to receive a copy of the teacher's outline in advance. Listening all day long can be very taxing, and children with hearing loss expend more effort focusing in class. Listening breaks should be scheduled throughout the day to allow the child to rest. The daily schedule should be organized so that the child with hearing loss does not have several critical listening subjects all in a row. It would be best if the day could be organized so that activities requiring critical listening are interspersed with those that do not (such as gym, art, or music). These common-sense recommendations can make the difference between a successful and a stressful school experience, and teachers should be coached in their implementation.

No child with hearing loss should be in a classroom without an FM system. Even if the hearing loss is mild, listening in a classroom is difficult. Parents frequently report that children with hearing loss come home exhausted at the end of the day. While the child may appear to be doing relatively well, it requires a great deal of work to listen.

An FM system will significantly reduce the level of effort the child expends just receiving instructional information, leaving the child with more cognitive capacity for thinking about the new concepts offered by the teacher (Anderson, 2011).

▪ Remote Microphone Technologies/Connectivity: Signal-to-Noise Ratio (SNR) Enhancing Technologies

It has long been recognized that a remote microphone improves the SNR for a listener. That is, a microphone worn by a talker that uses radio or light waves to send the talker's voice to the listener, who wears a receiver, makes the desired signal louder by overcoming distance and background noise. Numerous studies show that academics, literacy, attention, and behavior improve when children have better access to the desired signal (Smaldino & Flexer, 2012).

Personal-Wearable FM System

While primary technologies (hearing aids and cochlear implants) allow auditory brain access in quiet, close situations, it is obvious that any noisy situation requires a remote microphone to channel intelligible speech to neural centers. However, many other situations that do not appear to be noisy situations also will benefit from the use of a remote microphone. Children who are in the process of learning language need constant exposure to a good, clear acoustic signal. We know that children need to overhear conversations around them and distance hearing is critical to developing both auditory and language skills. Hart and Risley (1999) have demonstrated that the number of words that a child hears is directly related to their IQ, and IQ is related to language skills.

Frequency modulation (FM) and other types of wireless systems improve signal quality and intelligibility much more than any signal processing scheme located entirely within the hearing aid (Dillon, Ching, & Golding, 2008). A personal-worn FM unit is a wireless personal listening device that includes a remote microphone placed near the desired sound source (usually the speaker's mouth, but it could also be a CD player or TV) and a receiver for the listener, who can be situated anywhere within about 50 feet of the talker. No wires are required to connect the talker and listener, because the unit is really a small FM radio that transmits and receives on a single frequency. Personal FM systems, therefore, offer a direct communication connection between the talker and listener in any communication situation.

Because the talker wears the remote microphone within 6 inches of her mouth, the personal FM unit creates a listening situation that is comparable to a parent or teacher being within 6 inches of the child's ear at all times, thereby allowing a positive and constant SNR (Sexton, 2003). The amount of SNR benefit will vary depending on several factors, such as FM ratio (the relationship of the loudness of the FM signal compared with the loudness of the CI or hearing aid microphone signal), whether or not the hearing aid or CI microphone is activated, how well the personal technology is programmed, how well the FM microphone is physically placed on the talker, and how effectively the talker uses the FM transmitter. SNR improvement using the FM microphone can be as much as 20 dB (HAT, 2008). Personal FM units are essential for a child with any type and degree of hearing loss, from minimal to profound, who is in any classroom or group learning situation (Anderson, Goldstein, Colodzin, & Inglehart, 2005; ASHA, 2000; Flynn, Flynn, & Gregory, 2005). Several models of FM equipment are available. The most common styles currently used include one where the FM receiver is built into the ear-level hearing aid case, and another where a small FM receiver boot is attached directly to the bottom of the ear-level hearing aid or to a cochlear implant speech processor. This small, attachable FM receiver has the advantages of a clear signal and small size. Care needs to be exercised to avoid losing the small parts, especially when used by a young child.

Classroom Audio Distribution Systems (CADS)

Sound field technology, now referred to as CADS, is an effective educational tool that allows control of the acoustic environment in a classroom, thereby facilitating acoustic accessibility of teacher instruction for all children in the room (Crandell, Smaldino, & Flexer 2005). A sound field system looks like a wireless public address system, but it is designed specifically to ensure that the entire speech signal, including the weak high-frequency consonants, reaches every child in the room.

By using this technology, an entire classroom can be amplified through the use of one, two, three, or four wall- or ceiling-mounted loudspeakers. The teacher wears a wireless microphone transmitter, and her voice is sent via radio waves (FM), or light waves (infrared–IR) to an amplifier that is connected to the loudspeakers. There are no wires connecting the teacher with the equipment. The radio or light wave link allows the teacher to move about freely, unrestricted by wires. The loudspeakers are designed and positioned to uniformly improve the SNR throughout the areas where instruction occurs in the room.

A primary value of CADS is that the better SNR can focus the pupils and facilitate attention to relevant information. To that end, the clever use of the sound system's microphone can be a powerful teaching tool. Teacher's need to be in-serviced about how to use the microphone and their voice to create a listening attitude in the room; the purpose of the improved SNR is to quiet and focus the room, not to excite or distract the children.

In many instances, the best listening and learning environment for children with hearing difficulties can be created by using both a CADS and a personal-worn FM system at the same time. The CADS, appropriately installed in a mainstreamed classroom, improves acoustic access for all students in the classroom. For children especially challenged by the effects of poor SNR and reverberation, such as those with hearing loss or auditory processing problems, a personal FM system might be more effective. The teacher need wear only a single transmitter if the child's personal FM transmitter is coupled to the audio-out port of the CADS using an appropriate patch cord. Children with hearing loss or other auditory function disorder greatly benefit from having access to the two microphones of the CADS. They also benefit from having a quiet environment in the classroom and a specific auditory focus, as designated by the use of the remote microphone. Because of the added complexity of using two technologies, teachers do require in-servicing about both technologies, including how to troubleshoot them and how to use them appropriately.

Desktop Sound System

Desktop or totable sound field systems have been introduced to provide ideal sound field conditions for individual students. A small loudspeaker is placed on a student's desk. In some regions, students with exceptional listening needs, such as cochlear implant students or students with auditory processing problems, use this form of sound field amplification. Obviously, not all students in the room benefit from this kind of system because it does not provide uniform amplification throughout the classroom. Anderson and Goldstein (2004) found that desktop units and personal-worn FM systems provide better speech perception scores than CADS for some children with hearing aids and cochlear implants by providing a more effective SNR.

Loop Systems

Electromagnetic analog induction loop amplification systems, one of the oldest forms of room amplification, are not commonly used as classroom hearing assistance technologies today, although they are experiencing a resurgence in public places, especially in Europe (Kricos, 2010). In a loop system, a microphone is connected by hard wire or wirelessly to an amplifier. The amplifier transmits the electrical signal from the microphone to a length of insulated copper wire encircling the room, and the electrical current flowing through the wire creates an electromagnetic field that can be picked up by any device that uses a telecoil, typically a hearing aid or cochlear implant (Kricos, 2010). Hearing aids fit on children usually include a telecoil option.

Advantages to using a loop system in a classroom with one or more children with hearing loss include: loops tend to be the least expensive choice of all forms of room amplification; the loop system operates on a universal frequency; for students who have hearing aids with strong telecoils, no separate receiver or headset is required to receive the signal; and the looped signal is modified by the students' own hearing aids so it will be optimized for each individual, assuming that the hearing aids have been set appropriately for the child.

Some disadvantages to using a looped classroom are that the loop system requires children to have hearing aids or cochlear implants with a built-in telecoil or with a separate telecoil-enabled receiver to access the signal; children whose hearing aids or cochlear implants do not have an M+T option must choose either the acoustic or electromagnetic signal for listening; interference may occur when more than one loop system is used in nearby rooms; the signal quality (and therefore speech recognition) decreases the further a child moves from the induction loop; and induction loop systems are subject to interference from several sources, including fluorescent lighting and unshielded electrical power lines (Beck & Fabry, 2011).

Bluetooth Technologies: Wireless Connectivity

Wireless connectivity to the environment and to electronic devices is an evolving horizon for hearing aid wearers (Schum, 2010). Indeed, Bluetooth (BT) technologies are having a significant impact on development of wireless assistive devices (Levitt, 2004). Bluetooth is a proprietary open wireless technology standard for exchanging data using short wavelength radio transmissions in the 2.4 GHz frequency range to link computers and other digital devices together; it offers flexibility and increased access to multiple technologies (Beck & Fabry, 2011). Even though BT is the primary wireless technology used in cell phones and other electronics, BT wireless transmission poses a problem for hearing aids because the size of the transmitters and receivers is large compared with the components of hearing aids. In addition, BT transmission has high power requirements that exceed the capabilities of hearing aid-size batteries, and limited bandwidth relative to dedicated FM systems.

The current solution is to use a body-worn gateway device that accepts signals from various formats, such as BT, direct audio input, and FM, converts the input signal to a digital magnetic signal, and then sends the signal to a digital magnetic receiver that is integrated in the electronics of the hearing aid (Nyffeler & Dechant, 2010).

To overcome some of the BT limitations, the hearing aid industry has recently developed new dedicated wireless digital signal processing devices that allow hearing aids to communicate directly with a programming device, television, cell phone, or a second hearing aid worn on the opposite ear (Beck & Fabry, 2011). These technologies offer improved ease of use, more attractive cosmetics, and better performance, but still cause the hearing aid to have a shorter battery life, thereby increasing costs. Nevertheless, the vision is to provide a universal standard for connectivity that is low cost, easy to use, and effective.

Auditory Feedback Loop: Another Use for the FM Microphone for Acoustic Accessibility of the Child's Own Voice

The auditory feedback loop is the process of self-monitoring (input) and correcting one's own speech (output). Auditory feedback is crucial for the attainment of auditory goals and fluent speech (Perkell, 2008). That is, a child must be able to hear his or her own

speech clearly to produce clear speech sounds. Improving the SNR of the child's own speech can boost the salience of the speech signal.

Obtaining audibility of high-frequency sounds is important not just for perception of other people, but also to assist children in monitoring their own voice as they attempt to produce the sounds. Unfortunately, high-frequency sounds radiate from the mouth in a very directional manner, so despite the close proximity of a child's ear to his or her mouth, the level of high-frequency fricative sounds at the input to the hearing aid or cochlear implant may be relatively low (Pittman, Stelmachowicz, Lewis, & Hoover, 2003). Therefore, to facilitate development of the child's auditory feedback loop, place the microphone of the FM system within 6 inches of the child's mouth when she is speaking (especially during auditory-verbal therapy) or reading aloud. Because speaking and reading are interrelated, speaking into the FM microphone will highlight the child's speech and allow her to monitor and control her speaking and reading fluency.

■ Efficacy of Technology

Is the Technology Really Helping the Child?

The fact that a child has technology does not guarantee that the child is hearing well with the technology. If a child is using hearing aids or a cochlear implant, the first step is to know that the primary technology is providing the expected benefit. Even though an FM system will reduce the problems associated with distance and noise, the FM cannot compensate for poor hearing aid settings. While assessing speech perception in quiet at a comfortable level may provide sufficient information when checking technology in the clinic, it does not provide sufficient information about acoustic accessibility at home, in school, and in after-school activities. To measure accessibility in critical situations, it is important to test hearing aids and cochlear implants in the sound room, at normal and soft speech levels, in quiet and in competing noise (Madell, 2008a). For FM systems to work appropriately, it is critical that hearing aids be correctly selected and programmed (see Chapter 3 in this book). First, the hearing aid needs to meet the needs of the specific hearing loss. Benefit needs to be validated using aided thresholds to demonstrate hearing at sufficiently soft levels to be certain that, with technology, children have access to speech information throughout the frequency range, especially high frequencies (Anderson, 2011). Such testing will provide information about modification of hearing aid settings to permit children to hear what they need to hear (Dillon, Ching, & Golding, 2008; Madell, 2007, 2008a, 2008b; Stender, Appleby, & Hallenbeck, 2011).

Hearing Assistance Technology (HAT) Guidelines

The HAT guidelines identify fitting goals for hearing assistance technology to provide audibility and intelligibility of the following:

- Speech recognition that is commensurate with performance in ideal listening situations
- Full audibility of self and others
- Reduced effects of distance, noise, and reverberation

The guidelines describe full audibility as:

- Consistent signal from the talker regardless of head movement
- Technology that will be worn consistently by the individual, parent, or teacher
- Technology that will provide full audibility according to the listener group

Listener groups include children who use hearing aids, children who use cochlear implants, and children with normal hearing who do not use technology.

The guidelines discuss regulatory considerations and qualifications of personnel who fit and monitor FM systems. Standards by which HAT effectiveness should be evaluated are reviewed. FM systems (personal, individual, and classroom audio-distribution systems, infrared, and induction systems) are discussed in some detail. The guidelines describe the types of systems available, and discuss their advantages and disadvantages. Candidacy is reviewed as well as fitting and verification protocols. Validation, training, and use are reviewed. Monitoring and managing equipment are discussed in detail, including procedures for checking systems to be sure they are working. Strategies for implementing guidelines in the schools are offered. See the following website for the full HAT document: http://www.audiology.org/resources/document library/Documents/HATGuideline.pdf.

Verification and Validation of FM Benefit

It is essential to verify FM benefit. One should not assume that the FM is working simply because we plug it in. The FM needs to be tested when it is recommended and checked every morning. The fact that it worked yesterday does not mean it is working today. Verification is always recommended, following manufacturer's protocol, to ensure that the child is getting a consistent signal between the hearing aid and the FM system.

In addition to verification, validation is critical. Test booth validation should include performance with and without the FM systems. Testing should include aided thresholds, and also thresholds with the FM system. If aided thresholds are not providing sufficient gain, the hearing aids will need to be adjusted prior to proceeding. While the FM system can improve performance, it cannot make up for a poorly fit hearing aid. Speech perception testing should be performed using a speech perception test that is linguistically and age appropriate (Madell, 2008a). Testing should be conducted at normal (50 dB HL) and soft (35 dB HL) conversational levels in quiet, and at a normal conversational level with competing noise, preferably four talker babble (Madell, 2007, 2008a). See **Table 8.1** for an example of the type of test form that can be used to record test results.

Validation of FM Technology at Home and School

The need for FM use in a school setting has been documented for years (HAT, 2008). That is, FM use has been viewed primarily as a tool for use in classrooms. However, FM has many other uses that are often overlooked. The remote microphone (placed within 6 inches of the desired sound source) can improve signal clarity for virtually anyone, and certainly for everyone with a hearing loss who uses audition to receive spoken language.

Validation should be conducted in all situations in which the child is using the FM system, including home and school. At the very least, the system needs to be checked every day. It is not sufficient to ask the child if it is working. Many children with hearing loss are not able to accurately assess if the system is working. The person with the microphone (parent, teacher, scoutmaster) should stand several feet away from the child to be sure the child has to rely on the FM to hear the message, not the hearing aids. She may ask questions of the child to see if he is hearing. These should be questions that the child cannot anticipate and should be changed each day, such as *"What color are your shoes?"* Repeating the Ling sounds [m, a, e, oo, sh, s] in random order can also be used to test FM performance.

Testing also can be conducted in the classroom to assess HAT benefit. Johnson and Seaton (2012) suggest a test called the Functional Listening Evaluation (FLE), which assesses hearing up close and at a distance, with and without the FM system. This test can be conducted in a classroom setting and provides important information about performance. Please see the following website for the full version of the FLE: http://www.handsandvoices.org/pdf/func_eval.pdf.

Table 8.1   Test form for recording technology benefit

	Right technology	Left technology	Binaural	Binaural + FM
50 dB HL				
35 dB HL				
50 dB HL +5 SNR				

Test booth validation with personal technology (hearing aids, Baha, and/or cochlear implants) will provide important information that is useful in adapting the technology as well as in counseling. Demonstrating improved speech perception scores, especially for soft speech and for speech in noise, is very helpful in counseling children with hearing loss, their parents, and classroom teachers, all of whom would probably elect not to use the FM if given the choice.

Using Checklists for Verification of Acoustic Accessibility

In addition to the above testing, checklists provide very useful information about how a child performs in several different situations. Some of these tools are designed to be completed by parents, some by students, and some by the professionals who work with the child. It can be very useful to have forms completed by several different people to obtain a broad picture. When everyone scores the child's performance the same way, it is easy to determine what kind of educational remediation is needed. Different scores may indicate that not everyone is looking at the child the same way, that everyone does not have the same standards for the child, or that the child is performing differently in different situations. Results of rating scales are very helpful in counseling children and parents about school concerns. A description of several available checklists is itemized below, and many can be obtained from the following website: http://successforkidswithhearingloss.com.

- *Screening Instrument for Targeting Educational Risk (SIFTER)* (Anderson, 1989). Norm-referenced checklist comparing teachers' perceptions of classroom function for elementary-aged students with and without hearing loss. For example, "How distractible is the student compared to his or her peers?"
- *Preschool Screening Instrument for Targeting Educational Risk (Preschool SIFTER)* (Anderson & Matkin, 1996). Norm-referenced checklist comparing teachers' perceptions of classroom function for preschool-aged students with and without hearing loss. For example, "How well does the child understand basic concepts when compared to classmates?"

- *Secondary Screening Instrument for Targeting Educational Risk (Secondary SIFTER)* (Anderson, 2004). Norm-referenced checklist comparing teachers' perceptions of classroom function for secondary-aged students with and without hearing loss. For example, "How do the student's general foundation skills (i.e., reading level) compare to the difficulty of work expected in class?"
- *Listening Inventory For Education–Revised (LIFE–R)* (Anderson, Smaldino, & Spangler, 2011). Student self-rates ability to hear and understand in each of 15 listening situations. A separate form allows the teacher to evaluate listening difficulty. Sections include classroom listening situations and situations outside the classroom.
- *Children's Auditory Performance Scale (CHAPS)* (Smoski, Brunt, & Tannahill, 1992). A judgment of student attention in six listening conditions resulting in a score of normal or at-risk. Ages 5+.
- *FM Listening Evaluation* (Johnson & Seaton, 2012). This rating scale can be completed by a parent, a teacher, an audiologist, or other clinician working with the child. It rates distance at which a child can hear a variety of different stimuli in a variety of different conditions. For example, "Student responds to his name when spoken to in quiet at 3 feet, 10 feet; in noise at 3 feet, 10 feet."
- *Fisher's Auditory Problems Checklist* (Fisher, 1985, modified by Johnson & Seaton, 2012). Rates attention, comprehension, discrimination, speech in noise, localization, sensitivity, long- and short-term memory, speech, and language problems.

Use of Remote Microphones Outside of School

The use of FM systems and remote microphones in classrooms is well documented. Very little has been written about FM use outside of school settings, but clinicians who have used them in other settings have reported very positive results. The work of Hart and Risley (1999) has clearly demonstrated that the number of words children speak is directly related to the number of words spoken to the child. For a child with hearing loss, this is clearly an issue. If the primary speaker is not close to the child, the child hears fewer words. An FM system can significantly increase the number of words actually heard by a child with hearing loss, as reported by Moeller, Donaghy, Beauchaine, Lewis, and Stelmachowicz (1996), who found that more consistent auditory input can be obtained if FM systems are used in home as well as in school settings. Nguyen and Bentler (2011) found that children are more likely to practice their emerging spoken language with caregivers when using an FM system. One author's clinical experience (JRM) with infants and FM also has been excellent.

Parents report that wearing the microphone is a reminder for them to speak more. When the infant or preschooler is not close by, parents can still communicate easily. Parents uniformly report that the systems are easy to manage and that the children seem more attentive and more alert to sound when the FM is being used. FM use in the car or on the playground, or in difficult communication situations, provides additional listening time (Madell, 1992, 1996).

As children grow older and become involved in other activities, more opportunities for use develop. Children involved in sports can have a great deal of difficulty hearing on a playing field. If the coach uses an FM system, the child will have good acoustic access to directions. The transmitter will also be useful in ballet class, religious school, scouts, and on the playground. Friends, as well as adults, can learn to use the transmitter to assist in communication. Once people overcome apprehension about using the technology, most people are happy to have the improved communication available.

Appropriate FM Use

FM users need to be reminded of a few basic rules. When the primary talker is not speaking to the child wearing the FM receiver, the microphone could be set on "mute" to avoid having the child listen to information that is not relevant and that may interfere with the child's current task. This would be especially true in a school setting if the child is working on one thing and the teacher is speaking about something else with another child. On the other hand, there could be value in purposely letting the child "listen-in" to the back and forth exchange between family members and perhaps between the teacher and another student. This overhearing is a valuable way that typical children develop "theory of mind" (the capacity to understand that others are separate individuals with their own thoughts and emotions) and gain an understanding of the emotional exchanges between people. The

challenge is to determine how to enable "listening in" to other conversations without compromising the child's independent work. The point is, we may be removing the child's opportunity to learn from other conversations by always turning off the FM mic when the child is not the direct recipient of the conversation.

Users of FM systems need to be reminded about microphone placement. Ideally, the microphone should be a boom mic worn on the head and always in the correct position in front of the talker's mouth. If a clip-on or lavaliere microphone is used, it should be clipped in the middle of the shirt a few inches below the talker's mouth. Clipping the microphone to the side will result in a signal that is significantly reduced when the talker turns her head to the opposite side. Care should be taken to clip the mic in such a way that it does not slip under clothes or become tangled in jewelry.

▨ Summary and Conclusion

Auditory access is a multi-faceted model. The primary concept is ensuring that an optimal auditory signal is being delivered to infants and children with hearing loss in all life settings—home, school and playground, car, and afterschool activities. Said another way, the first step in attainable and sustainable listening and spoken language outcomes is acoustic accessibility of all auditory information. This chapter has discussed technological and environmental management strategies for achieving acoustic access to the child's brain for growth and development of neural centers. What is at stake is not just sound, but a vital bridge to their future, to help children with hearing loss become productive members of our society.

▨ References

Akhtar, N., Jipson, J., & Callanan, M. A. (2001). Learning words through overhearing. *Child Development, 72*(2), 416–430.

American Speech-Language-Hearing Association [ASHA] (2000). *Guidelines for fitting and monitoring FM systems* [Guidelines]. Available from http://www.asha.org/members/deskref-journals/deskref/default.

Anderson, K. L. (1989). *S.I.F.T.E.R.: Screening Instrument for Targeting Educational Risk*. Retrieved from http://successforkidswithhearingloss.com/catalog/sifters.

Anderson, K. L. (2001). Voicing concern about noisy classrooms. *Educational Leadership, 58*(7), 77–79.

Anderson, K. L. (2004). *Secondary S.I.F.T.E.R.: Screening Instrument for Targeting Educational Risk in secondary students*. Retrieved from http://successforkidswithhearingloss.com/catalog/sifters.

Anderson, K. L. (2011). Predicting speech audibility from the audiogram to advocate for listening and learning needs. *Hearing Review, 18*(10), 20–23.

Anderson, K. L., & Goldstein, H. (2004). Speech perception benefits of FM and infrared devices to children with hearing aids in a typical classroom. *Language, Speech, and Hearing Services in Schools, 35*(2), 169–184.

Anderson, K. L., Goldstein, H., Colodzin, L., & Inglehart, F. (2005). Benefit of S/N enhancing devices to speech perception of children listening in a typical classroom with hearing aids or a cochlear implant. *Journal of Educational Audiology, 12,* 14–28.

Anderson, K. L., & Matkin, N. (1996). *Preschool S.I.F.T.E.R.: Screening Instrument for Targeting Educational Risk in preschool children (age 3–kindergarten)*. Retrieved from http://successforkidswithhearingloss.com/catalog/sifters.

Anderson, K. L., Smaldino, J. J., & Spangler, C. (2011). *LIFE–R: Listening Inventory for Education-Revised* Retrieved from http://successforkidswithhearingloss.com/wp-content/uploads/2011/08/Teacher-LIFE-R.pdf

ANSI/ASA. (2002). *American National Standard: Acoustical performance criteria, design requirements, and guidelines for schools*. Melville, NY: Acoustical Society of America.

ANSI/ASA. (2010). *American National Standard: Acoustical performance criteria, design requirements, and guidelines for schools, part 1: Permanent schools*. Melville, NY: Acoustical Society of America. Retrieved from http://asa.aip.org.

Beck, D. L., & Fabry, D. (2011). Access America: It's about connectivity. *Audiology Today, 23*(1), 24–29.

Berlin, C. I., & Weyand, T. G. (2003). *The brain and sensory plasticity: Language acquisition and hearing*. Clifton Park, NY: Thomson Delmar Learning.

Bess, F. H., & Humes, L. E. (2003). *Audiology: The fundamentals* (3rd ed.). Philadelphia, PA: Lippincott Williams & Wilkins.

Bhatnagar, S. C. (2002). *Neuroscience for the study of communicative disorders* (2nd ed.). Philadelphia, PA: Lippincott Williams & Wilkins.

Boothroyd, A. (1997). Auditory development of the hearing child. *Scandinavian Audiology Supplement, 46*(Suppl. 46), 9–16.

Chermak, G. D., Bellis, T. J., & Musiek, F. E. (2007). Neurobiology, cognitive science, and intervention. In G. D. Chermak & F. E. Musiek (Eds.), *Handbook of (central) auditory processing disorder: Comprehensive intervention* (Vol. II, pp. 3–28). San Diego, CA: Plural.

Ching, T. Y. C., van Wanrooy, E., Dillon, H., & Carter, L. (2011). Spatial release from masking in normal-hearing children and children who use hearing aids. *The Journal of the Acoustical Society of America, 129*(1), 368–375.

Cole, E. B., & Flexer, C. (2011). *Children with hearing loss: Developing listening and talking, birth to six*. San Diego, CA: Plural Publishing, Inc.

Crandell, C. C., Smaldino, J. J., & Flexer, C. (2005). *Sound field amplification: Applications to speech perception and classroom acoustics* (2nd ed.). Clifton Park, NY: Thomson Delmar Learning.

Dillon, H., Ching, T., & Golding, M. (2008). Hearing aids for infants and children. In J. R. Madell & C. Flexer (Eds.), *Pediatric audiology: Diagnosis, technology, and management.* New York, NY: Thieme Medical Publishers.

Doidge, N. (2007). *The brain that changes itself: Stories of personal triumph from the frontiers of brain science.* New York, NY: Penguin Books.

Fisher, L. I. (1985). Learning disabilities and auditory processing. In R. J. Van Hattum (Ed.), *Administration of speech-language services in the schools* (pp. 231–292). San Diego, CA: College Hill Press.

Flynn, T. S., Flynn, M. C., & Gregory, M. (2005). The FM advantage in the real classroom. *Journal of Educational Audiology, 12,* 35–42.

Hart, B., & Risley, T. R. (1999). *The social world of children: Learning to talk.* Baltimore, MD: Paul H. Brookes.

HAT(2008). Hearing assistive technology. Retrieved from http://www.audiology.org/resources/documentlibrary/Documents/HATGuideline.pdf.

Johnson, C. D., & Seaton, J. B. (2012). *Educational audiology handbook* (2nd ed.). Clifton Park, NY: Delmar Cengage Learning.

Knightly, L. M., Jun, S. A., Oh, J. S., & Au, T. K. (2003). Production benefits of childhood overhearing. *The Journal of the Acoustical Society of America, 114*(1), 465–474.

Kricos, P. (2010). Looping America: One way to improve accessibility for people with hearing loss. *Audiology Today, 22,* 38–43.

Leavitt, R., & Flexer, C. (1991). Speech degradation as measured by the Rapid Speech Transmission Index (RASTI). *Ear and Hearing, 12*(2), 115–118.

Leibold, L. J., & Neff, D. L. (2011). Masking by a remote-frequency noise band in children and adults. *Ear and Hearing, 32*(5), 663–666.

Levitt, H. (2004). Assistive listening technology: What does the future hold? *Volta Voices, 11*(1), 18–21.

Ling, D. (2002). *Speech and the hearing-impaired child: Theory and practice* (2nd ed.). Washington, DC: Alexander Graham Bell Association for the Deaf and Hard of Hearing.

Madell, J. R. (1992). FM systems as primary amplification for children with profound hearing loss. *Ear and Hearing, 13*(2), 102–107.

Madell, J. R. (1996). FM systems: Beyond the classroom. *Hearing Journal, 30,* 44–46.

Madell, J. R. (2007). Using speech perception to maximize auditory function. *Volta Voices,* 16–20.

Madell, J. R. (2008a). Evaluation of speech perception in infants and children. In J. R. Madell & C. Flexer (Eds.), *Pediatric audiology: Diagnosis, technology,*

and management (pp. 89–105). New York, NY: Thieme Medical Publishers.

Madell, J. R. (2008b). Selecting appropriate technology: Hearing aids, FM, and cochlear implants. *The Hearing Journal, 61*(11), 42–47.

Moeller, M. P., Donaghy, K. F., Beauchaine, K. L., Lewis, D. E., & Stelmachowicz, P. G. (1996). Longitudinal study of FM system use in nonacademic settings: Effects on language development. *Ear and Hearing, 17*(1), 28–41.

Nelson, P. B., & Blaeser, S. B. (2010). Classroom acoustics: What possibly could be new? *The ASHA Leader, 15*(11), 16–19.

Nguyen, H., & Bentler, R. (2011). Optimizing FM systems: Verification of device function at fitting and follow-up preserves advantages of use. *The ASHA Leader, 16*(12), 5–6.

Nyffeler, M., & Dechant, S. (2010). The impact of new technology on mobile phone use. *Hearing Review, 17*(3), 42–49.

Perkell, J. S. (2008). *Auditory feedback and speech production in cochlear implant users and speakers with typical hearing.* Paper presented at the 2008 Research Symposium of the Alexander Graham Bell Association International Convention, Milwaukee, WI.

Pittman, A. L., Stelmachowicz, P. G., Lewis, D. E., & Hoover, B. M. (2003). Spectral characteristics of speech at the ear: Implications for amplification in children. *Journal of Speech, Language, and Hearing Research, 46*(3), 649–657.

Schum, D. J. (2010). Wireless connectivity for hearing aids. *Advance for Audiologists, 12*(2), 24–26.

Sexton, J. (2003). FM as a component of primary amplification. *Educational Audiology Review, 20*(4), 4–5.

Smaldino, J. J. (2011). New developments in classroom acoustics and amplification. *Audiology Today, 23*(1), 30–36.

Smaldino, J. J., & Flexer, C. (2012). *Handbook of acoustic accessibility: Best practices for listening, learning, and literacy in the classroom.* New York, NY: Thieme Medical Publishers.

Smoski, W. J., Brunt, M. A., & Tannahill, J. D. (1992). Listening characteristics of children with central auditory processing disorders. *Language, Speech, and Hearing Services in Schools, 23,* 145–152.

Stender, T., Appleby, R., & Hallenbeck, S. (2011). V & V and its impact on user satisfaction. *Hearing Review, 18*(4), 12–21.

Tallal, P. (2004). Improving language and literacy is a matter of time. *Nature Reviews Neuroscience, 5*(9), 721–728.

9 Listening and Spoken Language at School Age

For most children with hearing loss, the need for intervention to develop listening skills continues throughout their school years. This chapter presents the integration of listening and spoken language in school learning environments. Practical techniques aimed at continued progress in listening and language development, including social communication throughout the school years, are presented. This chapter highlights the essential contribution of school team members to a positive inclusion experience and continues to emphasize the important ongoing partnership with parents, drawing from recent research in this field. This chapter also describes intervention activities for children of school age.

◾ Inclusion in Regular Education Environments

What Is Inclusion?

The literature across the spectrum of education for children with various special needs proposes several definitions of inclusion. These definitions appear to embrace several common dimensions: inclusion involves helping children to reach their full potential, fosters a sense of belonging to a community (e.g., classroom, school, and society), and recognizes the diversity of learners. The following definition adopted by one educational jurisdiction is an example of a working definition that encompasses these characteristics:

> Inclusive education is about educating all students in a way that allows them to reach their full potential as valuable human beings while contributing to and enhancing their communities. It is a child-centered philosophy and approach that recognizes that every child has something positive to contribute to society and can reach his or her full potential if given appropriate opportunities and supports. Inclusive education is "an approach and not a place"; an approach that promotes the accommodation of all children into the learning experience in a way that maximizes their potential and fosters their self-esteem and sense of belonging to the school community and the larger society. It is about recognizing and celebrating the diversity of learners and providing an opportunity for them to be the best that they can be. (Mackay, 2007)

Two primary viewpoints regarding educational placement dominate the literature on education of children with hearing loss, one where students are educated in regular school settings and the other where they receive their education in special schools alongside peers with hearing loss (Spencer & Marschark, 2010). Historically, inclusion, which was often referred to as mainstreaming or integration, has been presented as part of a cascade model of services where children were placed in settings with peers with normal hearing on a part-time or full-time basis depending on their abilities (Deno, 1970). In current educational models, one of two situations generally exists: (1) the student is mainstreamed on a part-time basis in a regular classroom and pulled out to attend a special class where additional support is available, or (2) the student attends a regular classroom full-time. In the latter case, adaptations and accommodations are implemented to ensure academic success (Marschark, 2007). It is our premise that successful inclusion requires strong commitment from all stakeholders involved in the process.

Decisions about inclusion were and continue to be largely influenced by philosophy about how children with special needs should be educated both by legislation and by the availability of resources to support children's learning in classrooms in general education settings (Powers, 1996a, 1996b). Pioneers who advocated development of spoken language through hearing for children with hearing loss have long been proponents of inclusion in the regular school system (Ling & Ling, 1978; Pollack, 1977). Advocates have favored general education placements on the basis that children could develop more typical patterns of spoken language, social communication, and overall social functioning.

In this chapter and throughout the book, inclusion refers to full-time attendance and participation in a regular school program with peers with normal hearing. Since the advent of early detection and better access to sound through hearing technology, many more families choose general education programs for their children (Marschark, 2007). For example, in Australia, reports suggest that there has been a trend for some time to integrate the vast majority of students with hearing loss in the general school system (Power & Hyde, 2002, 2003). While less than 50% of students with hearing loss in the United States were integrated in regular school settings in the 1970s (Karchmer & Trybus, 1977), a new survey in 2001 revealed an important increase, in that more than two-thirds of American students with hearing loss were being educated full-time or part-time with hearing peers (Karchmer & Mitchell, 2003). The overwhelming majority of today's students who attend regular school systems are using listening and spoken language (Akamatsu, Mayer, & Hardy-Braz, 2008). In particular, in the last two decades cochlear implantation has had an important impact on the number of children with severe to profound hearing loss in regular educational settings (Archbold & Mayer, 2012; Archbold, Phil, & O'Donoghue, 2009; Geers, Strube, Tobey, Pisoni, & Moog, 2011).

Children with hearing loss enter school at various levels of auditory and spoken language functioning and require technological and intervention support to thrive alongside their peers with normal hearing. For various reasons, some children, despite preschool language intervention, enter school with language levels below that of their peers and are therefore at risk of having difficulty keeping up with the expectations of a typical classroom (Fitzpatrick, Crawford, Ni, & Durieux-Smith, 2011; Nicholas & Geers, 2007). On the other hand, many children who have received amplification and intervention in the first months of life are more likely to enter school with language, speech, and social skills at or near their peers' competencies (Yoshinaga-Itano, 2003). The following sections describe how inclusion can be practiced to foster development, that is, how hearing rehabilitation continues in the school system.

Benefits of Inclusion

Regular schools are by definition places in which listening and spoken language occur naturally and continuously. Students with hearing loss are expected to learn to listen in a variety of contexts and communicate through spoken language. The proposed advantages of inclusion for children include the opportunity to attend neighborhood schools and to learn effective ways of communicating alongside peers in settings where they have exposure to typical auditory and language experiences. With early intervention, the majority of students will have acquired language through typical developmental models. Identification and inclusion in the general education system from the beginning allow them to continue to expand their social, academic, and emotional learning in natural contexts. Attendance at a neighborhood school, rather than a special school for students with hearing loss, which is often located at some distance from the child's home, facilitates on-going support by family and friends. Research has shown positive spoken language outcomes for students attending general educational settings (Eriks-Brophy et al, 2006; Eriks-Brophy et al, 2012; Geers, Brenner, & Tobey, 2010). These settings not only incorporate opportunities for spoken communication but also enable children to acquire age-level academic skills needed to access post-secondary studies or work settings (Eriks-Brophy et al, 2012; Goldberg & Flexer, 2001). As elaborated below, being simply placed in a regular classroom is not sufficient, and the skills necessary to achieve age-appropriate language and academic functioning must continue to be developed. Several factors facilitate healthy development at school age, including a strong commitment to the whole process of inclusion, which requires parents, school professionals, and clinicians/teachers to work in partnership.

Challenges of Inclusion

As discussed in Chapter 8, one of the greatest challenges to learning in a regular school is the physical nature of the classroom itself, which presents acoustic barriers to optimal learning. The school setting consists of several other acoustically challenging environments, such as the gymnasium, cafeteria, and playground. These variables will impact the auditory attention and the opportunities for incidental learning by students with hearing loss in the classroom. As discussed in Chapter 8, different acoustic environments can be managed and how specific factors, such as distance, noise, and reverberation, can be reduced to optimize listening.

As noted above, some children arrive at school with considerable gaps in their listening, spoken language, and general knowledge skills. These fundamental skills are a prerequisite for literacy, for academic learning, and for establishing social relationships with peers (Marschark, 2007; Stinson & Antia, 1999). Learning in a regular classroom setting involves being exposed to complex linguistic input, which requires high-level cognitive processes to integrate the information received. As described by Easterbrooks and Estes (2007), hearing loss specifically results in delays in processing speed of the acoustic information (e.g., when the teacher is presenting new material) and delays in reading and other academic content areas, and interferes with social interaction, particularly in group settings. Even children who have age-appropriate language skills at school entry are at risk for some of these difficulties as they adapt to a fast-paced learning environment.

Recent work with school-based specialized teachers of the deaf and hard of hearing indicated that some parents are unprepared for the new realities of classroom learning and the new and challenging learning situations their children will face. Teachers suggested that both parents and clinicians/teachers would benefit from being more aware of the realities of a school environment (Fitzpatrick & Olds, submitted manuscript). In the teachers' words:

> They don't understand what happens in the outside world and what happens in the classroom. They really need to come and see, like it's a confusing place for some of these kids. It's a lot to deal with ... it's a lot of energy, ..., it's utter chaos. [Kids] know what's [happening] with their therapist one-on-one. That doesn't transfer to the real world.

Therefore, the school system is faced with the challenge of implementing programs that provide children with access to the conditions and specialized services required to optimize the inclusive experience.

▦ Supporting Inclusion through a Team Approach

School systems offer a variety of educational programs and specialized services for children with hearing loss included in the regular school setting. A team approach has been widely advocated and the team works with the family and student throughout the school years. In many education systems, clinicians/ teachers provide specialized services in listening and communication development for students with hearing loss from school entry through high school. Based on a needs assessment, a spectrum of services, from indirect to direct intervention, is generally provided for students in school settings.

Indirect Services

Indirect intervention refers to the monitoring of children with hearing loss who are expected to be able to follow the regular curriculum alongside their peers with normal hearing. This group often includes children with unilateral and milder forms of hearing loss as well as some children with more severe losses who have age-appropriate language skills. For these children, the clinician/teacher or an educational audiologist is involved in ensuring classroom acoustic accessibility through remote microphone systems (see Chapter 8) and in informing and coaching the classroom teacher about hearing loss, particularly in the early school period. Monitoring and follow-up to check progress are highly recommended to ensure that technology is functioning and that the child is keeping pace with peers. In this way, there is an opportunity to prevent difficulties from arising or at least to address them as they surface. Given the epidemiology of hearing loss, in a typical school population this type of follow-up might apply to 50% or more of the children with hearing loss (Fortnum, Summerfield, Marshall, Davis, & Bamford, 2001; Watkin & Baldwin, 2011).

Direct Services

Direct services refers to individualized intervention with children, most of whom experience some degree of language delay. As noted above, although children acquire language during the preschool years enabling them to attend regular classrooms, a substantial number have gaps in language structures, vocabulary, and social skills compared with their normal hearing peers (Fitzpatrick et al, 2012; Geers, Moog, Biedenstein, Brenner, & Hayes, 2009; Stinson & Antia, 1999). For these children, direct intervention services are typically recommended to support their development in an inclusive setting (Antia, Jones, Reed, & Kreimeyer, 2009).

In some school service models, direct intervention services may also be provided to children who have age-appropriate language skills as measured by standardized language assessments. Despite adequate language, some children may receive direct intervention services because expert opinion suggests that these children require ongoing therapy to maintain auditory and spoken language skills and to avoid falling behind their peers. Many practitioners consider that continuing intervention to advance the child's spoken language and literacy skills is justified and even necessary for children with hearing loss because they are at risk for difficulties in fast-paced classroom learning environments (Fitzpatrick & Doucet, in press). Providing these children with direct services at school entry may provide a "buffer" to help them adapt to classroom learning and actually prevent difficulties as classroom language and literacy become more complex. Accordingly, direct services for these children can be viewed as preventive care, essentially preparing the child and family with knowledge and skills to prevent delays in language, social function, and learning.

A partnership between educational professionals, parents, and the student seems to be the preferred model of care for children of school age. In the subsequent section, we briefly describe the roles and contributions of these various partners.

Partnerships in Service Delivery

Parents

Parents have important decisions to make regarding educational options for their child. While choices in rural areas may be limited, families in urban areas are often faced with multiple choices regarding type of school (e.g., private and public schools, alternative schools, open classroom arrangements) and specialized intervention services available. During this period, parents often require support and information from clinicians/teachers in preschool and school programs to make informed decisions. In some cases, these decisions can be very straightforward, but for others, because of religious, cultural, and other reasons, they can be stressful. For many reasons, the transition period from preschool to school services is a period that deserves attention. For some parents, it involves a discharge from intervention services and clinicians/teachers with whom they have developed relationships and confidence, while for others there may be a continuity of services with the same clinician/teacher from preschool to school. However, for all parents, starting school involves the shift from a home or preschool environment to a more formal learning setting. For all, regardless of whether the child has special needs or not, it represents an important milestone in the child's life, one that can be amplified for parents of children with hearing loss. It is both an exciting period in the life of a child and family and one that can be marked by some apprehension for parents of children with special needs. Our work with parents suggests that transition to school can be one of the most difficult periods associated with parenting a child with hearing loss.

During the school years, parents continue to play an important role in the continued development of their child's listening and spoken language skills. In a family-centered program, parents are a key ingredient to a successful inclusive experience. Similar to preschool services described in earlier chapters, parents and clinicians/teachers work closely together to optimize the child's listening and spoken language potential. One of the fundamental differences compared with the preschool period is that the child is now expected to acquire the skills necessary to thrive in a more formal and often structured learning environment that society has established. In this new structure, other professionals become essential partners.

Classroom Teacher

One of the most important professionals shaping the child's educational experience (and the parent's experience) is the classroom teacher. Teachers must manage a classroom with children who have a wide range of abilities and also understand the social and academic effects of hearing loss and the relationship between audition, language, and literacy acquisition. In addition, they must learn to use specialized hearing technology and learn new strategies to facilitate learning for children with hearing loss, some of whom have delayed speech and/or language. The classroom teacher supports inclusion by collaborating with the clinician/teacher and the parents and providing them, to some extent, with her insights into the child's needs based on her observations and assessments. After all, the teacher is in an ideal position to compare the student's functioning with that of his peers with normal hearing.

It is essential that clinicians/teachers provide regular classroom teachers, similar to the parents of a young child, with techniques to optimize the environment and specific teaching strategies that facilitate classroom learning and classroom participation. Providing an environment that makes communication possible for all students will facilitate the participation of the student with hearing loss. It is important therefore that teachers demonstrate a positive attitude toward the child with hearing loss and understand the impact of hearing loss with respect to the effects on distance and incidental learning, listening in noise and group interaction. While some teachers naturally adapt their teaching strategies, others require considerable coaching to adapt their teaching to maximize learning for a child with hearing loss. **Table 9.1** provides a list of guidelines that are commonly provided to teachers to facilitate classroom learning. Other strategies are provided in resources such as Smaldino and Flexer (2012) and Marschark (2007).

Table 9.1   Guidelines for regular classroom teachers

- Use the remote microphone system as appropriate for instruction of different subject areas
- Circulate a pass-around microphone for other students in the classroom
- Speak in a clear voice facing the student whenever possible
- Provide visual support, e.g., diagrams, notes on the board, to facilitate understanding
- Position yourself to facilitate speechreading (pay attention to lighting and position when speaking)
- Adjust the pace, particularly when presenting new material
- Check the student's comprehension of the material presented, e.g., by asking questions
- Encourage the student to take the responsibility of advocating for his needs, e.g., request repetition or clarification
- Use closed-caption materials when possible
- Provide written materials to support information presented using audio-visual media when possible

Student

From the start, the student with hearing loss must be encouraged to show initiative and participate fully in the classroom activities. As the child matures, the clinician/teacher and all other school professionals work together to facilitate the development of autonomy and self-advocacy. For example, the student must learn to manage her own hearing technology, including remote microphone system. To this end, an understanding of hearing loss and its implications for school learning becomes an important aspect of the intervention pro-gram. Students must learn to apply the rules of communication in a group, ask for clarifica-tions during communication breakdowns, and express the need for additional support. Con-sequently, it is important that students learn about the listening situations that are diffi-cult for them and learn strategies that can be helpful. Effectively, as we will see below, this becomes part of the intervention program with the student. The student's motivation and engagement can greatly enhance her learning experience.

Clinician/Teacher

In most school systems where inclusion is prac-ticed, clinicians/teachers play an essential role in continuing listening and spoken language development. The continued development or maintenance of these skills is aimed at equip-ping the child with the foundations necessary for literacy and academic and social develop-ment. As discussed in Chapter 3, this role can be assumed by specialists from different disci-plines. The particular discipline is often deter-mined by regional employment practices, the availability of trained specialists, and regulatory bodies. We continue to use the designation cli-nician/teacher to refer to the professional (e.g., teacher of the deaf and hard of hearing, audi-tory-verbal therapist, speech-language patholo-gist) who assumes the role of listening and spoken language specialist in the school system.

The clinician/teacher works closely with parents, teachers, and, of course, the student to ensure that optimal listening and learning environments, as well as educational strate-gies, are implemented to facilitate inclusion. The amount of direct intervention compared with consultation services varies accord-ing to the child's needs, the setting, and resources, and to some degree the philosophy of how services should be delivered. Services are frequently offered through a pull-out or withdrawal method where children receive individual listening, speech, and language intervention as well as additional instruction in literacy and academics according to their needs determined on the basis of a compre-hensive assessment (see section below). Some programs tend to prefer a "push-in" method, where specialized instruction occurs within the context of the classroom.

An important role of the clinician/teacher is to provide information and training to other students and school professionals about deaf-ness and its impact on communication and learning. Ongoing exchange of information with the classroom teacher (or teachers) will help establish successful communication that can facilitate understanding of the specific needs of the student with hearing loss (Stinson & Liu, 1999).

Educational Audiologist

Ideally, an educational audiologist is part of the school team and oversees all of the audiologic aspects of the child's hearing technology and classroom acoustics. The audiologist educates teachers, students, parents, and other school per-sonnel about hearing loss and its consequences. She also provides technical support to clinicians/ teachers, particularly related to technology and acoustic accessibility. The educational audiolo-gist can interpret clinical test results regarding the benefits of hearing aids or cochlear implants and help classroom teachers understand the limitations of hearing technology in various lis-tening conditions. Audiologists can also perform functional hearing evaluations to better identify school accessibility challenges and make recom-mendation for improving the listening environ-ment. Unfortunately, smaller school systems may not include school-based audiology services, in which case the clinician/teacher assumes the role of managing many of these important educational and practical aspects of the child's hearing care.

Other Educational Personnel

Educational assistants. Children with hearing loss who present severe gaps in language may not be able to follow a regular school curriculum and may require considerably more direct classroom support than a regular teacher can offer. In some cases, educational assistants are provided as part of the team services, primarily to assist the teacher in providing the support required for a child to continue in an inclusive environment. Educational assistants, because of their intense work with both teachers and students, often act as liaisons between the regular classroom teacher and the clinician/teacher who manages the child's spoken language intervention. These professionals can be an important asset for clinicians/teachers, in that they continue auditory and language stimulation and implement specific techniques to help children who have considerable important gaps in their language development. Frequently, these educators attend the individualized intervention sessions provided by the clinician/teacher so that they can learn auditory techniques and exchange information with the clinician/teacher about specific classroom learning challenges. In particular, the educational assistant notes difficulty with vocabulary, concepts, and new material presented in the classroom.

Other personnel. Depending on the individual child's circumstances, numerous other individuals may be included in the school team at various times. For example, children presenting additional disabilities may require supports from resource teachers, occupational therapists, and/or physiotherapists. Students and families may also benefit at various times from support from psychologists and social workers. In some cases, these services are not available through school services and need to be accessed through clinical programs.

■ Intervention at School Age

Transition from Preschool to School Services

As noted above, preparation for inclusion begins before the child starts school, in the form of guidance and information for both parents and teachers and other specialists in the regular school system who will be involved with the child. For parents, part of the coaching requires helping them to understand the multiple demands placed on a child in a fast-paced and noisy learning environment. To facilitate transition, several procedures before and at the beginning of the school year can be helpful:

- The child and family can visit the school to meet school personnel.
- The classroom teacher can observe an intervention session with the child. When possible, this can take place before the child starts school or in the early school period. This provides an early opportunity for the clinician/teacher to help the teacher understand the child's needs and establish a partnership from the outset.
- The classroom teacher should be provided with a good introduction to the hearing technology, particularly the remote microphone system, and receive considerable support in the early weeks of school to ensure it is appropriately used.
- The classroom teacher is provided with information about hearing loss and its impact on learning in school, and environmental modifications to facilitate the child's understanding. Teacher workshops where new teachers have the opportunity to interact with experienced teachers (who have taught children with hearing loss) are recommended. **Table 9.2** details a list of themes that can be presented during a teacher training workshop.

Table 9.2 Suggested topics for teacher training workshop

- Basic understanding of normal hearing and types and severity of hearing loss

- Listening and spoken language intervention—a team approach

- Collaboration between clinician/teacher and classroom teacher

- Roles of parents in child's continued language and social development

- Understanding hearing loss and its impact on school learning and participation

- Impact of hearing loss on vocabulary, language, and literacy

- Social implications of hearing loss

- Hearing technology: hearing aids, cochlear implants, remote microphone systems (e.g., FM systems)

- Environmental, instructional, and assessment accommodations

Assessment

Successful inclusion of children with hearing loss in regular settings involves an understanding of the individual needs of each child (Cawthorn, 2001). Intervention by the clinician/teacher requires a comprehensive assessment of the student's auditory, speech, language, academic and social needs. Given that the child is learning alongside his peers with normal hearing, it is important to use assessment tools that enable comparison with typically developing children.

Functional Hearing Assessment

Since the greatest barrier to the child's learning is the reduction in acoustic information directly related to the hearing loss, an evaluation of functional hearing is extremely important. Several tools have been developed to assist with understanding the student's ability to function in various listening conditions. These tools provide a more in-depth picture of the child's hearing abilities that extends beyond the degree of hearing loss presented on an audiogram. For example, for young children, the Children's Home Inventory of Listening Development (CHILD) (Anderson & Smaldino, 2011), among other things, helps the parent identify areas of concern and possible situations where listening difficulties might occur. Another tool, the Teacher's Evaluation of Aural/Oral Performance of Children (TEACH) consists of questions for teachers targeting the child's everyday listening environment (Ching & Hill, 2005). For older children, several other tools, such as the Listening Inventory for Education (LIFE) (Anderson, Smaldino, & Spangler, 2011), which has recently been revised, can help the student identify difficult listening situations in the school environment. For example, the LIFE presents students with situations like working in small groups, listening to school announcements, and attending a school assembly.

The advantages of these measures are that they are conducted in a typical school or social setting and provide meaningful information that can help guide intervention. These measures can also serve as discussion tools for counseling with parents and teachers to help them become aware of challenging situations for the student. Students themselves can also glean insights to help them understand and strategize with respect to difficulties encountered (Anderson & Arnoldi, 2011).

A more informal but valuable type of assessment involves observation of the student in the classroom. This serves many purposes, including an understanding of the student's participation and communication abilities in the classroom. It

also provides the clinician/teacher with a realistic understanding of the expectations and challenges of learning in a typical classroom setting.

Communication Assessment

Language assessments help situate the school-age child with respect to his peers with normal hearing, evaluate the child's progress, and help guide the focus of intervention. Usually, a battery of standardized tests, with normative data for typically developing children, is used to assess various receptive and expressive linguistic skills, including speech production and intelligibility, vocabulary, semantics, syntax, morphology, and pragmatics. See Paul and Norbury (2012) for a description of tests for school-age children. Other tests probing language-related areas can be added as deemed appropriate. As the child ages, other linguistic areas might be assessed, such as social communication and more advanced language processes.

In addition to standardized tests, other checklists, scales, and questionnaires can be included in the test battery to probe specific areas of language development. For example, if a child's speech skills are delayed at school age, the clinician/teacher might find tools such as the Ling Phonetic Level Evaluation and the Ling Phonologic Level Evaluation useful (Ling, 2002). These tools were specifically developed as remedial assessment tools to help clinicians/teachers establish speech teaching targets for children with hearing loss. Although many children now follow a developmental sequence in speech development, these tools can help define targets when systematic speech intervention is required.

Other criterion-referenced measures, some of which have been developed specifically for children with hearing loss, such as the Cottage Acquisition Scales for Listening, Language,

and Speech (CASLLS) (Wilkes, 2003), and other types of checklists, can guide the clinician/teacher in establishing specific intervention targets. Clinicians/teachers also develop their own tools to monitor progress and to probe specific language domains, which can help them refine teaching targets.

Spontaneous language samples are also highly recommended as a complement to the above measures as they provide a good indication of the student's language in a natural communication context. In this sense, they provide more meaningful information about how a child uses language compared with most standardized tests. Techniques to collect representative samples of a child's language have been well developed and described in the literature (Ling & Ling, 1978; Owens, 2008). It is important to set up situations to elicit a variety of language forms to obtain a good overview of the child's ability to use different types of discourse, such as conversation, description, narration, explanation, and questions (Ling & Ling, 1978). Systematic analysis can be conducted using various tools, such as the Developmental Sentence Scoring Reweighted Score (Lee, 1974) and the Assigning Structural Stage Procedure (Miller, 1981) or with the assistance of specialized software, such as Systematic Analysis of Language Transcription (Miller & Chapman, 2003) or Child Language Data Exchange System (CHILDES) (MacWhinney, 2000). Clinicians/teachers may also find language samples useful even if they carry out a less systematic analysis based on their experience to identify specific problem areas.

Social Language and Social Skills

Social development is one of the difficulties associated with hearing loss (Spencer & Marschark, 2010). Classrooms and schools in general are complex social settings and may present social and emotional challenges. Communication difficulties may impact the ability of students with hearing loss to make friends (Luckner, Schauermann, & Allen, 1994). Tools

have been developed permitting observation of social interactions in students with hearing loss to facilitate intervention. Examples of these tools, such as the Observation of Social Interactions—Preschool and Kindergarten and the Minnesota Social Skills Checklist, can be found in Anderson and Arnoldi (2011), as well as several other resources.

Literacy and Academics

At school age, to complete the assessment profile it is also essential to assess the child's literacy and academic abilities to compare the student's functioning with that of her peers. Literacy is addressed in Chapter 10 of this book. Academic assessment generally falls within the domain of the regular classroom teacher or resource teachers for children who experience difficulties. Clinicians/teachers may, at their discretion, administer standardized tests that probe academic skills. In some districts, standardized achievement tests are also administered to all students school-wide or even regionally to document performance.

Intervention with the Student

The assessment provides a profile of the student and assists in prioritizing areas of intervention and in discussing areas of strengths and weaknesses with parents, teachers, and students themselves. Following the comprehensive assessment, the clinician/teacher prepares an intervention plan for each individual student. In many school districts, a formal document, frequently referred to as an Individualized Education Plan, may also be mandated by the school jurisdiction. The amount (direct intervention hours) and specific delivery model vary in part according to the student's needs but many other factors may influence these decisions, such as availability of specialized resources, philosophy of school system, and amount of other school and home supports available.

Based on the assessments, individualized objectives can be specified in the various domains of listening and spoken language that should be specific, measurable, attainable, realistic, and time sensitive. From the long-term intervention plan, specific lesson plans can be detailed for the student. However, as discussed during the preschool years, a diagnostic intervention approach is favored to continually monitor the student's progress in natural communication contexts and to adjust intervention targets.

For school-age children, the essential components of intervention sessions are often categorized into the domains of listening skills, speech, language, and academics, with an emphasis on learning through audition (Estabrooks, 2006; Olmstead, Mischook, & Doucet, in press). This classification is more for organizational purposes in planning intervention, but intervention aims to incorporate all of these areas in activities and specific teaching tasks, all aimed at continued development and refinement of the child's auditory and spoken-language abilities. In addition to specific content, the clinician/teacher takes into account the child's age and cognitive level and interests in preparing specific teaching activities. Auditory rehabilitation, therefore, involves the use of specific techniques that focus on developing competencies in listening and language. For example, the student practices certain targets, such as understanding a story or following instructions (for a school assignment) in different acoustic conditions, such as with background music, at different distances, and with multiple speakers and different accents. **Table 9.3** presents examples of techniques used in promoting listening in intervention.

Integration of Academic Targets

Many students require additional support to achieve or maintain academic skills comparable to their peers. Additional services are usually available through general school resources for all children who lag behind. However, it is also common practice for clinicians/teachers to incorporate academic targets into their intervention sessions. Clinicians/teachers become familiar with school curriculum and grade-level standards. Ongoing collaboration between the clinician/teacher and classroom teacher helps with the integration of academic goals into intervention sessions. For example, if renewable energy is an upcoming topic in science, the clinician/teacher can present vocabulary and related concepts in an activity that also includes auditory memory targets or specific linguistic targets, such as sentence expansion. Speech production targets, for example, co-articulation, can also be prac-

Table 9.3   Techniques promoting listening

- Acoustic highlighting (emphasis placed on certain key elements of speech)

- Reduce background noise

- Present information through audition first before visual presentation of material

- Imitation

- Modeling

- Expansion

- Prompting

- Pausing

- The "auditory sandwich" technique—stimuli are presented through audition only first, then with vision, and again through audition only

- Closed-set versus open-set auditory tasks

- Sitting behind or beside the child

- Practice advanced auditory skills—auditory comprehension in noise and from a distance

ticed using academic content. The languages of mathematics, history, geography, chemistry, and biology provide a fertile source of vocabulary and concepts to develop auditory skills and advanced thinking skills and to expand the student's world knowledge.

Parent Guidance

As described above, parents are integral to the intervention process throughout the child's school years, building on their work in the early years. Therefore, the parent is fully included in the child's intervention. This involves attending sessions in which parents learn how to continue stimulating listening and spoken language and how to integrate the child's academic material with listening, speech, and language targets. For example, the parent can be shown how to take new vocabulary from a science class and use it in auditory-memory activity. Specific suggestions are provided for parents—in this case, a visit to the natural science museum. Inclusion of the parents in direct intervention sessions helps ensure that the parents are aware of the child's progress and gaps and provides parents with a realistic understanding of the demands of the school environment (Eriks-Brophy et al, 2006). When parents do not attend intervention sessions for various reasons, communication between the clinician/teacher and the parents is of utmost importance to support families in providing a rich learning environment outside school. In some cases, for example, in the case of adolescents, regular attendance at individual sessions may be reduced as the team works toward developing autonomy and self-determination. For further discussion, see Duncan, Rhoades, and Fitzpatrick (in press).

Social Communication and Skills

Social inclusion involves the development of friendships and interactions with peers (Stinson & Antia, 1999). The notion of social belonging preoccupies parents and children themselves, particularly adolescents (Eriks-Brophy et al, 2006, 2007). Studies suggest that children with hearing loss in regular school settings are at risk for difficulties in social development (Cappelli, Daniels, Durieux-Smith, McGrath, & Neuss, 1995; Kluwin & Stinson, 1993). Some of the studies that highlight the social difficulties of children with hearing loss were conducted prior to widespread use of cochlear implants and early intervention and may not always reflect the current context. More recent studies present more positive results related to social integration (Moog, Geers, Gustus, & Brenner, 2011). However, in general, there is concern about the social development of children with hearing loss in inclusive settings. One of the barriers to social integration is the child's competency in spoken language (Duncan, 1999; Most, 2007; Stinson & Whitmire, 2000) and the barriers created by the hearing loss itself related to distance listening, overhearing, and incidental learning (Cole & Flexer, 2011).

In addition to working on closing the gap in the child's listening and language skills, it is important to expose children to everyday functional language used by their peers. Because of reduced accessibility to sound and a poorer quality speech signal, students miss out on incidental and "cool" language, that is, popular language used by all kids (i.e., chill out, give me a break, put a sock in it). They also sometimes have difficulty with the use of humor, sarcasm, irony, and jokes. Therefore, although spoken language may be appropriate as measured by formal tests, clinicians/teachers continue to challenge and expand the child's auditory and language abilities so that she can more effec-tively communicate in everyday communica-tion contexts. As children mature, they learn to adjust and use different types of language with different communication partners, such as a teacher or school administrator versus a classmate.

Strategies for social development. Social language and skills can be taught in diverse situations, such as through role-playing and presentation of scenarios, as well as through group games and activities. Sports and other extracurricular activities provide excellent opportunities for socialization and learning age-appropriate skills, and parents are encour-aged to involve their young children in a range of activities. It is through these interactions that children develop appropriate self-advo-cacy skills, which are so important for chil-dren with hearing loss (Anderson & Arnoldi, 2011). The classroom and other school-specific activities, such as gym, also provide opportu-nities to learn social interaction. To this effect, classroom teachers can be encouraged to spe-cifically identify the needs of children with hearing loss and provide opportunities for practice. **Table 9.4** outlines examples of strat-egies for social development used in practice by clinicians/teachers, adapted from Olmstead, Mischook, and Doucet (in press).

Table 9.4 Examples of strategies for social development used in practice by clinicians/teachers

---

- Identify with student problematic situations (e.g., listening in noise) and set up together a series of helpful strategies and solutions

- Discuss social skills, such as rules of conversation, working in teams, responding to social cues, politeness, sensitivity to others, and how to make friends

- Demonstrate appropriate and inappropriate behaviors in role play for discussion

- Teach "cool" language

- Practice different types of communication, such as telephone, e-mail, text message, Skype, Facebook, and Twitter

- Invite peers to attend individualized session

- Organize social events with peers with hearing loss

- Teach specific vocabulary related to emotions and feelings

- Discuss humor and figurative language, idiomatic expressions, and sarcasm

- Teach communication breakdown repair strategies

- Discuss self-advocacy strategies

Source: Compiled from Olmstead et al (in press); Anderson & Arnoldi (2011).

Summary

Given the tremendous advancements in hearing technology and early intervention, today's children with hearing loss can be expected to complete regular education programs. Recent studies suggest that many, but not all, are developing age-appropriate spoken language skills and achieving academic outcomes comparable to their peers with normal hearing (Dornan, Hickson, Murdoch, Houston, & Constantinescu, 2010; Eriks-Brophy et al, 2012; Fitzpatrick et al, 2012; Geers & Hayes, 2011).

The trend is toward the inclusion of children with hearing loss in regular school programs. Schools are naturally rich in listening, spoken language, and social interactions, and, therefore, provide optimal opportunities for children to continue developing and practicing their auditory and communication skills. However, children are at risk for not achieving age-appropriate skills and require rehabilitation to maximize their potential in inclusive settings. Clinicians/teachers work in collaboration with parents, students, and many other professionals to identify individual needs and to facilitate opportunities for success.

Acknowledgments

Sections of this chapter were inspired by a previous collaboration with Tina Olmstead and Muriel Mischook for a book chapter titled "Communication auditive-verbale en pratique à l'école." In Fitzpatrick, E. M. and Doucet, S. P. (in press). *Apprendre à écouter et à parler: La déficience auditive chez l'enfant*. Ottawa, ON: Les Presses de l'Université d'Ottawa.

References

Akamatsu, C. T., Mayer, C., & Hardy-Braz, S. (2008). Why considerations of verbal aptitude are important in educating deaf and hard-of-hearing students. In M. Marschark & P. C. Hauser (Eds.), *Deaf cognition: Foundations and outcomes* (pp. 131–169). New York: Oxford University Press.

Anderson, K. L., & Arnoldi, K. A. (2011). *Building skills for success in the fast-paced classroom: Optimizing achievement for students with hearing loss*. Hillsboro, OR: Butte Publications.

Anderson, K. L., & Smaldino, J. J. (2011). *The Children's Home Inventory for Listening Difficulties (CHILD)*. Retrieved from http://successforkidswithhearingloss.com.

Anderson, K. L., Smaldino, J. J., & Spangler, C. (2011). *Listening Inventory for Education–Revised (LIFE–R)*. Retrieved from http://successforkidswithhearingloss.com.

Antia, S. D., Jones, P. B., Reed, S., & Kreimeyer, K. H. (2009). Academic status and progress of deaf and hard-of-hearing students in general education classrooms. *Journal of Deaf Studies and Deaf Education, 14*(3), 293–311.

Archbold, S., & Mayer, M. (2012). Deaf education: The impact of cochlear implantation? *Deafness & Education International, 14*(1), 2–15.

Archbold, S., Phil, M., & O'Donoghue, G. M. (2009). Education and childhood deafness: Changing choices and new challenges. In J. K. Niparko (Ed.), *Cochlear implants: Principles and practices* (2nd ed., pp. 313–321). Philadelphia, PA: Lippincott Williams & Wilkins.

Cappelli, M., Daniels, T., Durieux-Smith, A., McGrath, P., & Neuss, D. (1995). Social development of children with hearing impairments who are integrated into general education. *The Volta Review, 97*(3), 197.

Cawthorn. S. (2001). Teaching strategies in inclusive classrooms with deaf students. *Journal of Deaf Studies and Deaf Education, 6*(3), 2123–2225.

Ching, T. Y., & Hill, M. (2005). *Teacher's Evaluation of Aural/Oral Performance of Children (TEACH)*. Retrieved from http://www.outcomes.nal.gov.au/Assessments.

Cole, E. B., & Flexer, C. (2011). *Children with hearing loss: Developing listening and talking, birth to six* (2nd ed.). San Diego, CA: Plural Publishing, Inc.

Deno, E. (1970). Special education as developmental capital. *Exceptional Children, 37*(3), 229–237.

Dornan, D., Hickson, L., Murdoch, B., Houston, T., & Constantinescu, G. (2010). Is auditory-verbal therapy effective for children with hearing loss? *The Volta Review, 110*(3), 361–387.

Duncan, J. (1999). Conversational skills of children with hearing loss and children with normal hearing in an integrated setting. *The Volta Review, 101*(4), 193–211.

Duncan, J., Rhoades, E. A., & Fitzpatrick, E. M. (in press). *Auditory rehabilitation for adolescents with hearing loss*. New York: Oxford University Press.

Easterbrooks, S. R., & Estes, E. L. (2007). *Helping deaf and hard of hearing students to use spoken language*. Thousand Oaks, CA: Cowin Press.

Eriks-Brophy, A., Durieux-Smith, A., Olds, J., Fitzpatrick, E., Duquette, C., & Whittingham, J. (2006). Facilitators and barriers to the inclusion of orally educated children and youth with hearing loss in schools: Promoting partnerships to support inclusion. *The Volta Review, 106*(1), 53–88.

Eriks-Brophy, A., Durieux-Smith, A., Olds, J., Fitzpatrick, E., Duquette, C., & Whittingham, J. (2007). Facilitators and barriers to the inclusion of orally educated children and youth with hearing loss into their families and communities. *The Volta Review, 107*(1), 5–36.

Eriks-Brophy, A., Durieux-Smith, A., Olds, J., Fitzpatrick, E., Duquette, C., & Whittingham, J. (2012). Communication, academic, and social skills of young adults with hearing loss. *The Volta Review, 112*(1), 5–35.

Estabrooks, W. (Ed.) (2006). *Auditory-verbal therapy and practice*. Washington, DC: Alexander Graham Bell Association for the Deaf and Hard of Hearing.

Fitzpatrick, E. M., Crawford, L., Ni, A., & Durieux-Smith, A. (2011). A descriptive analysis of language and speech skills in 4- to 5-yr-old children with hearing loss. *Ear and Hearing, 32*(5), 605–616.

Fitzpatrick, E. M., & Doucet, S. P. (in press). *When should children be discharged from an auditory-verbal program?* In W. Estabrooks (Ed.), *101 FAQs about auditory-verbal practice*. Washington, DC: AG Bell Association.

Fitzpatrick, E. M., & Olds, J. (submitted manuscript). Beyond hearing: Perspectives from teachers on school functioning of children with cochlear implants.

Fitzpatrick, E. M., Olds, J., Gaboury, I., McCrae, R., Schramm, D., & Durieux-Smith, A. (2012). Comparison of outcomes in children with hearing aids and cochlear implants. *Cochlear Implants International, 13*(1), 5–15.

Fortnum, H. M., Summerfield, A. Q., Marshall, D. H., Davis, A. C., & Bamford, J. M. (2001). Prevalence of permanent childhood hearing impairment in the United Kingdom and implications for universal neonatal hearing screening: Questionnaire-based ascertainment study. *BMJ (Clinical Research Ed.), 323*(7312), 536–540.

Geers, A. E., Brenner, C. A., & Tobey, E. (2010). Long-term outcomes of cochlear implantation in early childhood: Sample characteristics and data collection. *Ear and Hearing, 32*, 2S–12S.

Geers, A. E., & Hayes, H. (2011). Reading, writing, and phonological processing skills of adolescents with 10 or more years of cochlear implant experience. *Ear and Hearing, 32*(Suppl. 1), 49S–59S.

Geers, A. E., Moog, J. S., Biedenstein, J., Brenner, C., & Hayes, H. (2009). Spoken language scores of children using cochlear implants compared to hearing age-mates at school entry. *Journal of Deaf Studies and Deaf Education, 14*(3), 371–385.

Geers, A. E., Strube, M. J., Tobey, E. A., Pisoni, D. B., & Moog, J. S. (2011). Epilogue: Factors contributing to long-term outcomes of cochlear implantation in early childhood. *Ear and Hearing, 32*(1, Suppl), 84S–92S.

Goldberg, D. M., & Flexer, C. (2001). Auditory-verbal graduates: Outcome survey of clinical efficacy. *Journal of the American Academy of Audiology, 12*(8), 406–414.

Karchmer, M. A., & Mitchell, R. E. (2003). Demographic and achievement characteristics of deaf and hard-of-hearing students. In M. Marschark & P. Spencer (Eds.), *Oxford handbook of deaf studies, language and education* (pp. 21–37). New York: Oxford University Press.

Karchmer, M. A., & Trybus, R. J. (1977). *Who are the deaf children in "mainstream" programs? (Series R, no. 4)*. Washington, DC: Gallaudet College, Office of Demographic Studies.

Kluwin, T. N., & Stinson, M. S. (1993). *Deaf students in local public high schools: Background, experiences, and outcomes*. Springfield, IL: Charles C Thomas.

Lee, L. (1974). *Developmental sentence analysis*. Evanston, IL: Northwestern University Press.

Ling, D. (2002). *Speech and the hearing-impaired child: Theory and practice* (2nd ed.). Washington, DC: Alexander Graham Bell Association for the Deaf.

Ling, D., & Ling, A. H. (1978). *Aural habilitation: The foundations of verbal learning in hearing-impaired children*. Washington, DC: Alexander Graham Bell Association for the Deaf, Inc.

Luckner, J. L., Schauermann, D., & Allen, R. (1994). Learning to be a friend. *Perspectives in Education and Deafness, 12*(5), 2–7.

Mackay, A. W. (2007). *Inclusion! What is inclusion anyway? Questions and answers about the Mackay report on inclusion*. Fredericton, NB: Department of Education, Government of New Brunswick.

MacWhinney, B. (2000). *The CHILDES project: Tools for analysing talk, volume 1: Transcription format and programs; volume 2: The database*. Mawah, NJ: Lawrence Erlbaum Associates.

Marschark, M. (2007). *Raising and educating a deaf child* (2nd ed.). New York: Oxford University Press.

Miller, J. F. (1981). *Assessing language production in children*. Boston, MA: Allyn & Bacon.

Miller, J. F., & Chapman, R. (2003). *Systematic Analysis of Language Transcripts (SALT)* [Computer porgram]. Madison, WI: University of WIsconsin–Madison.

Moog, J. S., Geers, A. E., Gustus, C. H., & Brenner, C. A. (2011). Psychosocial adjustment in adolescents who have used cochlear implants since preschool. *Ear and Hearing, 32*(1, Suppl), 75S–83S.

Most, T. (2007). Speech intelligibility, loneliness, and sense of coherence among deaf and hard-of-hearing children in individual inclusion and group inclusion. *Journal of Deaf Studies and Deaf Education, 12*(4), 495–503.

Nicholas, J. G., & Geers, A. E. (2007). Will they catch up? The role of age at cochlear implantation in the spoken language development of children with severe to profound hearing loss. *Journal of Speech, Language, and Hearing Research, 50*(4), 1048–1062.

Olmstead, T., Mischook, M., & Doucet, S. P. (in press). Communication auditive-verbale en pratique à l'école. In E. M. Fitzpatrick & S. P. Doucet (Eds.). *Apprendre à écouter et à parler: La déficience auditive chez l'enfant.* Ottawa, ON: Les Presses de l'Université d'Ottawa.

Owens, R. O. (2008). *Language development: An introduction* (7th ed.). Boston: Allyn & Bacon Publishers.

Paul, R., & Norbury, C. F. (2012). *Language disorders from infancy through adolescence: Listening, speaking, reading, writing, and communicating* (4th ed.). St. Louis, MO: Elsevier, Inc.

Pollack, D. (1977). *Educational audiology for the limited hearing infant* (4th ed.). Springfield, IL: Charles C Thomas Publisher.

Power, D., & Hyde, M. (2002). The characteristics and extent of participation of deaf and hard of hearing students in regular classes in Australian schools. *Journal of Deaf Studies and Deaf Education, 7*(4), 302–311.

Power, D., & Hyde, M. (2003). Itinerant teachers of the deaf and hard of hearing and their students in Australia: Some state comparisons. *International Journal of Disability Development and Education, 50*(4), 385–401.

Powers, S. (1996a). Inclusion is an attitude not a place: Part 1. *Journal of the British Association of the Teachers of the Deaf, 20*(2), 35–41.

Powers, S. (1996b). Inclusion is an attitude not a place: Part 2. *Journal of the British Association of the Teachers of the Deaf, 20*(3), 65–69.

Smaldino, J. J., & Flexer, C. (2012). *Handbook of acoustic accessibility: Best practices for listening, learning and literacy in the classroom.* New York: Thieme Medical Publishers.

Spencer, P. E., & Marschark, M. (2010). *Evidence-based practice in educating deaf and hard-of-hearing students.* New York: Oxford University Press.

Stinson, M. S., & Antia, S. D. (1999). Considerations in educating deaf and hard-of-hearing students in inclusive settings. *Journal of Deaf Studies and Deaf Education, 4*(3), 163–175.

Stinson, M. S., & Liu, Y. (1999). Participation of deaf and hard-of-hearing students in classes with hearing students. *Journal of Deaf Studies and Deaf Education, 4*(3), 191–202.

Stinson, M. S., & Whitmire, K. A. (2000). Adolescents who are deaf or hard of hearing: A communication perspective on educational placement. *Topics in Language Disorders, 20*(2), 58–72.

Watkin, P. M., & Baldwin, M. (2011). Identifying deafness in ealy childhood: Requirements after the newborn hearing screen. *Achives of Disorders in Childhood, 96,* 62–66.

Wilkes, E. (2003). *Cottage Acquisition Scales for Listening, Language and Speech (CASLLS).* San Antonio: TX: Sunshine Cottage.

Yoshinaga-Itano, C. (2003). From screening to early identification and intervention: Discovering predictors to successful outcomes for children with significant hearing loss. *Journal of Deaf Studies and Deaf Education, 8*(1), 11–30.

10   Literacy, Listening, and Spoken Language

Literacy for all children, including those affected with hearing loss, remains an important theme in education. Essential to full participation as an independent member of society is the ability to achieve a high level of competency in reading and writing. Illiteracy is a major economic cost for the individual, the family, and society (Maxwell & Teplova, 2007). We have seen in previous chapters that dramatic changes have occurred in the last decades, with the advance of hearing technologies providing children with hearing loss access to sound and enabling them to learn to listen and speak. However, the acquisition of competent literacy skills joins spoken language development as one of the major challenges for a child with hearing loss. This chapter highlights the relationship between audition, spoken language, and literacy and discusses the interaction between audition and spoken language. The impact of hearing loss on the typical acquisition of literacy skills is discussed, and practical intervention activities are described.

What Is Literacy?

Literacy has been defined in a variety of ways. The ABC Life Literacy Canada defines literacy as "the ability to understand and employ printed information in daily activities at home, at work, and in the community—to achieve one's goals, and to develop one's knowledge and potential" (Organization for Economic Co-operation and Development, Human Resources Development Canada, and Statistics Canada, 1997). Desjardins (2004) defined literacy in terms of intermediate outcomes, such as knowledge and skills, but mostly in terms of long-term outcomes, such as economic, physical, and social well-being for adults who use reading and learning in their personal and professional lives. Paul and Whitelaw (2011, p. 178) refer to reading more specifically as "a complex entity that involves language, cognitive, and affective factors."

Literacy and Hearing Loss

Historical Perspective

Literacy is not a new topic for children with hearing loss—as long as there have been concerns related to the education of children with hearing loss, there has been research and discussion about the best practices for developing reading and writing skills. In the early 1900s, Pintner (1918) published a series of research documenting the relationship between reading, language, and deafness. A century later, literacy is more then ever a preoccupation in the education of children with hearing loss. Since the early 1800s, with the opening of the first schools for the deaf in the United States, a plethora of communication approaches have been advocated for the development of language skills. Along with these diverse communication methods, many different techniques have been applied to teach children to read and write. Various models proposed for teaching reading to children with normal hearing are also used in developing reading skills in children with hearing loss (Paul & Whitelaw, 2011). Some models focus primarily on cognitive processes, leading to the reading of isolated words and the identification of letters and associated sounds, while other models focus on comprehension and on the similarities between language acquisition and reading acquisition.

Historically, children with prelingual deafness showed severe delays in the acquisition of literacy skills. The Babbidge (1965) report heightened awareness of major difficulties, revealing that students with hearing loss rarely achieved a reading level past the 3rd to 5th grade level at graduation from high school. Research has shown that as many as 50% of children with hearing loss achieve a median reading comprehension corresponding to about a 4th grade level for hearing students (Gallaudet Research Institute, 2003; Traxler, 2000). Over all, numerous studies have documented delayed literacy skills in children with hearing loss, including those in oral education programs. However, other studies have demonstrated that children with hearing loss who have had early access to amplification and who are learning in a regular school setting achieve better literacy outcomes (Antia, Jones, Reed, & Kreimeyer, 2009; Geers, Strube, Tobey, Pisoni, & Moog, 2011). For example, in the study by Geers et al (2011), children who received a cochlear implant before 2 years of age were more likely to show better results in language and literacy at high school than those who were implanted at 4 to 5 years of age.

Relationship between Language, Audition, and Literacy

Children with hearing loss appear to follow the same sequence of literacy development as their peers with normal hearing (Mayer, 2007; Williams, 2004). However, as mentioned previously, acquiring reading and writing skills has always been one of the main challenges for children with hearing loss. Recent research relates reading difficulties to langage delays, specifically difficulties in phonological processing, vocabulary, sentence structure, and conversation (Moeller, Tomblin, Yoshinaga-Itano, Connor, & Jerger, 2007; Perfetti & Sandak, 2000). Children with limited or late access to hearing in the preschool years miss out on the acoustic information underlying the foundations for developing age-appropriate language competencies, and are, therefore, at risk for delayed literacy skills (Robertson, 2009). For example, studies have shown a strong correlation between language and phonological awareness in preschoolers with normal hearing (Chaney, 1992; Perfetti & Sandak, 2000). Phonological awareness is the ability to segment sentences into words, to recognize and produce rhymes, to segment, isolate, and blend phonemes in spoken words, and to manipulate phonemes. In their study on children's use of phonology, Perfetti and Sandak (2000) exposed the contribution of strong spoken language foundations in accessing written language.

Research in children with normal hearing has identified three fundamental skills that form the foundation for literacy acquisition: vocabulary, phonological awareness, and alphabetic principle (Ehri et al, 2001). In addition, reading involves three main competencies: the ability to decode words, the ability to comprehend the meaning of written text, and reading fluency. These are influenced by the child's world knowledge and previous exposure to reading. Hearing difficulties can disrupt typical reading because reduced access to speech sounds interferes with decoding. Children, therefore, have more difficulty with written texts because of their limitations in various linguistic components, including phonology, morphology, syntax, and semantics (Marschark, 2007; Trezek, Wang, & Paul, 2010).

For children with hearing loss, there is strong evidence that being able to use phonological information while reading is a strong asset in literacy development (Colin, Magnan, Ecalle, & Leybaert, 2007; Perfetti & Sandak, 2000). As stated by Paul and Whitelaw (2011), the whole process of the development of the articulatory-auditory loop in young children with hearing loss is essential to the process of acquiring later literacy skills. Furthermore, the limited access to distance hearing and incidental hearing and learning can sometimes limit the development of conceptual knowledge, therefore interfering in the process of reading comprehension. When a child does not have the background knowledge about the subject matter of reading materials presented in the classroom, reading difficulties arise (Boisclair & Sirois, 2000; Robertson, 2009).

▪ Emergence of Literacy in Young Children

Guiding Parents

Literacy starts at birth and encompasses all of children's experiences with oral language, books, print, stories, and communication in general. Emergent literacy, as described by Williams (2004, p. 352), is the term most commonly used to represent a "new way of conceptualizing very young children's initial encounters with print and their early reading and writing development." This period is generally understood as the time before children learn to read and write conventionally.

With early identification and intervention, there are increased expectations that children with hearing loss will develop literacy skills comparable to their peers with normal hearing. However, since even a mild hearing loss can have an impact on the development of reading and writing skills (Antia et al, 2009), it is important to be aware that the early years are critical to ensure successful acquisition of later literacy skills. It is during the early years, through frequent access to books and stories, that children begin to understand the function of print and learn appropriate strategies to access the meaning of text.

Much of what we know about emergent literacy stems from an extensive body of research on children with typical hearing and spoken language development. This knowledge provides a useful structure for literacy intervention in young children with hearing loss who are using hearing to develop spoken language.

Evidence from research examining emergent literacy for children with hearing loss suggests that they follow the same path as their peers with normal hearing, that is, the same foundation skills seem to be important for both groups when learning to read (Spencer & Oleson, 2008; Williams, 2004).

Current reading models have evolved from an emphasis on reading readiness (e.g., letter identification, sound/letter associations, considered as prerequisites to learning to read), to a broader conception of literacy. Learning to read and write is now viewed as requiring the child's active participation in a series of literacy activities that starts very early in life. Oral language, reading, and writing are complementary and are learned concurrently in literacy-rich environments (Williams, 2004). It is now widely known that typically developing children enter formal learning with a considerable amount of literacy experience, including world knowledge and various literacy abilities. **Fig. 10.1** presents the main factors influencing literacy acquisition.

Promoting Literacy at Home

Knowledge of foundation skills in literacy will help the clinician/teacher support parents in stimulating these aspects in their young children. Parents need to develop an understanding of the relationship between audition, language,

and literacy. Armed with this knowledge, parents following early intervention programs can learn how to promote literacy skills at home by stimulating from a very early age the child's spoken language, concrete and abstract vocab-

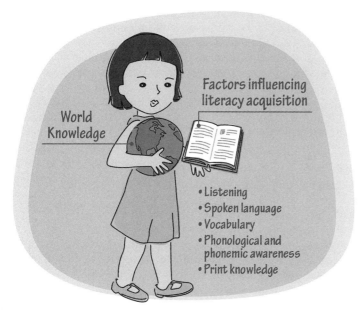

Fig. 10.1 Factors influencing literacy acquisition.

ulary, complex language structures, rhymes, and print awareness. Parents also need to be sensitized to the challenges that hearing loss creates for a child when learning to read and need to be guided on how to reduce the barriers to achieving competent reading skills.

From birth, parents should be encouraged to create literacy-rich environments to facilitate the acquisition of later reading and writing skills for their child. Since hearing loss affects incidental hearing and learning, children often do not overhear spontaneous conversations that take place during story reading. It is imperative to master the conversational forms of a language to facilitate later comprehension of the the the written form of a language (Trezek et al, 2010). In addition, because of their reduced hearing abilities,

children may miss common expressions and vocabulary associated with reading, such as the title, cover page, authors' names, and publishing information. To this effect, children benefit from being exposed to different types of print, such as newspapers, magazines, store flyers, pamphlets, cookbooks, and game rules. Components of a stimulating family environment for the promotion of literacy skills include the quality and quantity of spoken language, opportunities for conversations with adults to ensure exposure to complex and varied language models, access to a variety of books, and being read to aloud frequently (Robertson, 2009). Learning to read starts very early during the preschool years when cognitive and linguistic foundations are put into place (Snow, Burns, & Griffin, 1998).

Reading Aloud

Reading aloud has been identified as the single most important activity to build a knowledge base in children to ensure later competency in literacy (Anderson, Hiebert, Scott, & Wilkinson, 1985; Hoffman, Roser, & Battle, 1993). It is, therefore, essential that parents be encouraged and guided very early on to read aloud to their child. To compensate for reduced auditory input, it seems reasonable to conclude that children with hearing loss need more direct intervention and more frequent exposure to books and stories than their peers with normal hearing (Cole & Flexer, 2011; Robertson, 2009).

There are numerous benefits to reading aloud, as the practice helps establish the foundations necessary for later learning to read and write, that is, mastering the language of instruction and developing good conceptual and background knowledge while expanding vocabulary (Beck & McKewon, 2001). Other, very important advantages of reading aloud include establishing positive attitudes toward reading (Silvern, 1985), as well as developing auditory attention, imagination, creativity, inferencing from pictures and text, and problem solving skills (Trelease, 2006). Research has also shown that children improve their language and literacy skills when parents foster their active participation in story readings (Reese & Cox, 1999; Whitehurst et al, 1999). Guiding parents of children with hearing loss to read aloud daily ensures exposure to linguistic content that is at a more advanced level than spoken language heard in many every-

day environments. This practice facilitates lexical development and the comprehension of complex sentence structures. When reading aloud, parents can encourage their child to visualize and create mental images of the story. Different types of questions can be asked during the reading of a book, such as literal, inferential, and evaluative questions. Furthermore, learning to question oneself while reading helps develop interest and exercise different cognitive processes essential to developing good reading competencies (Gear, 2006). Developing the ability to respond to a range of question types teaches the child to question himself during reading, a practice that increases comprehension (Gear, 2006). **Table 10.1** shows examples of different types of questions that can be asked during and after reading a storybook.

Parents can be taught numerous specific techniques to facilitate emergent literacy. One useful technique is for parents to model strategies they themselves use to facilitate reading comprehension; this can help develop the child's thinking skills. The clinician/teacher should therefore help parents to recognize various strategies that can be used to develop thinking skills in their preschool age children, such as visualizing, questioning, and making connections with background knowledge. Parents of children with hearing loss should be taught how to maximize the reading aloud activity by talking about the characters, the pictures, the events, and the problems occur-

Table 10.1 Examples of different types of questions for the book "Making the Moose Out of Life" by Nicholas Oldland, Kids Can Press (Toronto, ON, 2010)

Literal questions (the answer is clearly taken from the text)

- Where did the moose live?
- Why did the moose not go skiing? Why did the moose not go with his friends?
- What animal did the moose meet on the deserted island?

Inferential questions (the answer is implicit in the text)

- Why did the moose feel he was missing something when not playing with his friends?
- Why did the moose decide to hop on the sailboat and go for a ride?
- What do you think happened to change the moose so that, at the end, he was not afraid anymore?

Evaluative questions (the child relates to his own experience to answer the questions)

- Why do you think the moose was always afraid of something at the beginning?
- Have you ever had a frightening experience?
- What do you do to avoid being afraid of something?

ring in the book. As Robertson (2009) stated, parents should read "with" the child and not "to" the child. To ensure acquisition of a range of competencies, such as vocabulary, print awareness, and sequencing, the child should be an active participant in the whole language and literacy experience (Mayer, 2007). Discussions about events in a story and about the different characters may also facilitate the development of social cognition and learning about the perspective of others, that is, theory of mind. The limited research on theory of mind in children with hearing loss suggests that even those who acquire spoken language demonstrate difficulties developing these skills (Figueras-Costa & Harris, 2001). Limited auditory access to conversation in the environment causes the child to miss incidental language and interaction that contribute to development of theory of mind. One way to help compensate for this lack of input is to provide the child with many opportunities to reflect on the mental and emotional states of characters in books and for parents to make connections between the experiences of the characters and those of the child.

The "Life Book" or "Language Experience Book"

Another extremely useful tool to help promote language and literacy skills in young children with hearing loss is the "life book," or what is more commonly known as the "language experience book." Not only does it help enrich the child's daily language experiences, but it can also be used to introduce new vocabulary, concepts, and complex sentence structures. When the child is very young, pictures of family members, familiar animals, and vehicles can be pasted in a scrapbook or notebook with the names written underneath the pictures. Action pictures can be added to ensure a variety of natural language, to enrich vocabulary, and to develop sentence structure. Any family activity, inside or outside the home, can be documented in the experience book, either by pasting pictures or making drawings from a recent visit somewhere.

Sharing the experience book with a young child offers many valuable opportunities to enhance conversational skills, promote the understanding of various types of explicit and implicit questions, and facilitate lexical acquisition (Robertson, 2009). Each entry in the experience book should have accompanying words or sentences. In early infancy, the written language should reflect the language used in the child's environment. Illustrated songs and nursery rhymes can also be included as a visual support when singing to the child. As the child ages, the language and concepts presented in the experience book become more complex, reflecting broader language and cognitive experiences that extend beyond the immediate environment. Pictures and drawings should represent events that are associated not only with the present, but also with the past and future. Writing about experiences and events offers opportunities to expand the child's linguistic and cognitive skills, including abstract thinking. When entries from the experience book are read to the child, she gradually understands the relationship between written and spoken language.

Experience books can be useful in developing narrative skills, for example, when retelling past events, such as a walk to the park or a visit to a zoo. Through pasting pictures in the book, talking about what happened, and then writing sentences describing the scenes, the child is given the opportunity to narrate the event and relate it to the written text in the experience book. Having good narrative skills has important implications for the development of imagination, as well as inferential and linguistic skills (Veneziano, 2010), which are associated with better reading abilities (Paris & Parish, 2003).

Numerous other activities can stimulate literacy and develop a child's interest in books and stories. **Table 10.2** present examples of literacy activities that can be performed at home with young children. All of these activities should take into account the participation of other family

Table 10.2 Experience book and invented stories—activities to promote literacy

The experience book—it can be started during the preschool years and continued throughout the school years:

During preschool, the experience book can be used to promote emergent literacy:
- Use of simple homemade stories that can be written and illustrated
- Illustrated sequence stories
- Drawing a picture after hearing a story read aloud
- Games with letters and letter sounds
- Illustrated rhymes
- Illustrations and texts for songs and nursery rhymes
- Expansion of vocabulary relating to a special topic taken from informative books (sea animals, space, children of the world, etc.)

During school years, the experience book can be used to expand literacy concepts:
- Follow-up activities after having read or heard a story (being a literary critic, answering questions related to the story, etc.)
- Writing of poems, short texts
- Follow-up writing exercise after a language activity (recipe, science experience, outing, etc.)
- Writing of messages to parents or to other family member
- Letters received from a friend or a family member

Invented stories and creation of books:

- During the preschool years, once the child has some expressive language, stories can be invented together.
- Writing and illustrating a story involve different processes, such as imagination, sequence, problem solving, visualization, and use of specific vocabulary.
- Many print concepts are taught, including author, illustrator, title page, back page, page number, letters, words, sentences, etc.
- The writing activity can be spread over a few days.
- Once the story is completed, the child draws the story (we start with very short stories when the child is younger, and as language is acquired, the story becomes longer and more complex).
- The language used in the story is based on the child's ideas, but written by the adult, always at a level higher than the child's receptive language to ensure the learning of new vocabulary, new concepts, and more complex sentence structures.
- Once the book is completed, the text and illustrations can be scanned to make more than one copy of the book. Those "books" can then be presented at daycare, shown to grandparents, etc.
- With school-age children, the same procedure is followed. The book can then be part of an oral presentation in class, with a copy given to the classroom and/or the school library.

members to promote enriched and varied natural spoken language interactions. Engaging the child with hearing loss, as well as all family members, in literacy enrichment will create a positive family atmosphere and constructive attitude toward stories, books, and print in general.

Supporting Literacy for School-Age Children

Literacy at school age requires a team effort for the child with hearing loss. The clinician/teacher encourages the continued involvement of the child's parents and establishes good collaboration with the classroom teacher. All members of the team should be aware of the impact of the child's hearing loss on the acquisition of literacy skills and take advantage of all learning situations to promote reading and writing. Reading competency is partially determined by the child's print and phonological awareness developed during the preschool years (Storch & Whitehurst, 2002). Phonological awareness is considered to be the best predictor of early literacy success for young readers (Wagner, Torgesen, & Rashotte, 1994; Whitehurst & Lonigan, 1998).

Problems Unique to School-Age Children with Hearing Loss

As discussed previously, the acquisition of literacy skills for children with hearng loss is similar to the process for children with normal hearing (Mayer, 2007; Paul, 2009; Williams, 2004). Children with normal hearing embark on reading at school having already had a wealth of language learning experience and opportunities to build world knowledge during the preschool years. In contrast, children with hearing loss have reduced incidental experience and a shorter learning period, placing them at risk for difficulties in the development of age-appropriate reading skills, including phonemic awareness, phonics, fluency, vocabulary, and text comprehension (National Reading Panel, 2000).

Paul (2009) contends that good knowledge of syntax is associated with good reading skills in students with hearing loss. Students who experience difficulty with the comprehension of a variety of syntactic structures can be expected to experience reading difficulties when these problematic sentence structures appear in text. Another characteristic observed in students with hearing loss is that, despite their ability to understand words or expressions in isolation, they often experience difficulties processing words when they are embedded in complex sentences (Paul, 2009). Weaknesses in spoken language translate to difficulties in reading acquisition as children are confronted with an enormous variety of written sentences. As discussed in Chapter 9, the clinician/teacher conducts a comprehensive language assessment to define the child's specific syntactic difficulties and target the linguistic skills that present challenges. Clinicians/teachers need to expose children, by reading aloud to them, from an early age, to a variety of texts that progress from simple to complex in both semantic and syntactic content, always slightly above the child's reading level, to advance her reading skills. As reported by Makdissi and Boisclair (2006), it is important that clinicians/teachers not oversimplify reading content by shortening texts or selecting written content that is comprised only of familiar words; such practices might interfere with the child's developing independent reading skills.

Writing Skills

Reading and writing are dependent on similar knowledge and cognitive processes, and strong relationships between the two have been reported (Fitzgerald & Shanahan, 2000; Shanahan, 2006). Because of this connection, parallel teaching of the two skills is recommended, and using writing to teach reading seems to lead to better results (Graham & Hebert, 2010; Tierney & Shanahan, 1991). At the same time, teaching writing through reading can help the child understand many aspects of the writing process, such as development of ideas, organization of ideas in text, and the use of specific vocabulary (Tierney & Shanahan, 1991).

Research on writing for students with hearing loss has not been as extensive as research in reading. For this population, learning to write, like reading, seems to rely on the same foundation skills of language and basic and conceptual knowledge (Boisclair & Sirois, 2000). Similar to reading, there is considerable variability in writing skills in students with hearing loss. Characteristic of students' writing is the use of shorter and much simpler sentences than their peers with normal hearing (Marschark, 2007). One study comparing students with cochlear implants to students with normal hearing showed specific difficulties for the children with hearing loss in the accurate use of syntactic structures in written sentences and production of fewer words in written narrative tasks (Spencer, Barker, & Tomblin, 2003). Taken together, studies report much lower levels of writing competencies for students with hearing loss relative to students with normal hearing (Marschark, 2007; Paul, 1998).

Intervention in Literacy

In recent years, considerable emphasis has been placed on identifying the characteristics of an efficient intervention program for children with normal hearing at risk for reading difficulties. Researchers have described several best practices in reading: early intervention of reading problems, individualized intervention taking into account the child's interests, provision of a wide variety of reading materials at home and in school, and teaching reading through meaningful text rather than teaching isolated reading strategies (Giasson, 2003; Saint-Laurent, Giasson, Simard, Dionne, & Royer, 1995; Torgeson, 2000). These practices have been found to be beneficial for children with normal hearing and can be implemented with children with hearing loss. Interventions in literacy with children with hearing loss at school age are drawn from practices with children with normal hearing. It is, therefore, of utmost importance that clinicians/teachers have knowledge of typical literacy acquisition to effectively adapt intervention strategies to address the specific needs of children with hearing loss (Trezek et al, 2010).

For the child with hearing loss, vocabulary development and syntactic abilities are often problematic areas (Marschark, 2007). The acquisition of vocabulary remains, with language acquisition and phonological and print awareness, a strong predictor of age-appropriate literacy skills (Kyle & Harris, 2006; Snow et al, 1998). In the early primary school grades, it is often stated that the child is learning to read, and that by grade three, she is reading to learn. To reach the stage of independent reading for learning, in addition to developing decoding skills, the child needs sufficient conceptual knowledge and vocabulary to access content and derive meaning from advanced texts. The clinician/teacher should take every opportunity to emphasize learning of new vocabulary and concepts through systematic teaching and encourage quality interactions with peers, parents, and other adults to develop strong foundations in vocabulary. Two methods for expanding vocabulary recommended by the National Reading Panel (2000) include specific word instruction and teaching word-learning strategies. Preteaching of new vocabulary and concepts from academic subjects can be another useful strategy to facilitate comprehension when the material is subsequently presented in class. Collaboration with regular classroom teachers is essential to find out in advance what topics will be presented. Books can be very useful tools for expanding the child's lexical and conceptual knowledge. **Table 10.3** presents a "literacy table activity" that can be used in individualized intervention to present and reinforce vocabulary and other literacy skills.

Another challenge for students with hearing loss is the comprehension of figurative language (figures of speech, metaphors, similes, and idiomatic expressions). Therefore, exposure to this type of lexical content from an early age is highly recommended, and some school-age children may require specific instruction (Luckner, Sebald, Cooney, Young, & Muir, 2006). Likewise, linguistic components, such as prefixes, suffixes, and compound words, can create difficulty for children. Presenting these types of lexical content in meaningful situations and in various contexts helps reinforce comprehension and retention.

In school, students with normal hearing continue to develop advanced thinking skills, such as complex questioning, visualizing, and inferring, to become competent readers (Gear, 2006). Students with hearing loss often require specific instruction to learn these strategies that will in turn promote and facilitate reading comprehension. Exposure to a range of reading

Table 10.3   Literacy tables

- Small table used to promote literacy activities on a certain topic (e.g., dinosaurs, friendship, the sea, spring, etc.). On the table and on the wall around the table, informative and narrative books, illustrations, and objects present information about a specific topic.

- It can be used at home or in school.

- The topic can be changed after one month and the child can help choose the next topic.

- Special activities are added to learn more about the books and objects that are on the table.

- Questions are written with the child about the topic and about areas of interest for the child. The answers to these questions are provided as we go forward in discovering the literacy table and its content.

- If the literacy table is a learning activity at school, the child is permitted to take the books home for reading and research.

- A story can be written together on the topic of the literacy table.

materials (e.g., books, magazines, newspapers, brochures) is important to provide opportunities to practice higher order thinking skills, such as cause-effect relationship, categorization, inference, and abstract thinking. It is important for students to learn not only thinking skills, but also metacognitive skills to help them understand and talk about these thinking strategies.

Students who show particular difficulty in acquiring age-appropriate reading and writing skills, despite good listening and language development, require specialized reading assessments and intervention. For example, in the case of a diagnosis such as dyslexia, a reading or other specialist frequently becomes involved in intervention and works with the school team. The inclusion of literacy experts in some school districts is a reflection of the importance currently attributed to literacy in all school-age children. Collaboration with these experts provides clinicians/teachers with opportunities to further develop knowledge and skillls that can be applied to individualized intervention sessions with students with hearing loss. Several useful resources in literacy are available in print and online. A short list of resources is presented at the end of this chapter.

Summary

Children with hearing loss are at risk for difficulties in literacy. There is a consensus that there are strong relationships between auditory and spoken language skills and literacy achievements. A fundamental theme of this chapter is that literacy development becomes an integral part of the intervention program as soon as the child's hearing loss is identified. Accordingly, the goal of audiologic rehabilitation is to guide parents to establish solid foundations in listening and spoken language to prevent later difficulties in reading and writing. Despite good spoken language, some children will require intensive and specific instruction to develop requisite skills, such as phonological awareness, vocabulary, and comprehension, to become competent readers. As discussed in Chapter 11, literacy has a long-term impact throughout the individual's life, from the early years to adulthood.

References

Anderson, R. C., Hiebert, E. H., Scott, J. A., & Wilkinson, I. A. G. (1985). *Becoming a nation of readers: The report of the commission on reading*. Champaign, IL: University of Illinois; National Academy of Education.

Antia, S. D., Jones, P. B., Reed, S., & Kreimeyer, K. H. (2009). Academic status and progress of deaf and hard-of-hearing students in general education classrooms. *Journal of Deaf Studies and Deaf Education, 14*(3), 293–311.

Babbidge, H. (1965). *Education of the deaf. A report to the Secretary of Health, Education, and Welfare by his Advisory Committee on the Education of the Deaf. Ref. No. 0–765–119*. Washington, DC: Government Printing Office.

Beck, I., & McKewon, M. G. (2001). Text talk: Capturing the benefits of read-aloud experiences for young children. *The Reading Teacher, 55,* 10–20.

Boisclair, A., & Sirois, P. (2000). L'émergence de la lecture et de l'écriture chez l'élève sourd. *Vivre le primaire, 13*(2), 34–38.

Chaney, C. (1992). Language development, metalinguistics skills, and print awareness in 3-year-old children. *Applied Psycholinguistics, 13*(4), 485–514.

Cole, E. B., & Flexer, C. (2011). *Children with hearing loss: Developing listening and talking, birth to six* (2nd ed.). San Diego, CA: Plural Publishing, Inc.

Colin, S., Magnan, A., Ecalle, J., & Leybaert, J. (2007). Relation between deaf children's phonological skills in kindergarten and word recognition performance in first grade. *Journal of Child Psychology and Psychiatry, and Allied Disciplines, 48*(2), 139–146.

Desjardins, R. (2004). *Learning for well-being: Studies using the International Adult Literacy Survey*. Stockholm, Sweden: Institute of Education, Stockholm University

Ehri, L. C., Nunes, S. R., Willows, D. M., Schuster, B. V., Yaghoub-Zadeh, Z., & Shanahan, T. (2001). Phonemic awareness instruction helps children learn to read: Evidence from the National Reading Panel's meta-analysis. *Reading Research Quarterly, 36*(3), 250–287.

Figueras-Costa, B., & Harris, P. (2001). Theory of mind development in deaf children: A nonverbal test of false-belief understanding. *Journal of Deaf Studies and Deaf Education, 6*(2), 92–102.

Fitzgerald, J., & Shanahan, T. (2000). Reading and writing relations and their development. *Educational Psychologist, 35,* 39–50.

Gallaudet Research Institute. (2003). Literacy and deaf students. Retrieved from http://www.gallaudet .edu/gallaudetresearchinstitute/publicationsand presentations/literacy.htm.

Gear, A. (2006). *Reading power: Teaching students to think while they read*. Markham, ON: Pembrooke.

Geers, A. E., Strube, M. J., Tobey, E. A., Pisoni, D. B., & Moog, J. S. (2011). Epilogue: Factors contributing to long-term outcomes of cochlear implantation in early childhood. *Ear and Hearing, 32*(1, Suppl), 84S–92S.

Giasson, J. (2003). *La lecture, de la théorie à la pratique* (2nd ed.). Montréal, PQ: Gaétan Morin éditeur.

Graham, S., & Hebert, M. (2010). *Writing to read: Evidence for how writing can improve reading*. A Report of Carnegie Corporation of New York, New York: Alliance for Excellent Education. Retrieved from http://carnegie.org/fileadmin/Media/Publications/ WritingToRead_01.pdf.

Hoffman, J. V., Roser, N. L., & Battle, J. (1993). Reading aloud in classrooms: From the modal toward the "model." *The Reading Teacher, 46,* 49–76.

Kyle, F. E., & Harris, M. (2006). Concurrent correlates and predictors of reading and spelling achievement in deaf and hearing school children. *Journal of Deaf Studies and Deaf Education, 11*(3), 273–288.

Luckner, J. L., Sebald, A. M., Cooney, J., Young, J., III, & Muir, S. G. (2006). An examination of the evidence-based literacy research in deaf education. *American Annals of the Deaf, 150*(5), 443–456.

Makdissi, H., & Boisclair, A. (2006). Modèle d'intervention pour l'émergence de la littératie. *Nouveaux cahiers de la recherche en éducation, 9*(2), 147–168.

Marschark, M. (2007). *Raising and educating a deaf child* (2nd ed.). New York: Oxford University Press.

Maxwell, J., & Teplova, T. (2007). Social consequence of low language/literacy skills. *Encyclopedia of Language and Literacy Development*. Retrieved from http://literacyencyclopedia.ca/pdfs/Social_Conse quence_of_Low_LanguageLiteracySkills.pdf.

Mayer, C. (2007). What really matters in the early literacy development of deaf children. *Journal of Deaf Studies and Deaf Education, 12*(4), 411–431.

Moeller, M. P., Tomblin, J. B., Yoshinaga-Itano, C., Connor, C. M., & Jerger, S. (2007). Current state of knowledge: Language and literacy of children with hearing impairment. *Ear and Hearing, 28*(6), 740–753.

National Reading Panel. (2000). *Report on the National Reading Panel: Teaching children to read: An evidence-based assessment of the scientific research literature on reading and its implications for reading instruction*. Jessup, MD: National Institute for Literacy at ED Pubs.

Organization for Economic Co-operation and Development, Human Resources Development Canada, and Statistics Canada. (1997). Literacy skills for the knowledge society: Further results from the international adult literacy survey. Retrieved from http://abclifeliteracy.ca/adult-literacy.

Paris, A. H., & Parish, G. S. G. (2003). Assessing narrative comprehension in young children. *Reading Research Quarterly, 38*(1), 36–76.

Paul, P. V. (1998). *Literacy and deafness: The development of reading, writing, and literate thought.* Needham Heights, MA: Allyn & Bacon.

Paul, P. V. (2009). *Language and deafness* (4th ed.). Sudbury, MA: Jones & Bartlett

Paul, P. V., & Whitelaw, G. M. (2011). *Hearing and deafness: An introduction for health and education professionals.* Sudbury, MA: Jones & Bartlett.

Perfetti, C. A., & Sandak, R. (2000). Reading optimally builds on spoken language: Implications for deaf readers. *Journal of Deaf Studies and Deaf Education, 5*(1), 32–50.

Pintner, R. (1918). The measurement of language ability and language progress of deaf children. *The Volta Review, 20,* 755–764.

Reese, E., & Cox, A. (1999). Quality of adult book reading affects children's emergent literacy. *Developmental Psychology, 35*(1), 20–28.

Robertson, L. (Ed.). (2009). *Literacy and deafness: Literacy and spoken language.* San Diego, CA: Plural Publishing.

Saint-Laurent, L., Giasson, J., Simard, C., Dionne, J. J., & Royer, É. (1995). *Programme d'intervention auprès d'élèves à risque: Une nouvelle option éducative.* Montréal: Gaetan Morin éditeur.

Shanahan, T. (2006). Relations among oral language, reading, and writing development. In C. MacArthur, S. Graham & J. Fitzpgerald (Eds.), *Handbook of writing research* (pp. 171–183). New York: Guilford.

Silvern, S. (1985). Parent involvement and reading achievement: A review of reseach and implications for practice. *Childhood Education, 62*(1), 46–50.

Snow, C. E., Burns, M. S., & Griffin, P. (Eds.). (1998). *Preventing reading difficulties in young children.* Washington, DC: National Academy Press.

Spencer, L. J., Barker, B. A., & Tomblin, J. B. (2003). Exploring the language and literacy outcomes of pediatric cochlear implant users. *Ear and Hearing, 24*(3), 236–247.

Spencer, L. J., & Oleson, J. J. (2008). Early listening and speaking skills predict later reading proficiency in pediatric cochlear implant users. *Ear and Hearing, 29*(2), 270–280.

Storch, S. A., & Whitehurst, G. J. (2002). Oral language and code-related precursors to reading: Evidence from a longitudinal structural model. *Developmental Psychology, 38*(6), 934–947.

Tierney, R. J., & Shanahan, T. (1991). Research on the reading-writing relationship: Interactions, transactions, and outcomes. In R. Barr, M. Kamil, P. Mosenthal & P. D. Pearson (Eds.), *Handbook of reading research 2* (pp. 246–280). New York: Longman.

Torgeson, J. K. (2000). Individual differences in response to early interventions in reading: The lingering problem of treatment resisters. *Learning Disabilities Research & Practice, 15*(1), 55–64.

Traxler, C. B. (2000). Measuring up to performance standards in reading and mathematics: Achievement of selected deaf and hard-of-hearing students in the national norming of the 9th edition Stanford Achievement Test. *Journal of Deaf Studies and Deaf Education, 5,* 337–348.

Trelease, J. (2006). *The read-aloud handbook* (6th ed.). New York: Penguin Group.

Trezek, B. J., Wang, Y., & Paul, P. V. (2010). *Reading and deafness: Theory, research, and practice.* Clifton Park, NY: Delmar Cengage Learning.

Veneziano, E. (2010). Peut-on aider l'enfant à mieux raconter? Les effets de deux méthodes d'intervention: Conversation sur les causes et modèle de récit. In H. Makdissi, A. Boisclair, & P. Sirois (Eds.), *La littératie au préscolaire: Une fenêtre ouverte vers la scolarisation* (pp. 107–144). Québec: Presses de l'Université du Québec.

Wagner, R. K., Torgesen, J. K., & Rashotte, C. A. (1994). Development of reading-related phonological processing abilities: New evidence of bidirectional causality from a latent variable longitudinal study. *Developmental Psychology, 30*(1), 73–87.

Whitehurst, G. J., Crone, D. A., Zevenbergen, A. A., Schultz, M. D., Velting, O. N., & Fishel, J. E. (1999). Outcomes of an emergent literacy intervention from Head Start through second grade. *Journal of Educational Psychology, 91,* 261–272.

Whitehurst, G. J., & Lonigan, C. J. (1998). Child development and emergent literacy. *Child Development, 69*(3), 848–872.

Williams, C. (2004). Emergent literacy of deaf children. *Journal of Deaf Studies and Deaf Education, 9*(4), 352–365.

■ Suggested Resources

Additional Resources Related to Literacy Activities and the Development of Literacy Skills in Children

The Hanen Centre resources:
  Preschool Language and Literacy Calendar
  ABC and Beyond: Building Emergent Literacy in Early Childhood Settings
  Eworkshop.on.ca—Online teaching resource: http://www.eworkshop.on.ca/edu/core.cfm?L=1

Children's storybooks online—http://www.magic keys.com/books/#yc

Canadian Language and Literacy Network—http://www.cllrnet.ca

Robertson, L. (Ed.). (2009). *Literacy and deafness: Literacy and spoken language.* San Diego, CA: Plural Publishing.

Trelease, J. (2006). *The read-aloud handbook* (6th ed.). New York: Penguin Group.

Trezek, B. J., Wang, Y., & Paul, P. V. (2010). *Reading and deafness: Theory, research, and practice.* Clifton Park, NY: Delmar Cengage Learning.

11 Transition to Living as an Adult with Hearing Loss

Transition from school to work and to postsecondary education has taken on increased importance in the general education system as a process to prepare students for adulthood. As demands from the workforce are constantly changing with technological and labor market transformations, educational systems are facing challenges to ensure easy transition from school to the postsecondary world (Feller, 2003). Adolescents with hearing loss are at risk for experiencing difficulties in making this transition because of the high-level demands for communication in postsecondary school and the workplace, the increasing requirement to work in teams, the rapid changes in the workplace, and the need to integrate into a knowledge society more generally. Preparing students with hearing loss for postsecondary education or work requires adequate intervention to build necessary skills throughout their preschool and school years.

This chapter identifies transitional periods and issues related to health and educational services, as well as work settings. Intervention practices designed to facilitate transition as children progress to new settings are discussed. An emphasis is placed on practical tools that are used to facilitate transition with this population of youth.

Transition to Adulthood

Throughout their lives, children with hearing loss and their families will experience different transitional periods—from preschool to school, primary school to secondary school, and, finally, to postsecondary education or the workplace. High school education is a time when adolescents are engaged in learning and experiencing social contexts that help prepare them for future education and workplace activities. Even for youth who have had an overall positive inclusion experience, life beyond high school, although one of the most exciting periods, is also one of the most challenging.

Essential Competencies

Essential competencies that facilitate the completion of postsecondary education and entry into work life have been defined by government agencies and educational systems and are increasingly integrated into school curricula as early as the elementary years. Competencies may be defined as "the knowledge, skills, abilities, and behaviors that employees use in performing their work" (http://www.tbs-sct.gc.ca/tal/comp-eng.asp). **Table 11.1** presents nine core competencies that are considered essential for the workplace based on a government survey of employment settings across Canada (http://www.edu.gov.mb.ca/tvi/my_poster.pdf). These skills have been identified as fundamental for any type of job, regardless of the level of complexity of the work, and provide a foundation for building new knowledge and skills. These competencies will enable young adults to be ready to adjust to change. Other competencies that have been identified as essential for ensuring easy transition to adulthood include a range of thinking skills, such as problem solving, decision making, and critical thinking. The clinician/teacher can make an important contribution to the development of these abilities in children. Practical activities, such as role playing and experience with real-life situations, can facilitate the learning and practice of different cognitive and thinking skills. These core competencies can be a useful starting point for the preparation of students with hearing loss for life beyond high school.

Table 11.1   List of nine essential competencies for postsecondary education and the workforce

Reading texts
Document use
Numeracy
Writing
Oral communication
Working with others
Computer use
Continuous learning
Thinking skills

Source: Retrieved from http://www.edu.gov.mb.ca/tvi/my_poster.pdf

Rationale for Transitional Support

Based on a review of studies related to transition, Punch, Hyde, and Creed (2004) concluded that transition from high school to postsecondary education and the workplace is more challenging for adolescents with hearing loss than for peers with normal hearing. Communication, academic, and social issues associated with hearing loss can create barriers to a smooth transition process (Bonds, 2003; Luckner, 2002). A major study undertaken across the United States suggested that individuals, particularly those with severe to profound hearing loss, achieved lower levels of postsecondary education, which lead to higher unemployment levels and significant societal costs (Mohr et al, 2000). This report provided an impetus for the importance of early access to hearing (e.g., through cochlear implants) for these individuals. Some research has also reported that parents had lower expectations for postsecondary education for their adolescents with hearing loss (Danermark, Antonson, & Lundström, 2001; Warick, 1994).

It is important to note that much of the literature on this topic includes a range of severity of hearing loss, and may not necessarily reflect the current or expected situation for today's young adults and newly identified children, who have greater access to early intervention and modern hearing aids and cochlear implant technologies. As noted by Geers (2006), current expectations for children with hearing loss are "a moving target," that is, given the continuing advances in technology and intervention, there is a risk that some research findings become rapidly outdated. For example, a recent study of 112 high school students who received cochlear implants before age 5 showed that 47 to 66% achieved scores on reading tests comparable to their peers with normal hearing (Geers & Hayes, 2011). Another study of 43 adolescents and young adults in Canada also reported encouraging results. At the time of the study, all were either attending high school (58%) or had graduated (42%) from high school. All but four of the young people who completed high school were in, or had undertaken, postsecondary studies (Eriks-Brophy et al, 2012). Goldberg and Flexer (1993, 2001) conducted two surveys with American and Canadian graduates of auditory-verbal programs to document their status. The results revealed that the vast majority were either studying or working in typical environments with hearing peers. The 2001 survey found that 91% of the respondents who were high school graduates or about to graduate had been fully integrated in regular high school, and all but three of them were pursuing postsecondary education. Nevertheless, over all, studies underscore the serious impact that hearing loss can have on educational and career opportunities.

▦ Supporting Transition to Adulthood

Impact of Hearing Loss on Transition

Hearing loss affects multiple aspects of the individuals' functioning. Research with adolescents suggests continued weaknesses in spoken language, working memory, and related areas (Geers & Hayes, 2011; Geers, Strube, Tobey, Pisoni, & Moog, 2011), all of which can be expected to have a negative effect on the acquisition of core competencies. While the concerns for a young child with hearing loss relate primarily to communication development, as the child matures, there are increasing concerns about the potential impact of hearing loss on numerous other aspects of life, including academic, social development, independence, and employment (Luckner, 2002). As Luckner pointed out, students with hearing loss need a wide variety of experiences in planning, exploring, problem solving, questioning, and discussing to be better prepared for postsecondary education and/or work. Some adolescents will, therefore, require additional support compared with their peers with normal hearing in making the transition to adulthood, specifically postsecondary education or workplace settings. Like their peers, adolescents with hearing loss need to receive training in developing learning skills, such as how to study, organize their time, take notes, and proofread their work (Luckner, 2002). Adolescents with hearing loss miss the incidental learning about career choices that normal-hearing adolescents naturally overhear through informal conversations and media sources, and, therefore, may need more direct instruction in that field. Again, the notion of incidental learning can affect children at all stages of their development and learning.

Punch et al (2004) recommend fostering career maturity that involves encouraging adolescents to explore a range of career options and make informed decisions. For example, exposure to specific activities that can prepare youth for the kind of collaboration required in the workplace can be beneficial. Examples of specific activities and experiences include short-term apprenticeships and internships, job shadowing, mentoring another student, and vocational high school programs. These activities generally involve partnerships between schools, postsecondary institutions, private and public employers, and community agencies (Bonds, 2003). Accordingly, the typical school team expands to include a type of "transition team" that includes vocational rehabilitation counselors, postsecondary educators, employers, and community support workers. All of these experiences can help students learn skills and communication that are used in employment settings. The clinician/teacher can assume the role of coordinator, ensuring that the student and family are aware of the various services available.

Parents who have been actively involved in their child's listening and spoken language acquisition and subsequent academic development continue to assume a critical role in helping their child make a successful transition. Preparation begins well before the youth graduates from high school. In focus group interviews, parents of youth with hearing loss and young adults themselves described strategies that were helpful with respect to integration into community life and that may facilitate transition from school to more independent decision making and living (Eriks-Brophy et al, 2007). For example, parents stressed the importance of ensuring that adolescents develop autonomy and are given opportunities for diverse experiences, such as social groups and part-time employment, to build skills and gain confidence in their own capabilities. Such experiences provide youth with opportunities where they are required to use different types of social language (e.g., serving customers) and social behavior.

Strategies to Facilitate Transition

Many school systems have well-developed programs aimed at developing essential competencies for adulthood. Even adolescents with normal hearing who have typical communication skills can benefit from this guidance. However, some school programs offer additional coaching and support for their students with hearing loss, with increased guidance for those who have gaps in communication or particular needs. This additional support is considered so important and a prerequisite to entering higher education or the workforce that some educational systems have implemented highly specific training programs, including an intensive "transition camp" during which students are presented with specific skills training. These experiences can provide an opportunity for exposure to other students with hearing loss who are experiencing the university or work environment, which has been proposed as one successful transitional strategy for adolescents (Flexer & Wray, 1990).

The following case describes the process that was undertaken in one school district for a youth who was at risk of having difficulties transitioning from high school to college. A consideration of each student's academic and functional abilities is required to help adolescents make realistic career choices. This evaluation extends beyond typical standardized language tests and should take into account the students' skills, interests, and potential for advanced education and/or integration into the workplace.

Simone is a 22-year-old young woman with bilateral severe sensorineural hearing loss. She has a twin sister with normal hearing. She was diagnosed at 3 years of age and fitted with bilateral hearing aids 2 months later. Listening and spoken language intervention were offered at home to Simone and her mother right after amplification. She attended her local school and continued receiving intervention services three times a week from a clinician/teacher. Her spoken language progressed at a slow rate, and in the primary grades she exhibited severe delays in vocabulary as well as difficulties in reading and writing. Throughout the school years, she continued to make some progress in receptive and expressive oral language, but her vocabulary remained severely delayed. Scores on the Peabody Picture Vocabulary Test, a receptive vocabulary measure, showed a 4-year delay at age 10, and later assessments indicated that she was not closing the gap. Although she attended a class with children with normal hearing, she received an individualized educational program throughout most of her schooling.

In high school, Simone was considered at risk for becoming a high school dropout. The results of a psychosocial evaluation at age 16 showed a mild cognitive delay and difficulties in the areas of social and emotional functioning. During the adolescent years, services in listening and language were increased to boost her oral communication skills. In addition, Simone was provided with specific services from a clinician/teacher who specialized in transition coaching to try to ensure school retention and to prepare her with specific skills for life after school. Part-time work in the community was organized during school hours (restaurant, residence for older people, pet grooming services). She also participated in weekend transition camps where she had the opportunity to meet other youth with hearing loss and to learn about many aspects of life as an adult. Transition services were maintained for an additional year after high school graduation to facilitate her successful integration into the community. Simone was enrolled in a program for individuals with intellectual delays and participated also in an independent daily living program, during which she stayed with a foster family in another community close to her home. She received services from a counselor who worked on independent living skills with individuals who have complex needs. Through this program she learned to use public transportation and other daily skills, such as banking. Simone's next big step is to attend the community college, where she plans to study early child education. Because of all her delays, a special program will be designed that involves a high number of practicum hours in child care placements so that she can obtain her certificate. Transition services for Simone have been critical in enabling her to finish high school and to successfully integrate into her community.

Transition Goals

An example of goals enumerated in one school district's transition program for youth with hearing loss is shown in **Table 11.2**. Although at first glance, these goals are common to all high school students, when providing support for youth with hearing loss, clinicians/ teachers often integrate these elements into their direct intervention services. For example, while working on telephone training, one can select vocabulary pertinent to a job application or create scenarios such as a work interview. When developing advanced writing skills, spe-

Table 11.2   Key elements to target in transition intervention

- Self-knowledge—interests, skills, aptitudes, learning styles

- Learning about careers—job responsibilities, training required, skills and competencies, salary, etc.

- Prerequisites for different jobs—compulsory high school courses, designated colleges and/or universities

- Understanding the job research process, resume, job application letter

- Financial literacy—budget, bank account, credit, income taxes, pension funds, etc.

- Assistive devices facilitating independence—fire alarms, doorbells, etc.

cific activities, such as an application letter and job resume, can be the material used to improve these skills. In essence, as described in Chapter 9, similar to integrating academic goals such as social science vocabulary, the clinicians/teachers aim to equip the adolescent with specific skills and knowledge while refining listening and spoken communication.

Another important aspect of career preparation for adolescents involves learning about the environmental and attitudinal barriers they might face as adults so that they can address them beyond high school. Studies have shown that adults with hearing loss are frequently uncomfortable discussing their hearing needs and making suggestions for accommodations with their employer or postsecondary program (Flexer & Wray, 1990; Laroche, Garcia, & Barrette, 2000). Previous research has also shown that adolescents arrive at college or university with limited information about their hearing loss, hearing aids, assistive listening devices, and the academic requirements at the postsecondary level (Flexer & Wray, 1990). Health literacy is, therefore, an important aspect of career preparation that clinicians/teachers can include in intervention programs. Very early on, students should learn that hearing and listening are their own responsibility, that they should monitor their own listening devices, and advise appropriate individuals (e.g., audiologist or teacher) of hearing difficulties they might encounter in school or other environments (Anderson & Arnoldi, 2011). They should also learn how to make communication partners aware of communication breakdowns. Harmer (1999) reported that

adults with hearing loss do not always possess the necessary self-advocacy skills to acquire information about the health care services they need, and do not know when to request appropriate services. In transitioning from pediatric to adult health care centers, youth and clinicians have reported that adapting can be difficult (Olds et al, 2012). For example, in some cases, parents continue to make health appointments for their adolescents and have difficulty allowing them to take responsibility for their hearing needs. Adolescents can be taught health and work literacy terminology as well as self-advocacy skills to help them find solutions to challenges in workplace, educational, and health settings. Our overall goal is to equip the youth with solid self-advocacy skills to be used in a variety of life situations in adulthood. For further discussion on self-advocacy and self-determination in adolescents with hearing loss, the reader is referred to Duncan, Rhoades, and Fitzpatrick (in press) and Anderson and Arnoldi (2011).

Students are also informed of resources for individuals with disabilities. These include financial supports (e.g., scholarships or special grants), associations and government programs that support the integration of people with disabilities into their communities (for example, special summer employment opportunities), as well as the availability of special services in postsecondary institutions. Very importantly, information is also provided about the utility of alerting and assistive devices beyond FM systems, such as visual alarm systems and various communication devices to encourage the youth to develop independence.

Summary

Academic preparation and counseling to facilitate the transition to postsecondary education or the workplace are an important component of support during the high school years. However, preparation for transition to adulthood should start long before high school and students with hearing loss need to be taught self-advocacy skills from early childhood. As we have seen previously, the development of literacy and communication skills is essential to ensure success in adulthood and should be part of transition intervention. Parents continue to play a very important role in the transition process and should be involved every step of the way, but their role changes as they aim to foster their child's autonomy. The clinician/teacher works in collaboration with the student, parents, and other school personnel to prepare the student for transition to adulthood. Resources and the approach to transitional support vary according to school policies and practices. Partnerships with community agencies that provide vocational programs and support individuals with hearing loss have been viewed as an important step in preparing youth for post high school educational and career choices.

Acknowledgments

We are grateful to Gisèle Desjardins, a specialized teacher for children with hearing loss, New Brunswick, Canada, for sharing many practical strategies applied in transition programs with youth.

References

Anderson, K. L., & Arnoldi, K. A. (2011). *Building skills for success in the fast-paced classroom: Optimizing achievement for students with hearing loss.* Hillsboro, OR: Butte Publications.

Bonds, B. G. (2003). School-to-work experiences: Curriculum as a bridge. *American Annals of the Deaf, 148*(1), 38–48.

Danermark, B., Antonson, S., & Lundström, I. (2001). Social inclusion and career development—transition from upper secondary school to work or post-secondary education among hard of hearing students. *Scandinavian Audiology. Supplementum, 30*(53), 120–128.

Duncan, J., Rhoades, E. A., & Fitzpatrick, E. M. (in press). *Auditory rehabilitation for adolescents with hearing loss.* New York: Oxford University Press.

Eriks-Brophy, A., Durieux-Smith, A., Olds, J., Fitzpatrick, E., Duquette, C., & Whittingham, J. (2007). Facilitators and barriers to the inclusion of orally educated children and youth with hearing loss into their families and communities. *The Volta Review, 107*(1), 5–36.

Eriks-Brophy, A., Durieux-Smith, A., Olds, J., Fitzpatrick, E., Duquette, C., & Whittingham, J. (2012). Communication, academic, and social skills of young adults with hearing loss. *The Volta Review, 112*(1), 5–35.

Feller, R. W. (2003). Aligning school counseling, the changing workplace, and career development assumptions. *Professional School Counseling, 6,* 262–271.

Flexer, C., & Wray, D. (1990). Post-secondary mainstreaming in a state college: Akron, Ohio. In M. Ross (Ed.), *Hearing-impaired children in the mainstream* (pp. 245–256). Parkton, MA: York Press, Inc.

Geers, A. E. (2006). Spoken language in children with cochlear implants. In P. E. Spencer & M. Marschark (Eds.), *Advances in the spoken language development of deaf and hard-of-hearing children.* New York: Oxford University Press.

Geers, A. E., & Hayes, H. (2011). Reading, writing, and phonological processing skills of adolescents with 10 or more years of cochlear implant experience. *Ear and Hearing, 32*(Suppl. 1), 49S–59S.

Geers, A. E., Strube, M. J., Tobey, E. A., Pisoni, D. B., & Moog, J. S. (2011). Epilogue: Factors contributing to long-term outcomes of cochlear implantation in early childhood. *Ear and Hearing, 32*(1, Suppl), 84S–92S.

Goldberg, D. M., & Flexer, C. (1993). Outcome survey of auditory-verbal graduates: Study of clinical efficacy. *Journal of the American Academy of Audiology, 4*(3), 189–200.

Goldberg, D. M., & Flexer, C. (2001). Auditory-verbal graduates: Outcome survey of clinical efficacy. *Journal of the American Academy of Audiology, 12*(8), 406–414.

Harmer, L. M. (1999). *Health care delivery and deaf people: Practice, problems, and recommendations for change.* New York: Oxford University Press.

Laroche, C., Garcia, L. J., & Barrette, J. (2000). Perceptions by persons with hearing impairment, audiologists, and employers of the obstacles to workplace integration. *Journal of the Academy of Rehabilitative Audiology, 33,* 61–90.

Luckner, J. L. (2002). *Facilitating the transition of students who are deaf or hard of hearing.* Austin, TX. PRO-ED, Inc.

Mohr, P. E., Feldman, J. J., Dunbar, J. L., McConkey-Robbins, A., Niparko, J. K., Rittenhouse, R. K., & Skinner, M. W. (2000). The societal costs of severe to profound hearing loss in the United States. *International Journal of Technology Assessment in Health Care, 16*(4), 1120–1135.

Olds, J., Fitzpatrick, E., Séguin, C., Moran, L., Whittingham, J., & Schramm, D. (2012). Facilitating the transition from the pediatric to adult cochlear implant setting: Perspectives of CI professionals *Cochlear Implants International,* 13, 5–15.

Punch, R., Hyde, M., & Creed, P. A. (2004). Issues in the school-to-work transition of hard of hearing adolescents. *American Annals of the Deaf, 149*(1), 28–38.

Warick, R. (1994). A profile of Canadian hard-of-hearing youth. *Canadian Journal of Speech-Language Pathology and Audiology, 18,* 253–259.

12 Audiologic Rehabilitation around the World

Contributions from Cindy Bell, Anita Bernstein, Cheryl Dickson, Dimity Dornan, Jill Duncan, Warren Estabrooks, Jasmine Gallant, Erin Gilbert, Donald M. Goldberg, Bruno Leprette, Sonia Leprette, Stephanie Lim, Mary McGinnis, Jean Sachar Moog, Jan North, Ellen A. Rhoades, Jacqueline Stokes

Throughout this book, we have attempted to assemble the best available evidence related to listening and spoken language development in children with hearing loss. Based on this evidence and our clinical experience, we have presented practical guidelines and strategies for developing spoken communication from infancy to adolescence. In this final chapter, it is important to underscore that no single model of care has been demonstrated to be "the best." Here, we take the reader "around the world" to highlight many different programs that have demonstrated positive outcomes in the development of spoken language in children.

Our goal is to profile different milieus and different types of service delivery models where prac-

titioners provide listening and spoken language services. We therefore invited colleagues who practice in different countries, work settings, and under different funding arrangements to identify the core ingredients of effective care. We selected practitioners who work with a range of children and families. Although we would have liked to present a snapshot of services at a country level, we knew that this would not be possible, given the differences in funding, philosophy, geography, and availability of trained professionals within a single country. We therefore opted to highlight a selection of diverse programs in several different countries. Finally, we also invited parents to share their perspectives on "what works" in developing listening and spoken language.

Perspectives from Around the World

Perspective of Practitioners

We invited practitioners from nine centers to contribute their views on audiologic rehabilitation. Specifically, individuals were asked to:

- Describe their service model: clinic, school, frequency of visits, home visiting, and funding arrangements (e.g., public health or education service, private practice, privately funded services).
- Present their expectations for children with hearing loss with respect to auditory, speech, and language functioning

at school entry. Since we were interested in exposing different perspectives, we requested that professionals provide outcome results based on data collected in their program when available and/or their clinical impressions, rather than a review of published literature.
- Describe the key ingredients of an effective program for audiologic rehabilitation.
- Identify the current issues and key challenges related to improving listening and spoken language outcomes in children.

From the Practitioners

In our presentation of the practitioners' summaries, rather than seek uniformity, we decided to respect the diversity and allow different viewpoints to emerge. Our goal is to present a "world" overview of perspectives of professionals and parents. A qualitative analysis of practitioners' contributions revealed several common themes.

Expectations. It is clear that today, professionals working in auditory rehabilitation expect that the vast majority of children with hearing loss can develop age-appropriate spoken language skills and attend general education programs alongside their peers with normal hearing. Spoken language for children with hearing loss has been a highly desirable goal for many decades (Ling & Ling, 1978; Pollack, 1977). These contributions indicate that, compared with 30 to 40 years ago, age-appropriate spoken language has become a worldwide norm for many typically developing children in countries where early identification and hearing technology are available. Furthermore, speech comparable to peers with normal hearing has become the expected outcome. As noted by several practitioners, when these outcomes are not achieved, it is due to other factors, such as developmental disabilities or specific environmental or family factors that prevent optimal access to technology and intervention.

Effective intervention. Through these practitioners' writings, quality pediatric audiology services and, particularly, a partnership between audiology and rehabilitation emerged as one of the core components of effective intervention. A closely related theme was the importance of monitoring and ensuring the very best hearing technology for children. Parent guid-

ance through specific auditory-based therapy was considered a key ingredient of care.

Challenges. The number of common concerns related to spoken language development across many different countries was striking. Key issues can be summarized in two main interrelated categories: (1) professional skills and training, and (2) delay to quality intervention, including difficulties with access to audiology, technology, and therapy services due to geographical or other region-specific barriers. It is also of interest to note some of the very specific issues that emerged. For example, in Australia, the vastness of the country was raised as a challenge to providing intervention services, and in Singapore, multicultural and multilinguistic needs were highlighted. In England, there was concern about organizational resistance to change related to rehabilitation services. Professionals in the United States noted lack of choice in intervention and expectations for auditory and spoken language development as key issues.

Dimity Dornan, Australia, Hear and Say

Hear and Say is a not-for-profit early intervention and implantable hearing technologies program based in Brisbane, Queensland, Australia, servicing over 520 children, and specializing in auditory-verbal therapy (AVT). The program follows the principles of listening and spoken language (LSLS). The program has seven LSLS certified auditory-verbal therapists. Full audiologic services are available, including diagnostics, cochlear implant program, troubleshooting, and regular monitoring of hearing aids and cochlear implants. All hearing aids are owned and fitted by Australian Hearing according to the National Acoustics Laboratory (NAL) protocol, and assessment follows the Alexander Graham Bell Academy for Listening and Spoken Language Recommended Audiologic Protocol. Children and at least one parent attend once per week for 1–1½ hours of AVT. Some children in outreach areas may receive the equivalent in short blocks of therapy.

Expectations for children with hearing loss. Expectations are based on a research study on outcomes of the AVT program at Hear and Say (Dornan, Hickson, Murdoch, Houston, & Constantinescu, 2010). The study had a matched group, repeated measures design, and was developed to measure outcomes for a group of 19 children aged 2 to 6 years educated with AVT. At the com-

mencement of the study, the AVT and TH (typical hearing) groups of children were matched for gender, language age, receptive vocabulary, and socioeconomic level. The children were tested at various time points, including the pretest (baseline), followed by posttests at 9, 21, 38, and 50 months from the start of the study. A battery of speech perception, language, and speech tests was devised to measure the speech perception, language, and speech outcomes for the two groups. The test battery included speech perception tests for the AVT group (live and recorded voice) and speech and language assessments for both groups of children. Reading, mathematics, and self-esteem assessments were added at the 38- and 50-month posttests for both the AVT and TH groups.

Results showed that the speech perception skills for the AVT group improved significantly (p < 0.05) from the pretest to the 38-months posttest for both the live and recorded voice measures. From the 38-months to the 50-months posttest, speech perception scores for live voice remained high and stable, and recorded voice scores were moderately high, indicating a good level of speech perception skills.

Over all, the total language, receptive vocabulary, and speech measures showed that significant progress was made for both the AVT and TH groups for the children who continued (*n* = 19) over the course of the study (pretest to 50 months). There were no significant differences in the rates of progress between the two groups for total language, receptive vocabulary, and speech skills from the pretest to the 50-months posttest. Mean total language score for the AVT group was only two months lower than the TH group at the 50-months posttest.

Preliminary results for reading and mathematics were based on the scores for a small number of pairs of AVT and TH group children (*n* = 7) who had reached school age and had scores for both the 38-months and 50-months posttests. The numbers in each group were considered too small for statistical comparison. However, the scores for the AVT and TH groups were comparable at both posttests. Parents rated their child's self-esteem as high, with no significant differences between the AVT and TH groups at both the 38-months and 50-months posttests.

These research outcomes mean that, at Hear and Say, we expect children to progress in listening and spoken language at a rate of 1 year of progress in 1 year of time, and if progress is slower than this, investigations are performed. Primary factors to investigate are whether the child's hearing device is optimal for the degree and type of hearing loss, and whether other educational, medical, family, or environmental factors could be causing the delay in development.

At Hear and Say, we believe that the key ingredients of an effective program include a family focus, with parents being educated simultaneously with children. Children learn spoken language through listening, and the auditory-verbal therapist guides and coaches parents to teach their child, with the goal of full inclusion into the mainstream.

Current issues and key challenges in improving speech and language outcomes for children include funding for listening and spoken language early intervention, parents being informed of all choices, access to listening and spoken language intervention for all children whose parents choose it, and access to optimal hearing technology (e.g., bilateral cochlear implants if children need them).

Jan North and Jill Duncan, Australia, Royal Institute for Deaf and Blind Children

The Royal Institute for Deaf and Blind Children (RIDBC), established in 1861, is one of Australia's oldest charitable organizations. Through flexible service delivery options, RIDBC provides evidence-based intervention to more than 1,000 children from birth to 18 years, their families, and their school communities throughout Australia.

RIDBC administers a range of schools and services for children with hearing loss, including: an early learning program (hearing impairment), reverse integrated preschools, special schools and support services in mainstream schools, an audiology center, a teleschool (distance program), a cochlear implant educational support service, an assessment unit, community support services, and therapy services (orthoptists, speech therapists, occupational therapists, physiotherapists, educational psychologists, audiologists, and a pediatrician). (Please see www.ridbc.org.au for detailed schools and services descriptions.)

RIDBC's underpinning philosophy embraces family centeredness throughout every primary and ancillary service, whereby families are the principal decision makers for their children. RIDBC is not aligned to one service delivery philosophy, but rather acknowledges that children and families require individualized programs. Practitioners are qualified to deliver all methods used to develop and support auditory-based spoken communication, such as auditory-verbal practice, auditory-oral education, and auditory training. Practitioners introduce sign support to a small number of children who require it.

For children with hearing loss whose families have chosen auditory-based spoken language, RIDBC practitioners aim to maximize individual child growth across the linguistic, cognitive, auditory, speech, and socioemotional developmental domains. Assessment and benchmarking are fundamental service delivery components that enable practitioners to measure child progress and to structure appropriate service delivery options. Children leaving the early intervention program and transitioning to school support services receive both direct face-to-face and indirect school consultancy intervention tailored to meet their individual needs. The extent of initial mainstream school integration depends on student and family needs. Approximately 70% of children enroll directly in mainstream schools, 15% are initially partially mainstreamed, and

15% (i.e., those who have significant additional disabilities) attend a full-time special school.

A purposeful scaffold of child and family support mechanisms ensures effective children's services management and optimal student learning outcomes. Practitioners base this scaffold on a clearly articulated model of assessment and planning. Service delivery is sufficiently flexible to allow practitioners the option of adding or changing support during high stress and transition periods, such as during cochlear implant candidacy, transitions from early intervention to school, or preparing for school leaving exams. Fundamental to successful child and student outcomes is the depth and breadth of service provision available via seamless communication between all practitioners.

RIDBC is committed to employing highly qualified practitioners. To this end, it co-administers a university graduate-level teacher of the deaf training program to ensure that children and students with hearing loss across Australia receive intervention from highly qualified practitioners. Further to this aim, RIDBC administers training and development for qualified professionals across the Asia Pacific. Additionally, RIDBC practitioners participate in weekly training.

More than 20% of RIDBC's children (and their families) are from a culturally and linguistically diverse background, including children from Aboriginal and Torres Strait Islander backgrounds. RIDBC endeavors to ensure equal access to services for these children and their families through a range of community support services.

A small percentage of school-age children have a disproportionate language deficit, whereby the student's actual rate of progress does not match the anticipated rate of progress. Determining the exact nature and cause of the delay continues to be a challenge. Practitioners use assessment protocols and intensive diagnostic processes to guarantee appropriate intervention, which leads to maximum development.

Australia has a very large landmass and a relatively small population, one-third of which live outside the major cities. RIDBC is committed to ensuring that children in regional and rural areas receive high-quality support services via a comprehensive telepractice program. RIDBC has developed advanced pedagogical skills to achieve the aims of this service.

Cheryl Dickson, New Zealand, Auditory-Verbal Consultancy

International service. Over the past 30 years, I have been providing listening and spoken language (auditory-verbal, AV) services in over 15 countries. I have worked with several providers, as well as running a private practice and founding a clinic in the Philippines. Some agencies were charitable trusts, while others were run by the government. I have provided services and have consulted with both private and public programs in the development of listening and spoken language services and training programs for staff working with children and families seeking spoken language outcomes.

Expectations. It is expected that every child whose family embraces listening and spoken language intervention methods will meet his or her own potential. For the average child with no additional challenges, this would result in age-appropriate speech and language and integration into the local school. For a child with additional conditions, the goal is specific to his or her own unique circumstances. Likewise, for a child with above

average capabilities, it is expected that he or she will achieve the highest level possible and continue on that course.

Key components of a successful program. An effective program requires comprehensive audiological services working in conjunction with the AV therapist and parents to ensure the child's technology is suited to the type and degree of hearing loss. It is essential to program the hearing aids or cochlear implant to ensure that access to the entire speech spectrum is a reality and not just a theory. The Alexander Graham Bell Academy for Listening and Spoken Language has published a best practices audiological protocol for children.

Once the audiology is completed, the most important aspect to a successful outcome is expert guidance for parents from a Certified Listening and Spoken Language Specialist. The practitioner guides parents in all aspects of teaching their child to listen and develop spoken language. The specialist is responsible for writing goals that are individual to each child and monitoring the progress made by each child to ensure it is adequate to reach age-appropriate speech and language, or the child's individual potential, in a timely manner.

Meeting the challenges. Throughout the world, AV practitioners are challenged in the area of monitoring and pinpointing a child's level of functioning at any given point in time. As I mentor professionals, I provide a system of comprehensive monitoring materials for preverbal and verbal children. These materials provide the framework for professionals to informally assess each child's current level of functioning in listening, speech, and language, and thus serve to inform the professional and the parents in setting appropriate goals in each area. They also provide the framework for monitoring the rate at which the child is achieving goals and moving through the developmental milestones necessary to reach age-appropriate speech and language or their individual potential.

Anita Bernstein, Canada, VOICE for Hearing Impaired Children

VOICE for Hearing Impaired Children is a Canadian not-for-profit organization whose four program areas include public education, parent support, advocacy, and an auditory-verbal (AV) program. The AV program, centered in Ontario, provides direct therapy services to children and their families in communities where AV is not a funded option. In addition, the AV Training and Mentorship Program provides professional development, training, and mentoring in the AV approach to school boards and other institutions that support children with hearing losses. The VOICE AV program is overseen by the VOICE director of therapy and training programs and is staffed by 18 contracted Listening and Spoken Language Specialists/Certified Auditory-Verbal Therapists (LSLS CERT AVTs). The VOICE AV program adheres to the principles and philosophy of AV practice as delineated by the Alexander G. Bell Academy for Listening and Spoken Language.

The VOICE AV therapy program has been in existence since the mid-1970s, and its goal was, and continues to be, to ensure that VOICE families, who could not otherwise access AV intervention through their local hospital or school, were able to receive this type of intervention in their own community. From its humble beginnings providing once-a-month itinerant services to a small number of families in several Ontario communities, the VOICE AV therapy program currently provides intervention to over 100 families. The VOICE organization and the families receiving intervention carry out fundraising collectively to support this service.

Children currently in the AV program range in age from infancy to late teens, have losses from mild to profound, and wear either conventional hearing aids or cochlear implants. The VOICE program follows a family-centered approach to AV intervention. Immediate and/or extended family members participate in therapy sessions to ensure a consistent home follow-up program. VOICE therapists work in collaboration with educators, audiologists, and other professionals in support of the children on their caseload. Children in the VOICE program receive AV intervention service on a weekly schedule until their auditory skills and receptive and expressive language are within normal limits and parents/caregivers are able to continue home follow-up and support. At this point, a transition program to reduced services is implemented, and yearly assessment is available as required. In the case of a child who has complex needs where hearing loss is not the primary concern, consultation services to the primary intervention team may be continued, on a reduced schedule, to ensure effective use of hearing and auditory skill development.

One of the challenges in ensuring accessibility to AV intervention has been the availability of qualified and certified LSLS professionals. This shortage was the impetus for the development of the VOICE AV Training and Mentorship Program, which has been in existence since 1994, and has provided training in 35 institutions. The goal of the VOICE AV Training and Mentorship Program is to ensure that families who would like a spoken language outcome for their child with hearing loss have access to qualified LSLS professionals during early intervention and in the school system.

In 2004, for VOICE's fortieth anniversary, an outcome study was conducted of VOICE adult alumni who learned to communicate by learning to listen and use spoken language through the AV. These young adults attended their neighborhood schools with their peers in full mainstream. Results gathered through a survey completed by 80 alumni were as follows:

- 100% completed or were finishing high school
- 60% attended college, of which 70% have their degree and 30% are still in college

- 48% have attended university (undergraduate), of which 47% have their degree and 53% are still in university
- 7.5% have attended graduate school, of which 60% have their degree and 40% are still in graduate studies
- 54% are working full- or part-time

Jasmine Gallant, Canada, New Brunswick Services for the Hearing Impaired (Francophone Sector), Department of Education and Early Childhood Development

The New Brunswick service for children with hearing loss (francophone sector) currently provides support for 208 children throughout the province from birth through high school. All services are funded publicly through the provincial Department of Education and Early Childhood. The province implemented a mandated universal newborn hearing screening program in 2003. The preschool intervention program is delivered through home visiting. Inclusion in regular education settings for all children has been a provincial mandate since 1987, and intervention services are typically provided on site at the child's neighborhood school. Special support is in place to facilitate transition from high school to postsecondary education or the workplace.

Intervention services are delivered using a listening and spoken language approach with expectations for age-appropriate communication and academic skills. Parents are integral partners in the intervention program throughout the preschool and school years. A systematic evaluation protocol has been implemented to monitor progress and guide intervention. However, to date, no systematic analysis of outcomes has been completed. Our results show that more than 90% of students complete their high school education, although a minority of children, generally with other disabilities, complete a modified program. More than 50% of students pursue postsecondary education.

Strengths of our program include the implementation of standard intervention protocols across specialized teachers, ongoing comprehensive assessments, and a continuity of service throughout the child's learning years. We have a well-established referral system and close communication with community audiology centers to ensure that children receive timely and appropriate audiologic care, as well as the services of an educational audiologist. All children have access to personal FM technology, and the majority of school systems provide both personal and soundfield technology. Professional training and mentoring are a requirement for all specialist teachers and are specifically defined objectives within the administrative plan and budgets.

Our challenges relate primarily to: (1) access to specialized teachers who are trained to provide services in a minority context, (2) availability of resources and intervention materials specifically related to hearing loss in French, and (3) geographical distance from audiological and other specialized health care services.

Jacqueline Stokes, England, Auditory Verbal[UK]

AV[UK] is a national charity and the UK's only specialist center dedicated to the delivery and training of auditory-verbal (AV) practice. We have two centers—one in the Midlands and the other in central London. Families travel from across the UK to one or the other center for an hour's therapy session once per fortnight and/ or receive AV sessions via Skype/Facetime. For some families, having face-to-face sessions involves a drive to the airport, a flight, the hire of a car, and a drive of an hour to the center, and then the return journey home. Most of the children also receive home visits from a teacher of the deaf and sometimes a speech and language therapist. These professionals vary in their knowledge of auditory-verbal therapy (AVT) and may prefer a visual-based system of communication. We are a preschool program and work with babies and infants from 2 months to 5 years.

A recent audit of the children who completed the program over the past 5 years showed that 80% of children left with listening and spoken language scores within normal limits; 36% of those had language that exceeded normal limits. Our outcomes are documented in two journal articles (Hogan, Stokes, & Weller, 2010; Hogan, Stokes, White, Tyszkiewicz, & Woolgar, 2008). The second of these papers looked at outcomes for children from low-income families. There was no significant difference in the spoken language outcomes for this group. Forty percent of our caseload has difficulties in addition to a hearing impairment. None currently has documented learning difficulties. Between a quarter and a third have English as an additional language. The 20% of children who do not acquire language within normal limits before entering school at 4 to 5 years of age typically have additional speech and communication difficulties (e.g., dyspraxia).

The key to successful auditory and spoken language outcomes for children is quality AVT. Our practitioners are all LSLS Cert AVTs who have specialized with the 0 to 5 age range. We are deliberate and proactive in functionally validating the child's technology when children first start with us and throughout the duration of the program. Parents are the focus of the therapy and they work in collaboration with the AV practitioner to drive their program forward. Children are motivated to learn through listening because adults have confidence in them as thinkers and problem solvers, and because it's fun.

There are at least two main barriers to improving listening and spoken language outcomes in children. The first is the 3 years needed to train professionals to work through audition. A practitioner intent on stimulating a child's auditory development first demonstrates what the child can access through technology, advocates for this to be optimized, shows how the child can develop understanding and use of language through listening, and relies on listening as the means to learn about the world. The second barrier is inertia, endemic in large organizations such as the National Health Service, which resists change. Change is rarely embraced, whether it is change in procedures or in outlook. Technological change in the field of hearing impairment is leading the way and challenging professionals to respond in innovative ways. We need practitioners to be inspired by the technology on offer and to work through audition to enable children who are deaf to become twenty-first century listeners.

Stephanie Lim, Singapore, Listen and Talk Program, Centre for Hearing and Ear Implants, Singapore General Hospital

The Listen and Talk Program is the early intervention arm of the Centre for Hearing and Ear Implants at the Department of Otorhinolaryngology at the Singapore General Hospital. Established in 2001, this center provides diagnosis, treatment, and evaluation of hearing disorders. Utilizing a listening and spoken language (auditory-verbal, AV) approach, parents and caregivers (domestic helpers, grandparents, and extended family members) are taught how to develop their child's listening and language skills by participating in weekly individualized parent guidance sessions. Therapy sessions may be partially funded by the government or fully paid by the families.

The center adopts a holistic model as ear, nose, and throat (ENT) surgeons, audiologists, AV therapists, medical social worker, and psychologist form the core group of professionals providing holistic care to our clients. During the course of intervention, the caregivers are provided with education, guidance, and family support by this team. When warranted, the AV therapist collaborates with physiotherapists, occupational therapists, speech therapists, and school educators in mainstream and/or special schools. This collaboration forms an integrated educational team that further supports the diagnostic role in listening and spoken language intervention to continuously assess each child on his or her progress and learning abilities. AV therapists visit schools to guide and support classroom teachers.

In any program, there are success stories, but not without challenges. Singapore is a multicultural and multilingual society. While most parents may use English as the main language spoken at home, many of these children are being looked after by their extended family, for example grandparents and aunties, and as most parents work full-time, their babies may be cared for by a nanny or a domestic helper who is usually a foreigner. There are even day-care centers for babies. With globalization and Singapore being a business hub, there is also an influx of foreigners, especially from China, Burma, and other countries around the world and Asia. This may pose challenges to therapists in guiding parents and/or caregivers and in understanding their culture and facilitating the assimilation of the families into the local culture and the language, as well as the education system.

We conducted a retrospective analysis of data from a cohort of children with bilateral severe to profound hearing loss and cochlear implants (Lam, Lim, Ong, & Low, 2009). We examined the effect of age of implantation and home language on school readiness. Using the Bracken's Basic Concept Scale, we analyzed the children's knowledge of colors, letters/sounds, numbers/counting, sizes/comparisons, and shapes. The results showed that children who were implanted prior to their third birthday performed significantly better than their

peers who were implanted at age 3 or older. Furthermore, children who speak English at home were also found to do significantly better when compared with their peers who speak a language/dialect other than English. Our conclusion was that children who are from English-speaking families and those who receive a cochlear implant before the age of 3 years were found to have conceptual knowledge comparable to their normal-hearing peers. The children who acquired the basic knowledge for formal schooling by the time they enter primary school would have a better chance to succeed in mainstream education.

The Listen and Talk Program at the Singapore General Hospital illustrates a good model of listening and spoken language practice in providing diagnosis and intervention and utilizing a holistic approach for the management of children with hearing impairment. A dedicated team, visionary leadership, and close collaboration between team members are important attributes of an effective program.

Mary McGinnis, United States, John Tracy Clinic

John Tracy Clinic was founded by a parent, and it continues to create and implement diagnostic and educational programs for families and their children with hearing loss from birth to age 5. A range of parent-centered programs is provided: distance learning courses for parents in English and Spanish, which reached 2,299 families around the world last year; demonstration home parent-infant services, serving 150 families last year; demonstration preschool, serving 24 families last year; auditory-verbal therapy for the preschool families; parent support groups; parent workshops; individual parent counseling; sibling camp, which includes support groups and workshops; audiological diagnostics and amplification counseling; developmental screenings; and consultation. Most programs are provided in English and Spanish. International Summer Sessions are provided in Spanish to families from Asia, Europe, and Latin America. Graduate students work with parents in a professional development school model as they participate in all of the parent-centered programs with families and their children at John Tracy Clinic.

All families who seek services for children from birth to age 3 are accepted into the demonstration home. The majority (80%) of the

~ 175 families that we serve on campus yearly are Spanish speaking and are classified as being low income. The majority of the children have severe to profound hearing loss and receive cochlear implants between 1 and 2 years of age. Many have multiple challenges (syndromes associated with hearing loss, sensory processing/modulation disorders, oral-motor, oral-sensory, and feeding issues, etc.). At age 3, many children, particularly those with multiple challenges, will continue services with their school district, while a small number (up to 24) will be accepted into the demonstration preschool for further development, and others will mainstream into their local preschool programs. In researching the progress of our bilingual English/Spanish-speaking children, we have found that, at all ages, they average 1 month's progress in 1 month's time in the development of both spoken languages.

John Tracy Clinic's approach to successful outcomes for the family is to provide family-centered support and education to assist the family in meeting its goals. Because of the Internet, many more families arrive in our parent-infant services having knowledge about options and immediately ask about cochlear implants and auditory-verbal therapy. All of our teaching staff are, or are being mentored to become, certified Listening and Spoken Language Specialists. To increase the number of qualified listening and spoken language specialists available to serve families, our training program graduates between 10 and 16 professionals a year with a teaching credential and master's degree.

Barriers to improving outcomes for families and their children continue to be (1) the lag from identification to intervention and amplification, (2) the lack of knowledge regarding research that supports the ability of children with hearing loss to learn two or more spoken languages, (3) the small number of qualified listening and spoken language specialists available to families, (4) the lack of mentorship in listening and spoken language once our graduate students enter the field, and (5) the lack of choice for families who seek listening and spoken language options for their children in schools.

Jean Sachar Moog, United States, Moog Center for Deaf Education

The Moog Center for Deaf Education provides audiological, educational, and support services to children with hearing loss from birth through the early elementary years. The Moog Center has a Family School program for children from birth to 3 years and their families, a preschool for children 3 to 5 years, and an early elementary program for children up to 8 years of age. In addition to our teaching/therapy staff, the Moog Center also has four pediatric audiologists who are experienced in fitting hearing aids on infants and in programming cochlear implants on very young children. Our goal is for our children to catch up with their hearing peers by kindergarten or first grade and to be mainstreamed as soon as they are ready.

There are over 50 families enrolled in our Family School birth-to-3 program. Of these, 70% of children were enrolled before they were 6 months old, and 90% before they were 1 year old. Our Family School program includes the following components: individual family sessions provided 3–4 times a month through a combination of home visits and center visits for children from birth to 18 months, toddler classes and individual therapy for children 18 months to 3 years, monthly parent support groups, weekly informational meetings, and on-site audiology.

The full-day preschool and early elementary programs provide a minimum of 2½ hours of focused instruction in groups of two to three children, and a preschool program in groups of 10 to 12 children, all of whom have hearing loss. Of the 34 children enrolled, 22 (65%) have cochlear implants and the rest use only hearing aids.

The key ingredient of an effective program for auditory habilitation and what really makes it all work is a true collaboration among competent audiologists, teachers, speech-language pathologists, parents, and others working with the child. For children to achieve their highest potential, all of those connected to the child must work together to support the child's development. A critical factor in the success of our children, in addition to knowledgeable and skilled teachers/therapists and supportive parents, is our very skilled on-site pediatric audiology staff who provide consistent access to sound through optimum device management.

Our expectations are for children to be caught up with their hearing peers by kindergarten in language skills and academics if they receive early intervention followed by preschool in an intensive, focused program such as the one at the Moog Center. A study of 5-year-olds at the Moog Center provides evidence that our children are meeting our expectations and demonstrate what is possible. Children who had been in our toddler program for more than 1 year and then in our preschool program for 2 to 3 years scored on tests standardized on children with typical hearing as follows at age 5 years: 93% scored within normal limits in vocabulary (PPVT and EOWPVT), with a mean standard score of 103, and 90% scored within normal limits in language (CELF-P), with a mean of 92 (Moog & Stein, 2008). In terms of listening skills, we expect our children to demonstrate the ability to understand spoken language and to converse at their language level through listening alone in quiet settings, and to score within the normal range on recorded open-set speech perception tests, and our test results support this outcome.

We believe many more children could be reaching these levels of achievement. The key challenges in improving listening and spoken language outcomes in children who are deaf or hard of hearing are (1) the critical shortage of professionals with the necessary skills in both audiology and in teaching, (2) delayed diagnosis resulting in children not being amplified by 3 months and provided intervention by 6 months, and (3) low expectations of professionals working with the children, as well as policy makers.

International Perspective

As described throughout this book, and by the clinicians/teachers who contributed their perspectives, there have been dramatic changes in the expected outcomes for today's children with hearing loss. However, for the most part, this represents a limited perspective based on research and practices in developed countries. Undoubtedly, the situation looks quite different for millions of children elsewhere in the world who do not have access to early identification and modern technology. We invited three professionals who have considerable experience in consulting, training, and developing programs around the world to share their global perspectives on listening and spoken language. We asked them to hone in on the developments they have observed and to highlight the key challenges in providing audiologic rehabilitation in developing countries. As indicated through these contributions, challenges on an international level include a need for training, access to technology, and delivering care in culturally diverse contexts.

Donald M. Goldberg, United States, President, Alexander Graham Bell Association for the Deaf

The past. The origin of listening and spoken language goes back to Victor Urbantschitsch, who wrote *Auditory Training for Deaf Mutism and Acquired Deafness* in 1895. Urbantschitsch's central argument was that the education and ultimately the emotional and social adjustment of profoundly deaf children could be facilitated by methodical and persistent auditory training (exercises) that exploited any remnant of residual hearing by stimulating what he termed a dormant auditory sense (Urbantschitsch, 1981, p. viii). Similarly, Max Goldstein, founder of the Central Institute for the Deaf in 1914, has been credited for creating the Acoustic Method (Goldstein, 1939) and advancing the notion regarding the power of audition. Goldstein worked with Urbantschitsch and was reportedly encouraged "to introduce his method to America and to convince all who would listen that congenitally deaf children could, by his approach, learn to talk intelligibly" (Urbantschitsch, 1981, p. x).

Goldstein, Emil Froeschels, and other Europeans who fled Nazi Germany arrived in the United States and planted the seed that would germinate into today's auditory-verbal practice (listening and spoken language). The idea that most "deaf" children had some remnant of residual hearing, coupled with the advent of wearable hearing aids in the 1940s, allowed the pioneers of auditory-verbal practice to begin exploring the belief that the use of amplified hearing might permit children who are deaf or hard of hearing to learn to listen, process, and communicate using spoken language. Pioneers of the auditory-verbal movement were Doreen Pollack, initially at Columbia Presbyterian Medical Center in New York City and later at the University of Denver and Porter Memorial Hospital in Denver, Colorado, and Helen Hulick Beebe in New York City and Easton, Pennsylvania. Other, later luminaries in the field included Dan Ling and Agnes ("Nan") Phillips, first in England and subsequently at the Montreal Oral School for the Deaf and McGill University in Montreal, Canada; Dr. Ciwa Griffiths in New York and later in California as founder of the Hear Center in Pasadena (Griffiths, 1974); and a variety of the colleagues and students of Ling, Pollack, and Beebe.

The future. Although challenges currently exist in facilitating a listening and spoken language outcome worldwide, notably in both the "developed" and "developing" regions and countries internationally, our futures in this changing landscape of deafness will likely include the following:

1. Younger and younger children identified throughout the world via universal newborn hearing screening
2. Continued advancements in hearing sensory technology (notably, affordable personal and group amplification systems and smaller-sized and implantable cochlear implants that will most likely be bilateral, implanted either simultaneously or sequentially)

3. Acceptance that parents are their children's most critically important change agent in learning to listen and in spoken language development.

Via coaching and teaching from a worldwide network of highly qualified providers—AG Bell's Listening and Spoken Language Specialists (LSLS) in Auditory-Verbal Therapy and Auditory-Verbal Education—the spoken language outcomes for these children will be even more impressive than current clinical research has already reported. Persons with access equal to that of their hearing peers to literacy, to educational opportunities at the postsecondary levels and beyond, to professional employment, and to the world, will be incredibly less encumbered than persons who were deaf in our past.

Conclusion. Today, both professionals and parents around the world are indebted to all the pioneers of auditory-verbal practice. The seeds of listening and spoken language development were planted about 75 years ago. They set the standard by even suggesting there was power in hearing and that it was indeed possible for a child who is deaf or hard of hearing to learn to communicate using spoken language learned primarily through listening. When reflecting about the pioneers of auditory-verbal practice who focused on "training the ear" and "training hearing," we now know that, based on current brain research (Moucha & Kilgard, 2006; Sharma et al, 2005), the pioneers were the first to be "training the brain." By accessing, stimulating, and growing neural connections in the auditory centers of the brain through intensive, meaningful, and cumulative practice, these auditory leaders were actually involved in brain development and training. Thousands of infants and children who are deaf or hard of hearing and their families have benefited immeasurably from their wisdom, knowledge, and nonwavering belief in the "power of hearing" and the "power of the brain."

Ellen A. Rhoades, United States, Independent Consultant

Globally, we are united in the desire to minimize potentially handicapping ramifications of hearing loss for all children. However, I often find a dichotomous situation that can present difficulties more problematic than those typically found in the more historically developed countries of North America and Europe. This disparity reflects sociocultural conditions.

The first situation has to do with financial impoverishment and its obvious outcomes. Many governments are unable to provide sufficient funds for:

- Current audiological equipment or diagnostic materials, hearing devices, or educational services that are geographically and financially accessible to rural families and their children
- Appropriate practitioner training, since some teachers have limited knowledge of hearing technology, child development, and strategies that facilitate listening and spoken language skills, as well as active parent participation
- Ongoing security measures to reduce local graft and theft that negatively impact service delivery

Particularly when impoverished parents are illiterate or do not have access to the Internet, insufficient practitioner knowledge bodes poorly for children with hearing loss.

At the other extreme, in some of these same countries across Latin America, Africa, Asia, and the Middle East, there are affluent families with a sense of entitlement. For some families on this end of the class divide, the sociocultural norm is to have considerable household help. This may mean at least a chauffeur, a nanny who sleeps in the family's home and travels with them, and another person who cleans and cooks for the family.

These circumstances may interfere with the child having consistent rich exposure to the native language. Nannies are sometimes older adolescents or young uneducated adults who, if they speak the family's native language, may speak it poorly and with a heavy accent or in a different dialect. For example, a Singaporean family who speak Chinese may have a young nanny speaking a Malaysian dialect. During household chores, the child with hearing loss may be kept occupied with television programs. The language spoken in that television program could be Chinese, Malay, English, or Singlish. Consequently, linguistic input may be potentially confusing as well as quite restricted.

Although access to current hearing technology is typically not an issue for affluent families, linguistic and child-rearing issues can present significant barriers in their quest to provide optimal language and learning experiences for children with hearing loss. For example, a nanny in Guatemala may do everything possible for the children of the household. This can include dressing and feeding the children every morning. While the children attend school, the domestic help shops, cleans, and washes and irons clothing. Consequently, some of these children do not have sufficient opportunities either to independently develop problem-solving skills or to learn the language of verbs that typically accompany the execution of household routines. Compounding the prob-

lem is that many nannies see to every whim of the families they serve, sometimes resulting in children who do not have opportunities to strengthen self-regulation capacities.

Aside from these sociocultural matters, the lack of normed spoken language milestones can pose difficulties for those parts of the world that do not speak English or Spanish. For example, although Arabic is one of the world's most frequently spoken languages, there are innumerable dialects spoken across the Arab Gulf region, and standard Arabic may not be heard until children attend school. The dearth of norm-referenced assessment instruments or speech and language developmental scales in Arabic is problematic for practitioners entrusted with providing optimal intervention services to Arabic families. Rectifying this necessitates a great deal of research and time, as well as cooperation across Arabic nations.

Warren Estabrooks, Canada, WE Listen International, Inc.

As a global consultant and international ambassador of the A. G. Bell Association for the Deaf and Hard of Hearing, I have been honored to train professionals on every continent. The primary mission is to work with professionals who commit to "pay it forward" by training other professionals. This work is now being done in South Africa, the Middle East, Portugal, Italy, Turkey, the UK, Poland, Sweden, Italy, Norway, Denmark, Southeast Asia, India, Brazil, Chile, Argentina, Japan, and others. In these countries, there is substantial interest from all sectors of the professional community to improve the outcomes of children with hearing loss. Most recently in South Africa, our group has developed its own national training program, which has been embraced by Stellenbosch University.

Around the world, the ongoing pursuit of science and artful listening and spoken language practices continues to yield greater possibilities than ever before for children who are born with hearing loss or who acquire hearing loss in early childhood. These children and their parents are transforming lives that might have been silent into personal worlds of sound. Most of these children are learning to listen to their own voices, listen to the voices of others, and listen to all the other sounds of life. By learning to listen, they are learning to talk. By learning to listen and talk, they are learning to communicate in spoken conversations. By learning to listen and talk, they are learning to read and write. By learning to listen and talk, they are achieving the dreams of an abundant academic and social life held for them by their parents.

Perspective of Parents

We also invited contributions from three parents from different countries whose four children developed spoken language through hearing. As evidenced in the descriptions of their experiences, some children had the benefit of early identification and intervention and others did not; some had access to services focused on listening and spoken language and some did not. Despite very different experiences, these par-

ents all invested in and succeeded in developing listening and spoken language development.

Parents were asked to respond to three questions:

- What worked for you and your child in achieving spoken language acquisition?
- What were the main challenges?
- What are your top three or four suggestions for parents?

Sonia and Bruno Leprette, France

What worked for you and your child in achieving spoken language acquisition?

- Early diagnosis and amplification. Our son, Matthieu, was diagnosed profoundly deaf at 3 months of age, received hearing aids shortly afterward, and had a cochlear implant at 14 months. This was a milestone so that his brain could receive the early auditory input. We strived to ensure that he had access to the best possible hearing through his technology.
- Daily experiences and exposure to language. We wanted him to have the best possible experiences in everyday activities and to be exposed to new vocabulary and interesting subjects. Realistic everyday experiences enabled him to learn new words for the things and activities that were most interesting to him.
- Telling stories or reading with him from his personal experience book. He was and is still fond of stories, and reading develops his concentration in listening and his imagination. We almost never go to bed without reading a story.
- The support of his older sister, the best auditory-verbal (AV) therapist. Julie was so spontaneous in talking, singing, and playing games with him. She forgot his deafness and talked with him as if he had normal hearing.
- Information about deafness, therapy, and programming of the cochlear implant. We spent time reading books about AV therapy, surfing the Internet for information from the cochlear implant manufacturers, and exchanging e-mails with AV therapists abroad, since the approach is not used in France. Fortunately, we found helpful and professional therapists who could provide us with counseling and literature and make occasional visits to our home in France.

What were the main challenges?

- Our biggest challenge was to find an AV therapist and an audiologist who shared our vision, because AV therapy is not currently standard practice in France. We felt that there were serious misunderstandings on the part of some professionals related to the effects of AV therapy on children, the limited effectiveness of AV therapy, and the strong emphasis on parental involvement in therapy sessions. We would have preferred to receive weekly therapy and coaching in our home area, but we felt the need to seek specialist services abroad in Germany, Switzerland, Canada, the United States, and Spain.
- One of our main challenges was, therefore, to remain committed to our goals and beliefs of what our child needed to develop listening and spoken language in spite of the lack of local support for our choices.
- It was often difficult to remain optimistic when we did not get the results we hoped for in terms of our son's language development. We had to remain confident and psychologically strong.

What are your top three or four suggestions for parents?

- Believe in the potential of your child. Do not set limits on your child because he is deaf; he has the same brain as his hearing peers and you should treat him as a normal child. It will give him confidence. He should have the opportunity to go to a regular school and choose his friends because of common interests and not because they are deaf!
- Be informed about the technology. We are lucky that our children were born at this time. The cochlear implant is a wonderful tool and enables them easy access to the speech banana (speech sounds). So provide your child with the latest and best hearing aids and/or cochlear implant.

- Be your child's best advocate. A young child must have the support of his parents because he cannot advocate for his own learning needs and services.
- Find some time to relax alone or as a couple in order not to focus only on deafness. Your journey will be a marathon and you need to manage your energy. Be involved with your child, but do not forget siblings and your husband or wife. Breaks are necessary to keep on going.

Cindy Bell, Malaysia

What worked for you and your child in achieving spoken language acquisition?

- The cochlear implant would have to be the biggest factor in helping Louis to achieve spoken language as it gave him the ability to hear consistently.
- Although he was diagnosed with hearing impairment when he was 2 days old, aided when he was 10 weeks old, and tested regularly to check that he had access to the spectrum of speech sounds, at the point where Louis was implanted he basically only had two-word sentences. I could understand what he was saying or trying to communicate, but looking back, most other people couldn't. While we thought he had access to the speech spectrum, he wasn't actually hearing the words consistently, because of numerous ear infections and his LVAS (which we were unaware of at the time).
- Once he had been implanted at 3 years and 10 months, the transformation in his speech and communication was amazing. It wasn't just the vocabulary and sentence structure that flourished, it was also the clarity in his speech. He now talks nonstop and is clearly understood.
- While the implant was probably our savior, his speech acquisition would also not have been possible without a lot of auditory-verbal therapy. I cannot overemphasize the importance of therapy in giving me the tools and support to help Louis learn.
- Also, talking or reading to Louis as much as I could helped immensely. I took every opportunity I could to give him access to spoken language.

What were the main challenges?

The challenges were mainly when he was younger, as follows:

- Trying to keep the hearing aids on when he was a baby. He was constantly pulling them off and I spent most of my time putting them back on.
- He had ear infection after ear infection (which may have been a symptom of living in Vietnam where we all suffered from one bug to the next), but we think that the infections added to the inconsistency in hearing.
- Our professional support team (ENT, audiologist, auditory-verbal therapist) were situated in another country (we moved when Louis was 2½), so we were fairly isolated. I travelled to Singapore with Louis every 6 weeks or so for checkups, testing, and therapy sessions.
- Equipment failure—again, living away from professional help meant that if we had equipment failure we couldn't get the apparatus fixed immediately.

What are your top three or four suggestions for parents?

- Talk, read, and sing to your child as much as you can. There were some days when I was just too tired for therapy or almost too tired to talk, but I would pick up a book and read, just to ensure that he was hearing words and new vocabulary. Reading also gave him a broader vocabulary and I would often read rhyming books or books with rhythmic text to help with intonation. I would also sing him songs, despite my terrible voice.

- Repeat, repeat, repeat the words that you are focusing on. For example, if you want your child to say "shoe/s" I would say, "Let's put your shoes on, oh there are your shoes, let's put your left shoe on, there you go your left shoe is on, let's put your right shoe on..."
- Buy the best equipment that you can possibly afford, maintain it consistently, and make sure that your child wears the aids and implant as much as possible.

If they cannot hear, then they cannot learn to talk.

- Surround yourself with a good team of people who can give you, as the parent, the support you need. People that you feel comfortable with, people whose judgment you trust; and go to/provide therapy as often as you can.
- If your child is borderline for an implant, push to have him implanted. The consistency in sound that it provided for us was invaluable—I often forget that he has a hearing problem at all.

Erin Gilbert, Canada

What worked for you and your child in achieving spoken language acquisition?

Our two preschool-aged boys (Tom and Ian) were both diagnosed with hearing loss at birth. Receiving this shocking news (as there is no history of hearing loss on either side of our families) was overwhelming, to say the least. Thankfully, the province of Ontario came to our rescue, first by identifying through newborn screening that our boys were not hearing normally and then by having the Infant Hearing Program hold our hand and guide us through our first paces of hearing tests, language options, and available services. As we gained knowledge of this new world, we were excited to learn that our boys could be expected to use oral language in their everyday lives.

At about 6 months of age, both of our boys began wearing hearing aids during their waking hours. They started biweekly visits to the Children's Hospital of Eastern Ontario (CHEO), where they participated in hour-long audio-verbal therapy sessions. Both boys *love* the games and activities that they take part in during this time. Here our sons were able to learn to listen and practice their speech in a fun environment. This practice has allowed them to develop skills to do their best work when their hearing is tested. These sessions also gave us (as parents) an opportunity to learn about age-appropriate sounds that we should expect our children to be making and to further understand what phonetics would pose as challenges to our boys due to their hearing

loss. Areas of difficulty would be reinforced both at home and in therapy. Within this timeframe, we were also introduced to preschool teachers from Sir James Whitney School for the Deaf, who were available to visit our home on a biweekly basis. These visits tie into what the boys are already taking away from their therapy session at CHEO, but more informally in the home environment. The goal is to help the children develop their skills and make a smooth transition into junior kindergarten. Both intervention programs do regular assessments of the boy's receptive and expressive abilities (in comparison to their fully hearing peers). This is always a bit nerve wracking, but so encouraging to see that they are meeting the expectations. This testing also gives us a chance to see what is expected, and what our next steps should be to keep the boys headed in the right direction as they get older (for example, working on rhymes, counting to ten, etc.).

We have also made an effort to take part in some of the groups that are established in our community for hearing-impaired children. Getting together with families through VOICE and Hands and Voices has allowed us to chat with other parents and has given our boys the chance to play with children who wear hearing aids/cochlear implants like themselves. Seeing the successes of the older children in these groups is truly thrilling, making them wonderful role models.

What were the main challenges?

In terms of challenges, I feel that we have been quite lucky. Our youngest son (Ian) did not like (hated) wearing his hearing aids as a baby. He required a bonnet that tied under his chin to keep them on. It was emotional to have to have this regular fight with such a sweet, innocent baby, but well worth it in the end. Our oldest son (Tom) has a hearing loss that proved to be progressive and rapid, showing drops in almost every hearing test he did. This was difficult in that once we had finally gotten our head around hearing aids and expectations for a certain degree of hearing loss, it would all change, to the point where he required cochlear implant surgery at age 3. Being accepting of this quick drop in hearing (from mild-moderate to moderate-profound) took some time. Now, seeing his ever-growing abilities, only 5 months after his surgery, is astounding and we are so grateful. I am currently facing the challenge of giving up some of the control/habits that I have developed as a mother of two hearing-impaired children. When they were babies, I always repeated things to the boys and narrated their lives to ensure they weren't missing anything and to reinforce language-building opportunities. Now, as our oldest prepares for school in the fall, I am often catching myself doing too much of the talking at a time when he needs to be becoming more independent.

What are your top three or four suggestions for parents?

Despite having a rather full schedule, I would strongly urge parents to take advantage of all of the wonderful (and free) services that are available for hearing-impaired children and their families. I would also remind parents to listen to the advice of the professionals they are working with, even when it is difficult. Finally, taking the time to connect with other families/children with hearing losses can be truly inspiring and a learning experience within itself.

As exemplified by these brief reflections, parents encounter very different experiences in making choices for their children. In some regions, listening and spoken language approaches to rehabilitation have become one of the standard options available, while in others, approaches such as cued speech and sign language are favored in developing communication. Due to these controversies and the lack of clear evidence for the effectiveness of various intervention approaches, parents can find themselves in conflicting situations, and accordingly, their experiences and needs can vary considerably. However, all parents credit their children's positive spoken language development to hearing technology and the parental guidance they received. Regardless of parents' experiences, their advice for other families is remarkably similar. Common parent-to-parent themes include treating a child like any typical child first and foremost, keeping up-to-date with new technology, and, finally, taking time for oneself and for family.

▪ Summary

This chapter provided a brief snapshot of diverse services in several different countries, as well as international perspectives about the current status of listening and spoken language for children with hearing loss. The chapter also briefly presented parents' perceptions of what makes listening and spoken language possible for children with hearing loss. Key issues in audiologic rehabilitation include the need for further training and delayed access to quality intervention services. Effective ingredients were consistent with the theme of this book and can be summarized as audiology and rehabilitation services working in concert to provide the very best access to hearing. In summary, both practitioners and parents expect that children, regardless of severity of hearing loss, will achieve age-appropriate spoken language and be able to fully participate in learning and social experiences with their peers.

References

Dornan, D., Hickson, L., Murdoch, B., Houston, T., & Constantinescu, G. (2010). Is auditory-verbal therapy effective for children with hearing loss? *The Volta Review, 110*(3), 361–387.

Goldstein, M. (1939). *The acoustic method*. St. Louis: Laryngoscope Press.

Griffiths, C. (Ed.). (1974). *Proceedings of the international conference on auditory techniques*. Springfield, IL: Charles C Thomas.

Hogan, S., Stokes, J., & Weller, I. (2010). Language outcomes for children of low-income families enrolled in auditory verbal therapy. *Deafness & Education International, 12*(4), 204–216.

Hogan, S., Stokes, J., White, C., Tyszkiewicz, E., & Woolgar, A. (2008). An evaluation of auditory verbal therapy using the rate of early language development as an outcome measure. *Deafness & Education International, 10*(3), 143–167.

Lam, S., Lim, S. Y. C., Ong, C. S., & Low, W. K. (2009). *Effect of age of implantation and home language on school readiness*. Paper presented at the the 7th Asia Pacific Symposium on Cochlear Implants and Related Sciences, 2009, Singapore.

Ling, D., & Ling, A. H. (1978). *Aural habilitation: The foundations of verbal learning in hearing-impaired children*. Washington, DC: Alexander Graham Bell Association of the Deaf, Inc.

Moog, J. S., & Stein, K. K. (2008). Teaching deaf children to talk. *Contemporary Issues in Communication Science and Disorders, 35,* 133–142.

Moucha, R., & Kilgard, M. P. (2006). Cortical plasticity and rehabilitation. *Progress in Brain Research, 157,* 111–122.

Pollack, D. (1977). *Educational audiology for the limited hearing infant* (4th ed.). Springfield, IL: Charles C Thomas Publisher.

Sharma, A. E., Martin, K., Roland, P., Bauer, P., Sweeney, M. H., Gilley, P., & Dorman, M. (2005). P1 latency as a biomarker for central auditory development in children with hearing impairment. *Journal of the American Academy of Audiology, 16*(8), 564–573.

Urbantschitsch, V. (1981). *Auditory training for deaf mutism and acquired deafness. (S.R. Silverman, Trans.)* Washington, DC: Alexander Graham Bell Association for the Deaf. (Original work published 1895).

Compilation of References

Akamatsu, C. T., Mayer, C., & Hardy-Braz, S. (2008). Why considerations of verbal aptitude are important in educating deaf and hard-of-hearing students. In M. Marschark & P. C. Hauser (Eds.), *Deaf cognition: Foundations and outcomes* (pp. 131–169). New York: Oxford University Press.

Akhtar, N., Jipson, J., & Callanan, M. A. (2001). Learning words through overhearing. *Child Development, 72*(2), 416–430.

Akhtar, N. (2005). The robustness of learning through overhearing. *Developmental Science, 8*(2), 199–209.

Almond, M., & Brown, D. J. (2009). The pathology and etiology of sensorineural hearing loss and implications for cochlear implantation. In J. K. Niparko (Ed.), *Cochlear implants: Principles and practices* (2nd ed., pp. 43–87). Philadelphia, PA: Lippincott Williams & Wilkins.

American National Standards Institute [ANSI]. (S3.5–1997 R2007). *Methods for the calculation of the speech intelligibility index.* New York: Acoustical Society of America.

American National Standards Institute [ANSI]. (S12. 60–2010). *Acoustical performance criteria, design requirements, and guidelines for schools, part 1: Permanent schools.* Melville, NY: Acoustical Society of America.

American Speech-Language-Hearing Association [ASHA] (2000). *Guidelines for fitting and monitoring FM systems* [Guidelines]. Available from http://www.asha.org/members/deskref-journals/deskref/default.

American Speech-Language-Hearing Association (ASHA). (2011). Type, degree, and configuration of hearing loss. *Audiology Information Series 7976–16.* Retrieved from http://www.asha.org/uploadedFiles/AIS-Hearing-Loss-Types-Degree-Configuration.pdf

Anderson, K. L. (1989). *S.I.F.T.E.R.: Screening Instrument for Targeting Educational Risk.* Retrieved from http://successforkidswithhearingloss.com/catalog/sifters.

Anderson, K. L. (2001). Voicing concern about noisy classrooms. *Educational Leadership, 58*(7), 77–79.

Anderson, K. L. (2004). *Secondary S.I.F.T.E.R.: Screening Instrument for Targeting Educational Risk in secondary students.* Retrieved from http://successforkidswithhearingloss.com/catalog/sifters.

Anderson, K. L. (2011). Predicting speech audibility from the audiogram to advocate for listening and learning needs. *Hearing Review, 18*(10), 20–23.

Anderson, K. L., & Arnoldi, K. A. (2011). *Building skills for success in the fast-paced classroom: Optimizing achievement for students with hearing loss.* Hillsboro, OR: Butte Publications.

Anderson, K. L., & Goldstein, H. (2004). Speech perception benefits of FM and infrared devices to children with hearing aids in a typical classroom. *Language, Speech, and Hearing Services in Schools, 35*(2), 169–184.

Anderson, K. L., Goldstein, H., Colodzin, L., & Inglehart, F. (2005). Benefit of S/N enhancing devices to speech perception of children listening in a typical classroom with hearing aids or a cochlear implant. *Journal of Educational Audiology, 12,* 14–28.

Anderson, R. C., Hiebert, E. H., Scott, J. A., & Wilkinson, I. A. G. (1985). *Becoming a nation of readers: The report of the commission on reading.* Champaign, IL: University of Illinois; National Academy of Education.

Anderson, K. L., & Matkin, N. (1996). *Preschool S.I.F.T.E.R.: Screening Instrument for Targeting Educational Risk in preschool children (age 3–kindergarten).* Retrieved from http://successforkidswithhearingloss.com/catalog/sifters

Anderson, K. L., & Smaldino, J. J. (2011). *The Children's Home Inventory for Listening Difficulties (CHILD).* Retrieved from http://successforkidswithhearingloss.com.

Anderson, K. L., Smaldino, J. J., & Spangler, C. (2011). *LIFE–R: Listening Inventory for Education-Revised* Retrieved from http://successforkidswithhearingloss.com/wp-content/uploads/2011/08/Teacher-LIFE-R.pdf.

Antia, S. D., Jones, P. B., Reed, S., & Kreimeyer, K. H. (2009). Academic status and progress of deaf and hard-of-hearing students in general education classrooms. *Journal of Deaf Studies and Deaf Education, 14*(3), 293–311.

ANSI/ASA. (2002). *American National Standard: Acoustical performance criteria, design requirements, and guidelines for schools.* Melville, NY: Acoustical Society of America.

ANSI/ASA. (2010). *American National Standard: Acoustical performance criteria, design requirements, and guidelines for schools, part 1: Permanent schools.* Melville, NY: Acoustical Society of America. Retrieved from http://asa.aip.org.

Archbold, S., & Mayer, M. (2012). Deaf education: The impact of cochlear implantation? *Deafness & Education International, 14*(1), 2–15.

Archbold, S. M., Nikolopoulos, T. P., Lutman, M. E., & O'Donoghue, G. M. (2002). The educational settings of profoundly deaf children with cochlear implants compared with age-matched peers with hearing aids: Implications for management. *International Journal of Audiology, 41*(3), 157–161.

Archbold, S., Phil, M., & O'Donoghue, G. M. (2009). Education and childhood deafness: Changing choices and new challenges. In J. K. Niparko (Ed.), *Cochlear implants: Principles and practices* (2nd ed., pp. 313–321). Philadelphia, PA: Lippincott Williams & Wilkins.

Arisi, E., Forti, S., Pagani, D., Todini, L., Torretta, S., Ambrosetti, U., & Pignataro, L. (2010). Cochlear implantation in adolescents with prelinguistic deafness. *Otolaryngology—Head and Neck Surgery, 142*(6), 804–808.

Babbidge, H. (1965). *Education of the deaf. A report to the Secretary of Health, Education, and Welfare by his Advisory Committee on the Education of the Deaf. Ref. No. 0–765–119.* Washington, DC: Government Printing Office.

Bagatto, M., Moodie, S., Scollie, S., Seewald, R., Moodie, S., Pumford, J., & Liu, R. (2005). Clinical protocols for hearing instrument fitting in the Desired Sensation Level method. *Trends in Amplification, 9*(4), 199–226.

Bagatto, M. P., Moodie, S. T., Seewald, R. C., Bartlett, D. J., & Scollie, S. D. (2011). A critical review of audiological outcome measures for infants and children. *Trends in Amplification, 15*(1), 23–33.

Bagatto, M., Scollie, S. D., Hyde, M., & Seewald, R. (2010). Protocol for the provision of amplification within the Ontario Infant Hearing Program. *International Journal of Audiology, 49*(Suppl. 1), S70–S79. 10.3109/14992020903080751.

Bagatto, M. P., Moodie, S. T., Malandrino, A. C., Richert, F. M., Clench, D. A., & Scollie, S. D. (2011). The University of Western Ontario Pediatric Audiological Monitoring Protocol (UWO PedAMP). *Trends in Amplification, 15*(1), 57–76.

Bagatto, M. P., Moodie, S. T., Seewald, R. C., Bartlett, D. J., & Scollie, S. D. (2011). A critical review of audiological outcome measures for infants and children. *Trends in Amplification, 15*(1), 57–76. 10.1177/1084713811420304.

Beck, D. L., & Fabry, D. (2011). Access America: It's about connectivity. *Audiology Today, 23*(1), 24–29.

Beck, I., & McKewon, M. G. (2001). Text talk: Capturing the benefits of read-aloud experiences for young children. *The Reading Teacher, 55,* 10–20.

Beebe, H. (1953). *A guide to help the severely hard of hearing child.* New York: Karger.

Beggs, W. D. A., & Foreman, D. L. (1980). Sound localization and early binaural experience in the deaf. *British Journal of Audiology, 14*(2), 41–48.

Belzner, K. A., & Seal, B. C. (2009). Children with cochlear implants: A review of demographics and communication outcomes. *American Annals of the Deaf, 154*(3), 311–333.

Berlin, C. I., Hood, L. J., Morlet, T., Wilensky, D., Li, L., Mattingly, K. R., . . . Frisch, S. A. (2010). Multisite diagnosis and management of 260 patients with auditory neuropathy/dyssynchrony (auditory neuropathy spectrum disorder). *International Journal of Audiology, 49*(1), 30–43 10.3109/14992020903160892.

Berlin, C. I., Morlet, T., & Hood, L. J. (2003). Auditory neuropathy/dyssynchrony: Its diagnosis and management. *Pediatric Clinics of North America, 50*(2), 331–340, vii–viii.

Berlin, C. I., & Weyand, T. G. (2003). *The brain and sensory plasticity: Language acquisition and hearing.* Clifton Park, NY: Thomson Delmar Learning.

Bernstein, A., & Eriks-Brophy, A. (2010). Supporting families. In E. A. Rhoades & J. Duncan (Eds.), *Auditory-verbal practice: Toward a family-centered approach* (pp. 225–257). Springfield, IL: Charles C Thomas.

Bess, F. H., Chase, P. A., Gravel, J. S., Seewald, R. C., Stelmachowicz, P. G., Tharpe, A. M., & Hedley-Williams, A. (1996). Amplification for infants and children with hearing loss. *American Journal of Audiology, 5*(1), 53–68.

Bess, F. H., Dodd-Murphy, J., & Parker, R. A. (1998). Children with minimal sensorineural hearing loss: Prevalence, educational performance, and functional status. *Ear and Hearing, 19*(5), 339–354.

Bess, F. H., & Humes, L. E. (2003). *Audiology: The fundamentals* (3rd ed.). Philadelphia, PA: Lippincott Williams & Wilkins.

Bhatnagar, S. C. (2002). *Neuroscience for the study of communicative disorders* (2nd ed.). Philadelphia, PA: Lippincott Williams & Wilkins.

Biernath, K. R., Reefhuis, J., Whitney, C. G., Mann, E. A., Costa, P., Eichwald, J., & Boyle, C. (2006). Bacterial meningitis among children with cochlear implants beyond 24 months after implantation. *Pediatrics, 117*(2), 284–289.

Blauert, J. (1997). *Spatial hearing: The psychophysics of human sound localization.* Cambridge, MA: The MIT Press.

Boisclair, A., & Sirois, P. (2000). L'émergence de la lecture et de l'écriture chez l'élève sourd. *Vivre le primaire, 13*(2), 34–38.

Bonds, B. G. (2003). School-to-work experiences: Curriculum as a bridge. *American Annals of the Deaf, 148*(1), 38–48.

Boothroyd, A. (1997). Auditory development of the hearing child. *Scandinavian Audiology Supplement, 46*(Suppl. 46), 9–16.

Boothroyd, A. (2008). The acoustic speech signal. In J. R. Madell & C. Flexer (Eds.), *Pediatric audiology: Diagnosis, technology, and management* (pp. 161–169). New York: Thieme Medical Publishers.

Boothroyd, A., & Eran, O. (1994). Auditory speech perception capacity of child implant users expressed as equivalent hearing loss. *Volta Review, 96*(5), 151–167.

Borden, G. J., Harris, K. S., & Raphael, L. J. (2003). *Speech science primer: Physiology, acoustics and perception of speech.* Baltimore, MD: Lippincott Williams & Wilkins.

Borg, E., Risberg, A., McAllister, B., Undermar, B. M., & Edquist, G. (2002). Language development in hearing-impaired children: Establishment of a reference material for a "Language test for hearing-impaired children," LATHIC. *International Journal of Pediatric Otorhinolaryngology, 65,* 15–26.

Boyle, C. A., Boulet, S., Schieve, L. A., Cohen, R. A., Blumberg, S. J., Yeargin-Allsopp, M., . . . Kogan, M. D. (2011). Trends in the prevalence of developmental disabilities in US children, 1997–2008. *Pediatrics, 127*(6), 1034–1042.

Bradley, J. S., Sato, H., & Picard, M. (2003). On the importance of early reflections for speech in rooms. *Journal of the Acoustical Society of America, 113*(6), 3233–3244.

Brown, C. J., Hughes, M. L., Luk, B., Abbas, P. J., Wolaver, A. A., & Gervais, J. P. (2000). The relationship between EAP and EABR thresholds and levels used to program the nucleus 24 speech processor: Data from adults. *Ear and Hearing, 21*(2), 151–163.

Brown, K. D., & Balkany, T. J. (2007). Benefits of bilateral cochlear implantation: A review. *Current Opinion in Otolaryngology and Head & Neck Surgery, 15*(5), 315–318.

Buchman, C. A., Adunka, O. F., Zdanski, C. J., & Pillsbury, H. C. (2011). Medical considerations for infants and children with hearing loss: The otologists' perspective. In R. Seewald & A.-M. Tharpe (Eds.), *Comprehensive handbook of pediatric audiology*. San Diego, CA: Plural Publishing, Inc.

Burger, T., Spahn, C., Richter, B., Eissele, S., Löhle, E., & Bengel, J. (2005). Parental distress: The initial phase of hearing aid and cochlear implant fitting. *American Annals of the Deaf, 150*(1), 5–10.

Byrne, D. (1983). Word familiarity in speech perception testing of children. *Australian and New Zealand Journal of Audiology, 5*(2), 77–80.

Byrne, D. (1986). Effects of frequency response characteristics on speech discrimination and perceived intelligibility and pleasantness of speech for hearing-impaired listeners. *Journal of the Acoustical Society of America, 80*(2), 494–504.

Byrne, D., & Ching, T. Y. C. (1997). Optimising amplification for hearing impaired children: I. Issues and procedures. *Australian Journal of Education of the Deaf, 3*(1), 21–28.

Byrne, D., Dillon, H., Ching, T. Y. C., Katsch, R., & Keidser, G. (2001). NAL-NL1 procedure for fitting nonlinear hearing aids: Characteristics and comparisons with other procedures. *Journal of the American Academy of Audiology, 12*(1), 37–51.

Canadian Working Group on Childhood Hearing. (2005). *Early hearing and communication development: Canadian Working Group on Childhood Hearing (CWGCH) resource document*. Ottawa.

Cappelli, M., Daniels, T., Durieux-Smith, A., McGrath, P., & Neuss, D. (1995). Social development of children with hearing impairments who are integrated into general education. *The Volta Review, 97*(3), 197.

Cawthorn. S. (2001). Teaching strategies in inclusive classrooms with deaf students. *Journal of Deaf Studies and Deaf Education, 6*(3), 2123–2225.

Cervera-Paz, F. J., & Manrique, M. J. (2005). Traditional and emerging indications in cochlear and auditory brainstem implants. *Revue de Laryngologie—Otologie—Rhinologie, 126*(4), 287–292.

Chaney, C. (1992). Language development, metalinguistic skills, and print awareness in 3-year-old children. *Applied Psycholinguistics, 13*(4), 485–514.

Chermak, G. D., Bellis, T. J., & Musiek, F. E. (2007). Neurobiology, cognitive science, and intervention. In G. D. Chermak & F. E. Musiek (Eds.), *Handbook of (central) auditory processing disorder: Comprehensive intervention* (Vol. II, pp. 3–28). San Diego, CA: Plural.

Ching, T. Y. C. (2011). Acoustic cues for consonant perception with combined acoustic and electric hearing in children. *Seminars in Hearing, 32*(1), 32–41.

Ching, T. Y. C. (2012). Hearing aids for children. In L. Wong & L. Hickson (Eds.), *Evidence based practice in audiologic intervention* (pp. 93–118). San Diego: Plural Publishing.

Ching, T. Y. C. (2012). Predicting developmental outcomes of early-and-late-identified children with hearing impairment, including those with special needs: Findings from a population study. Paper presented at the Newborn Hearing Screening 2012, Cernobbio, Italy.

Ching, T. Y. C., Crowe, K., Martin, V., Day, J., Mahler, N., Youn, S., . . . Orsini, J. (2010). Language development and everyday functioning of children with hearing loss assessed at 3 years of age. *International Journal of Speech-Language Pathology, 12*(2), 124–131 10.3109/17549500903577022.

Ching, T. Y. C., & Dillon, H. (2003). Prescribing amplification for children: Adult-equivalent hearing loss, real-ear aided gain, and NAL-NL1. *Trends in Amplification, 7*(1), 1–9.

Ching, T. Y. C., Dillon, H., & Byrne, D. (1998). Speech recognition of hearing-impaired listeners: Predictions from audibility and the limited role of high-frequency amplification. *Journal of the Acoustical Society of America, 103*(2), 1128–1140.

Ching, T. Y. C., Dillon, H., Day, J., & Crowe, K. (2007). The NAL study on longitudinal outcomes of hearing-impaired children: Interim findings on language of early and later-identified children at 6 months after hearing aid fitting. Paper presented at the A Sound Foundation Through Early Amplification: Fourth International Conference, Stafa, Switzerland.

Ching, T. Y. C., Dillon, H., Day, J., Crowe, K., Close, L., Chisholm, K., & Hopkins, T. (2009). Early language outcomes of children with cochlear implants: Interim findings of the NAL study on longitudinal outcomes of children with hearing impairment. *Cochlear Implants International, 10*(Suppl. 1), 28–32.

Ching, T. Y. C., Dillon, H., Hou, S., Zhang, V., Day, J., Crowe, K., . . . Thomson, J. (Early online). A randomised controlled comparison of NAL and DSL prescriptions for young children: Hearing aid characteristics and performance outcomes at 3 years of age. *International Journal of Audiology*.

Ching, T. Y. C., Dillon, H., Katsch, R., & Byrne, D. (2001). Maximizing effective audibility in hearing aid fitting. *Ear and Hearing, 22*(3), 212–224.

Ching, T. Y. C., Dillon, H., Marnane, V., Hou, S., Day, D., Seeto, M., . . . Hopkins, K. (Submitted). Outcomes of early-and-late-identified children at 3 years of age: Findings from a prospective population-based study. *Ear and Hearing*.

Ching, T. Y. C., Gardner-Berry, K., Day, J., Dillon, H., & Seeto, M. (In preparation). Outcomes of children with auditory neuropathy spectrum disorder at 3 years of age. *International Journal of Audiology*.

Ching, T. Y., & Hill, M. (2005). *Teacher's Evaluation of Aural/ Oral Performance of Children (TEACH)*. Retrieved from http://www.outcomes.nal.gov.au/ Assessments.

Ching, T. Y. C., & Hill, M. (2007). The Parents' Evaluation of Aural/Oral Performance of Children (PEACH) scale: Normative data. *Journal of the American Academy of Audiology, 18*(3), 220–235.

Ching, T. Y. C., Hill, M., Birtles, G., & Beecham, L. (1999). Clinical use of paired comparisons to evaluate hearing aid fitting of severely/profoundly hearing impaired children. *Australian and New Zealand Journal of Audiology, 21*(2), 51–63.

Ching, T. Y. C., Hill, M., & Dillon, H. (2008). Effect of variations in hearing-aid frequency response on real-life functional performance of children with severe or profound hearing loss. *International Journal of Audiology, 47*(8), 461–475.

Ching, T. Y. C., Hill, M., Van Wanrooy, E., & Agung, K. (2004). The advantages of wide-dynamic-range compression over linear amplification for children. *National Acoustic Laboratories Annual Report, 2003/2004*, 45–49.

Ching, T. Y. C., & Incerti, P. (2012). Bimodal fitting or bilateral cochlear implantation? In L. Wong & L. Hickson (Eds.), *Evidence based practice in audiologic intervention* (pp. 213–233). San Diego: Plural Publishing.

Ching, T. Y., Incerti, P., Hill, M., & van Wanrooy, E. (2006). An overview of binaural advantages for children and adults who use binaural/bimodal hearing devices. *Audiology & Neuro-Otology, 11*(Suppl. 1), 6–11.

Ching, T. Y. C., Johnson, E. E., Hou, S., Dillon, H., Zhang, V., Burns, L., . . . Flynn, C. (Submitted). A comparison of NAL and DSL prescriptive methods for paediatric hearing aid fitting: Estimates of loudness and speech intelligibility. *International Journal of Audiology*.

Ching, T. Y. C., O'Brien, A., Dillon, H., Chalupper, J., Hartley, L., Hartley, D., . . . Hain, J. (2009). Directional effects on infants and young children in real life: Implications for amplification. *Joural of*

Speech, Language, and Hearing Research, 52(5), 1241–1254.

Ching, T. Y. C., Scollie, S. D., Dillon, H., & Seewald, R. (2010). A cross-over, double-blind comparison of the NAL-NL1 and the DSL v4.1 prescriptions for children with mild to moderately severe hearing loss. *International Journal of Audiology, 49*(Suppl. 1), S4–S15 10.3109/14992020903148020.

Ching, T. Y. C., Scollie, S. D., Dillon, H., Seewald, R., Britton, L., & Steinberg, J. (2010). Prescribed real-ear and achieved real-life differences in children's hearing aids adjusted according to the NAL-NL1 and the DSL v.4.1 prescriptions. *International Journal of Audiology, 49*(Suppl. 1), S16–S25.

Ching, T. Y. C., van Wanrooy, E., & Dillon, H. (2007). Binaural-bimodal fitting or bilateral implantation for managing severe to profound deafness: A review. *Trends in Amplification, 11*(3), 161–192.

Ching, T. Y. C., van Wanrooy, E., Dillon, H., & Carter, L. (2011). Spatial release from masking in normal-hearing children and children who use hearing aids. *Journal of the Acoustical Society of America, 129*(1), 368–375.

Cole, E. B. (1992). *Listening and talking: A guide to promoting spoken language in young hearing-impaired children*. Washington, DC: Alexander Graham Bell Association for the Deaf.

Cole, E. B., & Flexer, C. (2011). *Children with hearing loss: Developing listening and talking, birth to six* (2nd ed.). San Diego, CA: Plural Publishing, Inc.

Cone-Wesson, B., & Wunderlich, J. (2003). Auditory evoked potentials from the cortex: Audiology applications. *Current Opinion on Otolaryngology and Head Neck Surgery, 11*(5), 372–377.

Chu, W. T., & Warnock, A.C.C. (2002). Detailed directivity of sound fields around human talkers (Report IRC-RR-104). *NRC Institute for Research in Construction: Research Report*. Retrieved from http://www.nrc-cnrc.gc.ca/obj/irc/doc/pubs/rr/ rr104/rr104.pdf

Colin, S., Magnan, A., Ecalle, J., & Leybaert, J. (2007). Relation between deaf children's phonological skills in kindergarten and word recognition performance in first grade. *Journal of Child Psychology and Psychiatry, and Allied Disciplines, 48*(2), 139–146.

Colletti, V., Carner, M., Miorelli, V., Guida, M., Colletti, L., & Fiorino, F. (2005). Auditory brainstem implant (ABI): New frontiers in adults and children. *Otolaryngology—Head and Neck Surgery, 133*(1), 126–138.

Colletti, V., Fiorino, F. G., Carner, M., Miorelli, V., Guida, M., & Colletti, L. (2004). Auditory brainstem implant as a salvage treatment after unsuccessful cochlear implantation. *Otology Neurotology, 25*(4), 485–496, discussion 496.

Coninx, F., Weichbold, V., Tsiakpini, L., Autrique, E., Bescond, G., Tamas, L., . . . Brachmaier, J. (2009). Validation of the LittlEARS Auditory Questionnaire in children with normal hearing. *International Journal of Pediatric Otorhinolaryngology, 73*(12), 1761–1768.

Cooper, R. P., & Aslin, R. N. (1989). The language environment of the young infant: Implications for early perceptual development. *Canadian Journal of Psychology, 43*(2), 247–265.

Coticchia, J. M., Gokhale, A., Waltonen, J., & Sumer, B. (2006). Characteristics of sensorineural hearing loss in children with inner ear anomalies. *American Journal of Otolaryngology, 27*(1), 33–38.

Crandell, C. C., & Smaldino, J. J. (2000). Classroom acoustics for children with normal hearing and with hearing impairment. *Language, Speech, and Hearing Services in Schools, 31,* 362–370.

Crandell, C. C., Smaldino, J. J., & Flexer, C. (2005). *Sound field amplification: Applications to speech perception and classroom acoustics* (2nd ed.). Clifton Park, NY: Thomson Delmar Learning.

Crockett, R., Baker, H., Uus, K., Bamford, J., & Marteau, T. M. (2005). Maternal anxiety and satisfaction following infant hearing screening: A comparison of the health visitor distraction test and newborn hearing screening. *Journal of Medical Screening, 12*(2), 78–82.

Danermark, B., Antonson, S., & Lundström, I. (2001). Social inclusion and career development—transition from upper secondary school to work or post-secondary education among hard of hearing students. *Scandinavian Audiology. Supplementum, 30*(53), 120–128.

Daya, H., Figueirido, J. C., Gordon, K. A., Twitchell, K., Gysin, C., & Papsin, B. C. (1999). The role of a graded profile analysis in determining candidacy and outcome for cochlear implantation in children. *International Journal of Pediatric Otorhinolaryngology, 49*(2), 135–142.

De Boysson-Bardies, B. (1996). *Comment la parole vient aux enfants.* Paris: Editions Odile Jacob.

DeCasper, A. J., & Fifer, W. P. (1980). Of human bonding: Humans prefer their mother's voices. *Science, 6*(208), 1174–1176.

DeCasper, A. J., & Spence, M. J. (1986). Prenatal maternal speech influences newborns' perception of speech sounds. *Infant Behavior and Development, 9*(2), 133–150.

Dehaene, S. (2009). *Reading in the brain: The new science of how we read.* New York: Penguin Books.

Deno, E. (1970). Special education as developmental capital. *Exceptional Children, 37*(3), 229–237.

Desjardins, R. (2004). *Learning for well-being: Studies using the International Adult Literacy Survey.* Stockholm, Sweden: Institute of Education, Stockholm University

Dettman, S. J., D'Costa, W. A., Dowell, R. C., Winton, E. J., Hill, K. L., & Williams, S. S. (2004). Cochlear implants for children with significant residual hearing. *Archives of Otolaryngology—Head and Neck Surgery, 130*(5), 612–618.

Dettman, S. J., Pinder, D., Briggs, R. J., Dowell, R. C., & Leigh, J. R. (2007). Communication development in children who receive the cochlear implant younger than 12 months: Risks versus benefits. *Ear and Hearing, 28*(Suppl. 1), 11S–18S.

Dillon, H., Ching, T., & Golding, M. (2008). Hearing aids for infants and children. In J. R. Madell & C. Flexer (Eds.), *Pediatric audiology: Diagnosis, technology, and management.* New York, NY: Thieme Medical Publishers.

Dillon, H., Keidser, G., Ching, T. Y. C., Flax, M., & Brewer, S. (2011). The NAL-NL2 prescription procedure. *Focus (San Francisco, CA), 40,* 1–10.

Doidge, N. (2007). *The brain that changes itself: Stories of personal triumph from the frontiers of brain science.* New York, NY: Penguin Books.

Donaldson, A. I., Heavner, K. S., & Zwolan, T. A. (2004). Measuring progress in children with autism spectrum disorder who have cochlear implants. *Archives of Otolaryngology—Head & Neck Surgery, 130*(5), 666–671.

Donegan, P. (2002). Normal vowel development. In M. J. Ball & F. E. Gibbon (Eds.), *Vowel disorders* (pp. 1–35). Woburn, MA: Butterworth-Heinemann.

Dornan, D., Hickson, L., Murdoch, B., Houston, T., & Constantinescu, G. (2010). Is auditory-verbal therapy effective for children with hearing loss? *The Volta Review, 110*(3), 361–387.

Dumon, T., Gratacap, B., Firmin, F., Vincent, R., Pialoux, R., Casse, B., & Firmin, B. (2009). Vibrant Soundbridge middle ear implant in mixed hearing loss: Indications, techniques, results. *Revue de Laryngologie—Otologie—Rhinologie, 130*(2), 75–81.

Duncan, J. (1999). Conversational skills of children with hearing loss and children with normal hearing in an integrated setting. *The Volta Review, 101*(4), 193–211.

Duncan, J., Rhoades, E. A., & Fitzpatrick, E. M. (in press). *Auditory rehabilitation for adolescents with hearing loss.* New York: Oxford University Press.

Dunn, C. D., Yost, W., Noble, W. G., Tyler, R. S., & Witt, S. A. (2006). Advantages of binaural hearing. In S. B. Waltzman & J. T. J. Roland (Eds.), *Cochlear implants* (pp. 205–221). New York: Thieme Medical Publishers.

Durieux-Smith, A., Fitzpatrick, E., & Whittingham, J. (2008). Universal newborn hearing screening: A question of evidence. *International Journal of Audiology, 47*(1), 1–10.

Easterbrooks, S. R., & Estes, E. L. (2007). *Helping deaf and hard of hearing students to use spoken language.* Thousand Oaks, CA: Cowin Press.

Edwards, L. C. (2007). Children with cochlear implants and complex needs: A review of outcome research and psychological practice. *Journal of Deaf Studies and Deaf Education, 12*(3), 258–268.

Edwards, L. C., Frost, R., & Witham, F. (2006). Developmental delay and outcomes in pediatric cochlear implantation: Implications for candidacy. *International Journal of Pediatric Otorhinolaryngology, 70*(9), 1593–1600.

Ehri, L. C., Nunes, S. R., Willows, D. M., Schuster, B. V., Yaghoub-Zadeh, Z., & Shanahan, T. (2001). Phonemic awareness instruction helps children learn to read: Evidence from the National Reading Panel's meta-analysis. *Reading Research Quarterly, 36*(3), 250–287.

Eisenberg, L. S., & Levitt, H. (1991). Paired comparison judgments for hearing aid selection in children. *Ear and Hearing, 12*(6), 417–430.

Eisenberg, L. S., Martinez, A. S., Sennaroglu, G., & Osberger, M. J. (2000). Establishing new criteria in selecting children for a cochlear implant: Performance of "platinum" hearing aid users. *Annals of Otology, Rhinology, and Laryngology, 185*(12, Suppl. 185), 30–33.

Elfenbein, J. (2000). Batteries required: Instructing families on the use of hearing instruments. In R. Seewald (Ed.), *A sound foundation through early amplification: Proceedings of an international conference* (pp. 141–149). Stafa, Switzerland: Phonak.

Erber, N. (1982). *Auditory training.* Washington, DC: A.G. Bell Association.

Erenberg, A., Lemons, J., Sia, C., Trunkel, D., & Ziring, P.; American Academy of Pediatrics. (1999). Newborn and infant hearing loss: Detection and intervention. American Academy of Pediatrics. Task Force on Newborn and Infant Hearing, 1998–1999. *Pediatrics, 103*(2), 527–530.

Eriks-Brophy, A., Durieux-Smith, A., Olds, J., Fitzpatrick, E., Duquette, C., & Whittingham, J. (2012). Communication, academic, and social skills of young adults with hearing loss. *Volta Review, 112*(1), 5–35.

Eriks-Brophy, A., Durieux-Smith, A., Olds, J., Fitzpatrick, E., Duquette, C., & Whittingham, J. (2006). Facilitators and barriers to the inclusion of orally educated children and youth with hearing loss in schools: Promoting partnerships to support inclusion. *The Volta Review, 106*(1), 53–88.

Estabrooks, W. (Ed.). (2006). *Auditory-verbal therapy and practice.* Washington, DC: Alexander Graham Bell Association for the Deaf and Hard of Hearing.

Estabrooks, W. (Ed.). (1998). *Cochlear implants for kids.* Washington, DC: Alexander Graham Bell Association for the Deaf.

Feller, R. W. (2003). Aligning school counseling, the changing workplace, and career development assumptions. *Professional School Counseling, 6,* 262–271.

Fenson, L., Dale, P. S., Reznick, J. S., Bates, E., Thal, D. J., & Pethick, S. J. (1994). Variability in early communicative development. *Monographs of the Society for Research in Child Development, 59*(5), 1–173, discussion 174–185.

Ferrand, C. T. (2007). *Speech science: An integrated approach to theory and clinical practice.* Boston, MA: Pearson Education, Allyn & Bacon.

Figueras-Costa, B., & Harris, P. (2001). Theory of mind development in deaf children: A nonverbal test of false-belief understanding. *Journal of Deaf Studies and Deaf Education, 6*(2), 92–102.

Fisher, L. I. (1985). Learning disabilities and auditory processing. In R. J. Van Hattum (Ed.), *Administration of speech-language services in the schools* (pp. 231–292). San Diego, CA: College Hill Press.

Fitzpatrick, E. (2007). Population infant hearing screening to intervention: Determinants of outcome from the parents' perspective. Doctoral thesis, University of Ottawa, Ottawa.

Fitzpatrick, E. (2010). A framework for research and practice in infant hearing. *Canadian Journal of Speech-Language Pathology and Audiology, 34*(1), 25–32.

Fitzpatrick, E., Angus, D., Durieux-Smith, A., Graham, I. D., & Coyle, D. (2008). Parents' needs following identification of childhood hearing loss. *American Journal of Audiology, 17*(1), 38–49.

Fitzpatrick, E., & Brewster, L. (2008). Pediatric cochlear implantation in Canada: Results of a survey. *Canadian Journal of Speech-Language Pathology and Audiology, 32*(1), 29–35.

Fitzpatrick, E., Coyle, D. E., Durieux-Smith, A., Graham, I. D., Angus, D. E., & Gaboury, I. (2007). Parents' preferences for services for children with hearing loss: A conjoint analysis study. *Ear and Hearing, 28*(6), 842–849.

Fitzpatrick, E., Durieux-Smith, A., Eriks-Brophy, A., Olds, J., & Gaines, R. (2007). The impact of newborn hearing screening on communication development. *Journal of Medical Screening, 14*(3), 123–131.

Fitzpatrick, E., Graham, I. D., Durieux-Smith, A., Angus, D., & Coyle, D. (2007). Parents' perspectives on the impact of the early diagnosis of childhood hearing loss. *International Journal of Audiology, 46*(2), 97–106.

Fitzpatrick, E. M. (2011a). *Defining typical development for children with hearing loss.* Paper presented at Australasian Newborn Hearing Screening Conference 2011, Perth, Australia.

Fitzpatrick, E. M. (2011b). *New challenges from newborn hearing screening: Children with mild bilateral and unilateral hearing loss.* Paper presented at the Australasian Newborn Hearing Screening Conference 2011, Perth, Australia.

Fitzpatrick, E. M. (2011c). *Newborn hearing screening: Making it work.* Paper presented at the Canadian Association of Speech-Language Pathology and Audiology Conference 2011, Montreal, Canada.

Fitzpatrick, E. M. (2011). Newborn hearing screening: Making it work. Paper presented at the Canadian Association of Speech-Language Pathology and Audiology Conference 2011, Montreal, Canada.

Fitzpatrick, E. M., Crawford, L., Ni, A., & Durieux-Smith, A. (2011). A descriptive analysis of language and speech skills in 4- to 5-yr-old children with hearing loss. *Ear and Hearing, 32*(5), 605–616.

Fitzpatrick, E. M., & Doucet, S. P. (In press). When should children be discharged from an auditory-verbal program? In W. Estabrooks (Ed.), *101 FAQs about auditory-verbal*

Fitzpatrick, E. M., Durieux-Smith, A., & Whittingham, J. (2010). Clinical practice for children with mild bilateral and unilateral hearing loss. *Ear and Hearing, 31*(3), 392–400.

Fitzpatrick, E. M., Jacques, J., & Neuss, D. (2011). Parental perspectives on decision-making and outcomes in pediatric bilateral cochlear implantation. *International Journal of Audiology, 50*(10), 679–687.

Fitzpatrick, E. M., Johnson, E., & Durieux-Smith, A. (2011). Exploring factors that affect the age of cochlear implantation in children. *International Journal of Pediatric Otorhinolaryngology, 75*(9), 1082–1087.

Fitzpatrick, E., McCrae, R., & Schramm, D. (2006). Cochlear implantation in children with residual hearing [Electronic]. *BMC Ear Nose and Throat Journal 6*(7).

Fitzpatrick, E. M., & Olds, J. (submitted manuscript). Beyond hearing: Perspectives from teachers on school functioning of children with cochlear implants.

Fitzpatrick, E. M., Olds, J., Gaboury, I., McCrae, R., Schramm, D., & Durieux-Smith, A. (2012). Comparison of outcomes in children with hearing aids and cochlear implants. *Cochlear Implants International, 13*(1), 5–15.

Fitzpatrick, E. M., & Whittingham, J. (Submitted manuscript). Mild bilateral and unilateral hearing loss in children: A 20-year view of characteristics and practices.

Fitzpatrick, E. M., Whittingham, J., & Durieux-Smith, A. (submitted manuscript). Mild bilateral and unilateral hearing loss in children: A 20-year view of characteristics and practices.

Fitzpatrick, E., Olds, J., McCrae, R., Durieux-Smith, A., Gaboury, I., & Schramm, D. (2009). Pediatric cochlear implantation: How much hearing is too much? *International Journal of Audiology, 48,* 101–107.

Fitzpatrick, E., Séguin, C., & Schramm, D. (2004). Cochlear implantation in adolescents and adults with prelinguistic deafness: Outcomes and candidacy issues. *International Congress Series, 1273,* 269–272.

Fitzgerald, J., & Shanahan, T. (2000). Reading and writing relations and their development. *Educational Psychologist, 35,* 39–50.

Flexer, C. (2004). Classroom amplification systems. In R. J. Roeser & M. P. Downs (Eds.), *Auditory disorders in school children* (pp. 284–305). New York: Thieme Medical Publishers.

Flexer, C. (1999). *Faciliating hearing and listening in young children.* San Diego, CA: Singular.

Flexer, C., & Wray, D. (1990). Post-secondary mainstreaming in a state college: Akron, Ohio. In M. Ross (Ed.), *Hearing-impaired children in the mainstream* (pp. 245–256). Parkton, MA: York Press, Inc.

Flynn, T. S., Flynn, M. C., & Gregory, M. (2005). The FM advantage in the real classroom. *Journal of Educational Audiology, 12,* 35–42.

Fortnum, H. M., Summerfield, A. Q., Marshall, D. H., Davis, A. C., & Bamford, J. M. (2001). Prevalence of permanent childhood hearing impairment in the United Kingdom and implications for universal neonatal hearing screening: Questionnaire based ascertainment study. *BMJ (Clinical Research Ed.), 323*(7312), 536–540.

Friedland, D. R., Venick, H. S., & Niparko, J. K. (2003). Choice of ear for cochlear implantation: The effect of history and residual hearing on predicted postoperative performance. *Otology Neurotology, 24*(4), 582–589.

Fryauf-Bertschy, H., Tyler, R. S., Kelsay, D. M., Gantz, B. J., & Woodworth, G. G. (1997). Cochlear implant use by prelingually deafened children: The influences of age at implant and length of device use. *Journal of Speech, Language, and Hearing Research, 40*(1), 183–199. Fucci, D. J., & Lass, N. J. (1999). *Fundamentals of speech science.* Needham Heights, MA: Allyn & Bacon.

Gallaudet Research Institute. (2003). Literacy and deaf students. Retrieved from http://www.gallaudet.edu/gallaudetresearchinstitute/publicationsandpresentations/ literacy.htm.

Gallaudet Research Institute. (2009). *Regional and national summary report of data from the 2007–2008 Annual Survey of Deaf and Hard of Hearing Children and Youth.* Washington, DC: Gallaudet University.

Galvin, K. L., Mok, M., Dowell, R. C., & Briggs, R. J. (2008). Speech detection and localization results and clinical outcomes for children receiving sequential bilateral cochlear implants before four years of age. *International Journal of Audiology, 47*(10), 636–646.

Gantz, B. J., & Turner, C. W. (2003). Combining acoustic and electrical hearing. *Laryngoscope, 113*(10), 1726–1730.

Gantz, B. J., Turner, C. W., Gfeller, K. E., & Lowder, M. W. (2005). Preservation of hearing in cochlear implant surgery: Advantages of combined electrical and acoustical speech processing. *Laryngoscope, 115*(5), 796–802.

Gardner-Berry, K., Ching, T. Y. C., & Day, J. (In preparation). Cortical evoked potentials and outcomes of children with auditory neuropathy spectrum disorders at 3 years of age. *International Journal of Audiology.*

Gear, A. (2006). *Reading power: Teaching students to think while they read.* Markham, ON: Pembrooke.

Geers, A. E. (2006). Spoken language in children with cochlear implants. In P. E. Spencer & M. Marschark (Eds.), *Advances in the spoken language development of deaf and hard-of-hearing children.* New York: Oxford University Press.

Geers, A. E., Brenner, C. A., & Tobey, E. (2010). Long-term outcomes of cochlear implantation in early childhood: Sample characteristics and data collection. *Ear and Hearing, 32,* 2S–12S.

Geers, A. E., & Hayes, H. (2011). Reading, writing, and phonological processing skills of adolescents with 10 or more years of cochlear implant experience. *Ear and Hearing, 32*(Suppl. 1), 49S–59S.

Geers, A. E., Moog, J. S., Biedenstein, J., Brenner, C., & Hayes, H. (2009). Spoken language scores of children using cochlear implants compared to hearing age-mates at school entry. *Journal of Deaf Studies and Deaf Education, 14*(3), 371–385.

Geers, A. E., Strube, M. J., Tobey, E. A., Pisoni, D. B., & Moog, J. S. (2011). Epilogue: Factors contributing to long-term outcomes of cochlear implantation in early childhood. *Ear and Hearing, 32*(Suppl. 2), 84S–92S.

Giasson, J. (2003). *La lecture, de la théorie à la pratique* (2nd ed.). Montréal, PQ: Gaétan Morin éditeur.

Gibson, W. P., & Sanli, H. (2007). Auditory neuropathy: An update. *Ear and Hearing, 28*(2, Suppl.), 102S–106S.

Gifford, R. H., Dorman, M. F., McKarns, S. A., & Spahr, A. J. (2007). Combined electric and contralateral acoustic hearing: Word and sentence recognition with bimodal hearing. *Journal of Speech, Language, and Hearing Research, 50*(4), 835–843.

Gilliver, M., Ching, T. Y. C., & Sjahalam-King, J. (Submitted). When expectation meets experience: Parents' recollections and experiences of a child with hearing impairment. *International Journal of Audiology*.

Goldberg, D. M., & Flexer, C. (2001). Auditory-verbal graduates: Outcome survey of clinical efficacy. *Journal of the American Academy of Audiology, 12*(8), 406–414.

Goldberg, D. M., & Flexer, C. (1993). Outcome survey of auditory-verbal graduates: Study of clinical efficacy. *Journal of the American Academy of Audiology, 4*(3), 189–200.

Golding, M., Pearce, W., Seymour, J., Cooper, A., Ching, T., & Dillon, H. (2007). The relationship between obligatory cortical auditory evoked potentials (CAEPs) and functional measures in young infants. *Journal of the American Academy of Audiology, 18*(2), 117–125.

Goldstein, M. (1939). *The acoustic method*. St. Louis: Laryngoscope Press.

Gomaa, N. A., Rubinstein, J. T., Lowder, M. W., Tyler, R. S., & Gantz, B. J. (2003). Residual speech perception and cochlear implant performance in postlingually deafened adults. *Ear and Hearing, 24*(6), 539–544.

Gordon, K. A., & Harrison, R. V. (2005). Hearing research forum: Changes in human central auditory development caused by deafness in early childhood. *Hearsay, 17*, 28–34.

Gordon, K. A., & Papsin, B. C. (2009). Benefits of short interimplant delays in children receiving bilateral cochlear implants. *Otology & Neurotology, 30*(3), 319–331.

Gordon, K. A., Papsin, B. C., & Harrison, R. V. (2006). An evoked potential study of the developmental time course of the auditory nerve and brainstem in children using cochlear implants. *Audiology & Neuro-Otology, 11*(1), 7–23.

Gordon, K. A., Twitchell, K. A., Papsin, B. C., & Harrison, R. V. (2001). Effect of residual hearing prior to cochlear implantation on speech perception in children. *Journal of Otolaryngology, 30*(4), 216–223.

Gordon, K. A., Valero, J., van Hoesel, R., & Papsin, B. C. (2008). Abnormal timing delays in auditory brainstem responses evoked by bilateral cochlear implant use in children. *Otology & Neurotology, 29*(2), 193–198.

Govaerts, P. J., Casselman, J., Daemers, K., De Ceulaer, G., Somers, T., & Offeciers, F. E. (1999). Audiological findings in large vestibular aqueduct syndrome. *International Journal of Pediatric Otorhinolaryngology, 51*(3), 157–164.

Graham, S., & Hebert, M. (2010). *Writing to read: Evidence for how writing can improve reading*. A Report of Carnegie Corporation of New York, New York: Alliance for Excellent Education. Retrieved from http://carnegie.org/fileadmin/Media/Publications/ WritingToRead_01.pdf.

Gravel, J. S., Fausel, N., Liskow, C., & Chobot, J. (1999). Children's speech recognition in noise using omni-directional and dual-microphone hearing aid technology. *Ear and Hearing, 20*(1), 1–11.

Griffiths, C. (Ed.). (1974). *Proceedings of the international conference on auditory techniques*. Springfield, IL: Charles C Thomas.

Gstoettner, W. K., Helbig, S., Maier, N., Kiefer, J., Radeloff, A., & Adunka, O. F. (2006). Ipsilateral electric acoustic stimulation of the auditory system: Results of long-term hearing preservation. *Audiology & Neuro-Otology, 11*(Suppl. 1), 49–56.

Guardino, C. A. (2008). Identification and placement for deaf students with multiple disabilities: Choosing the path less followed. *American Annals of the Deaf, 153*(1), 55–64.

Guidelines for Identification and Management of Infants and Young Children with Auditory Neuropathy Spectrum Disorder. (2008). Retrieved from http://www.childrenscolorado.org/pdf/Guidelines%20for%20Auditory%20Neuropathy%20-%20BDCCH.pdf.

Harmer, L. M. (1999). *Health care delivery and deaf people: Practice, problems, and recommendations for change*. New York: Oxford University Press.

Harrison, R. V. (2011). Development of the auditory system from periphery to cortex. In R. Seewald & A.-M. Tharpe (Eds.), *Comprehensive handbook of pediatric audiology*. San Diego, CA: Plural Publishing, Inc.

Harrison, R. V., Nagasawa, A., Smith, D. W., Stanton, S., & Mount, R. J. (1991). Reorganization of auditory cortex after neonatal high frequency cochlear hearing loss. *Hearing Research, 54*(1), 11–19.

Hart, B., & Risley, T. R. (1995). *Meaningful differences in the everyday experience of young American children*. Baltimore, MD: Paul H. Brookes Publishing Co.

Hart, B., & Risley, T. R. (1999). *The social world of children learning to talk*. Baltimore, MD: Paul H. Brookes Publishing Co.

Hashisaki, G. T., & Rubel, E. W. (1989). Effects of unilateral cochlea removal on anteroventral cochlear nucleus neurons in developing gerbils. *Journal of Comparative Neurology, 283*(4), 5–73.

HAT(2008). Hearing assistive technology. Retrieved from http://www.audiology.org/resources/docu mentlibrary/Documents/HATGuideline.pdf.

Hattori, H. (1993). Ear dominance for nonsense-syllable recognition ability in sensorineural hearing-impaired children: Monaural versus binaural amplification. *Journal of the American Academy of Audiology, 4*(5), 319–330.

Hawkins, D. B. (2004). Limitations and uses of the aided audiogram. *Seminars in Hearing, 25*(1), 51–62.

Hayes, H., Geers, A. E., Treiman, R., & Moog, J. S. (2009). Receptive vocabulary development in deaf children with cochlear implants: Achievement in an intensive auditory-oral educational setting. *Ear and Hearing, 30*(1), 128–135.

Hellman, S. A., Chute, P. M., Kretschmer, R. E., Nevins, M. E., Parisier, S. C., & Thurston, L. C. (1991). The development of a Children's Implant Profile. *American Annals of the Deaf, 136*(2), 77–81.

Hepper, P. G., & Shahidullah, B. S. (1994). Development of fetal hearing. *Archives of Disease in Childhood, 71*(2), F81–F87.

Hinojosa, R., & Marion, M. (1983). Histopathology of profound sensorineural deafness. *Annals of the New York Academy of Sciences, 405*, 459–484.

Hixon, T. J., Weismer, G., & Hoit, J. D. (2008). *Preclinical speech science: Anatomy, physiology, acoustics, and perception.* San Diego, CA: Plural.

Hodges, A. V., Balkany, T. J., Ruth, R. A., Lambert, P. R., Dolan-Ash, S., & Schloffman, J. J. (1997). Electrical middle ear muscle reflex: Use in cochlear implant programming. *Otolaryngology—Head and Neck Surgery, 117*(3 Pt 1), 255–261.

Hodgetts, B. (2011). Other implantable devices: Bone-anchored hearing aids. In R. Seewald & A.-M. Tharpe (Eds.), *Comprehensive handbook of pediatric audiology* (pp. 585–598). San Diego, CA: Plural Publishing, Inc.

Hoffman, J. V., Roser, N. L., & Battle, J. (1993). Reading aloud in classrooms: From the modal toward the "model." *The Reading Teacher, 46*, 49–76.

Hogan, S., Stokes, J., & Weller, I. (2010). Language outcomes for children of low-income families enrolled in auditory verbal therapy. *Deafness & Education International, 12*(4), 204–216.

Hogan, S., Stokes, J., White, C., Tyszkiewicz, E., & Woolgar, A. (2008). An evaluation of auditory verbal therapy using the rate of early language development as an outcome measure. *Deafness & Education International, 10*(3), 143–167.

Holt, R. F., & Kirk, K. I. (2005). Speech and language development in cognitively delayed children with cochlear implants. *Ear and Hearing, 26*(2), 132–148.

Hood, L. J. (1999). A review of objective methods of evaluating auditory neural pathways. *Laryngoscope, 109*(11), 1745–1748.

Hood, L. J., & Keats, B. J. B. (2011). Genetics of childhood hearing loss. In R. Seewald & A.-M. Tharpe (Eds.), *Comprehensive handbook of pediatric audiology.* San Diego, CA: Plural Publishing, Inc.

Hughes, M. L. (2006). Fundamentals of clinical ECAP measures in cochlear implant. Part 1: Use of the ECAP in speech processor programming. *Audiology Online.* Retrieved from http://www.audiologyonline.com/articles/article_detail.asp?article_id=1569.

Hughes, M. L., Brown, C. J., Abbas, P. J., Wolaver, A. A., & Gervais, J. P. (2000). Comparison of EAP thresholds with MAP levels in the nucleus 24 cochlear implant: Data from children. *Ear and Hearing, 21*(2), 164–174.

Hyde, M. (2011). Principles and methods of population screening in EDHI. In R. Seewald & A.-M. Tharpe (Eds.), *Comprehensive handbook of pediatric audiology* (pp. 283–337). San Diego, CA: Plural Publishing, Inc.

Hyde, M. L. (2005). Newborn hearing screening programs: Overview. *Journal of Otolaryngology, 34*(Suppl. 2), S70–S78.

Hyde, M., Punch, R., & Grimbeek, P. (2011). Factors predicting functional outcomes of cochlear implants in children. *Cochlear Implants International, 12*(2), 94–104.

Hyde, M., Punch, R., & Komesaroff, L. (2010). Coming to a decision about cochlear implantation: Parents making choices for their deaf children. *Journal of Deaf Studies and Deaf Education, 15*(2), 162–178 10.1093/deafed/enq004.

Ireton, H. (1992). *Child development inventories.* Minneapolis, MN: Behavior Science Systems, Inc.

Jackler, R. K., Luxford, W. M., & House, W. F. (1987). Congenital malformations of the inner ear: A classification based on embryogenesis. *Laryngoscope, 97*(3 Pt. 2, Suppl. 40), 2–14.

Johansen, I. R., Hauch, A. M., Christensen, B., & Parving, A. (2004). Longitudinal study of hearing impairment in children. *International Journal of Pediatric Otorhinolaryngology, 68*(9), 1157–1165.

Johnson, C. D., & Seaton, J. B. (2012). *Educational audiology handbook* (2nd ed.). Clifton Park, NY: Delmar Cengage Learning.

Johnson, J. L., White, K. R., Widen, J. E., Gravel, J. S., James, M., Kennalley, T., . . . Holstrum, J. (2005). A multicenter evaluation of how many infants with permanent hearing loss pass a two-stage otoacoustic emissions/automated auditory brainstem response newborn hearing screening protocol. *Pediatrics, 116*(3), 663–672.

Johnston, J. C., Durieux-Smith, A., Angus, D., O'Connor, A., & Fitzpatrick, E. (2009). Bilateral paediatric cochlear implants: A critical review. *International Journal of Audiology, 48*(9), 601–617.

Johnston, J. C., Durieux-Smith, A., O'Connor, A., Benzies, K., Fitzpatrick, E. M., & Angus, D. (2009). The development and piloting of a decision aid for parents considering sequential bilateral cochlear implantation for their child with hearing loss. *Volta Review, 109*(2-3), 121–141.

Johnston, J. C., Durieux-Smith, A., Fitzpatrick, E., O'Connor, A., Benzies, K., & Angus, D. (2008). An assessment of parents' decision-making regarding paediatric cochlear implants. *Canadian Journal of Speech-Language Pathology and Audiology, 32*(4), 169–182.

Joint Committee on Infant Hearing, American Academy of Pediatrics. (2007). *Year 2007 position statement: Principles and guidelines for early hearing detection and intervention programs. Pediatrics, 120*(4), 898–921.

Jones, E. G., & Pons, T. P. (1998). Thalamic and brainstem contributions to large-scale plasticity of primate somatosensory cortex. *Science, 282*(5391), 1121–1125.

Karchmer, M. A., & Mitchell, R. E. (2003). Demographic and achievement characteristics of deaf and hard-of-hearing students. In M. Marschark & P. Spencer (Eds.), *Oxford handbook of deaf studies, language and education* (pp. 21–37). New York: Oxford University Press.

Karchmer, M. A., & Trybus, R. J. (1977). *Who are the deaf children in "mainstream" programs? (Series R, no. 4)*. Washington, DC: Gallaudet College, Office of Demographic Studies.

Kawell, M. E., Kopun, J. G., & Stelmachowicz, P. G. (1988). Loudness discomfort levels in children. *Ear and Hearing, 9*(3), 133–136.

Keller, W. D., & Bundy, R. S. (1980). Effects of unilateral hearing loss upon educational achievement. *Child: Care, Health and Development, 6*(2), 93–100.

Kennedy, C. R., McCann, D. C., Campbell, M. J., Law, C. M., Mullee, M. A., Petrou, S., . . . Stevenson, J. (2006). Language ability after early detection of permanent childhood hearing impairment. *New England Journal of Medicine, 354*(20), 2131–2141.

Kent, R. D. (1997). *The speech sciences*. San Diego, CA: Singular.

Kiese-Himmel, C. (2002). Unilateral sensorineural hearing impairment in childhood: Analysis of 31 consecutive cases. *International Journal of Audiology, 41*(1), 57–63.

King, A. M. (2010). The national protocol for paediatric amplification in Australia. *International Journal of Audiology, 49*(Suppl. 1), S64–S69.

Kirk, K. I., Miyamoto, R. T., Lento, C. L., Ying, E., O'Neill, T., & Fears, B. (2002). Effects of age at implantation in young children. *Annals of Otology, Rhinology & Laryngology*, (Suppl. 189), 69–73.

Kishon-Rabin, L., Taitelbaum-Swead, R., Ezrati-Vinacour, R., & Hildesheimer, M. (2005). Prelexical vocalization in normal hearing and hearing-impaired infants before and after cochlear implantation and its relation to early auditory skills. *Ear and Hearing, 26*(4, Suppl.), 17S–29S.

Klee, T. M., & Davis-Dansky, E. (1986). A comparison of unilaterally hearing-impaired children and normal-hearing children on a battery of standardized language tests. *Ear and Hearing, 7*(1), 27–37.

Kluwin, T. N., & Stinson, M. S. (1993). *Deaf students in local public high schools: Background, experiences, and outcomes.* Springfield, IL: Charles C Thomas.

Knightly, L. M., Jun, S. A., Oh, J. S., & Au, T. K. (2003). Production benefits of childhood overhearing. *The Journal of the Acoustical Society of America, 114*(1), 465–474.

Korczak, P. A., Kurtzberg, D., & Stapells, D. R. (2005). Effects of sensorineural hearing loss and personal hearing aids on cortical event-related potential and behavioral measures of speech-sound processing. *Ear and Hearing, 26*(2), 165–185.

Korver, A. M. H., Konings, S., Dekker, F. W., Beers, M., Wever, C. C., Frijns, J. H. M., & Oudesluys-Murphy, A. M.; DECIBEL Collaborative Study Group. (2010). Newborn hearing screening vs. later hearing screening and developmental outcomes in children with permanent childhood hearing impairment. *JAMA, 304*(15), 1701–1708 [Journal article].

Kricos, P. (2010). Looping America: One way to improve accessibility for people with hearing loss. *Audiology Today, 22,* 38–43.

Kruger, B. (1987). An update on the external ear resonance in infants and young children. *Ear and Hearing, 8*(6), 333–336.

Kurtzberg, D. (1989). Cortical event-related potential assessment of auditory system function. *Seminars in Hearing, 10,* 252–262.

Kyle, F. E., & Harris, M. (2006). Concurrent correlates and predictors of reading and spelling achievement in deaf and hearing school children. *Journal of Deaf Studies and Deaf Education, 11*(3), 273–288.

Lam, S., Lim, S. Y. C., Ong, C. S., & Low, W. K. (2009). *Effect of age of implantation and home language on school readiness.* Paper presented at the the the 7th Asia Pacific Symposium on Cochlear Implants and Related Sciences, 2009, Singapore.

Langdon, H. W., & Wiig, E. H. (2009). Multicultural issues in test interpretation. *Seminars in Speech and Language, 30*(4), 261–278.

Laroche, C., Garcia, L. J., & Barrette, J. (2000). Perceptions by persons with hearing impairment, audiologists, and employers of the obstacles to workplace integration. *Journal of the Academy of Rehabilitative Audiology, 33,* 61–90.

Leavitt, R., & Flexer, C. (1991). Speech degradation as measured by the Rapid Speech Transmission Index (RASTI). *Ear and Hearing, 12*(2), 115–118.

Lee, L. (1974). *Developmental sentence analysis.* Evanston, IL: Northwestern University Press.

Levitt, H. (2004). Assistive listening technology: What does the future hold? *Volta Voices, 11*(1), 18–21.

Leibold, L. J., & Neff, D. L. (2011). Masking by a remote-frequency noise band in children and adults. *Ear and Hearing, 32*(5), 663–666.

Leibold, L. J., Yarnell Bonino, A., & Fleenor, L. (2007). The importance of establishing a time course for typical auditory development. In R. Seewald (Ed.), *Phonak Conference* (pp. 35–42). Chicago: Phonak.

Leigh, J., Dettman, S., Dowell, R., & Sarant, J. (2011). Evidence-based approach for making cochlear implant recommendations for infants with residual hearing. *Ear and Hearing, 32*(3), 313–322 10.1097/AUD.0b013e3182008b1c.

Leijon, A., Lindkvist, A., Ringdahl, A., & Israelsson, B. (1990). Preferred hearing aid gain in everyday use after prescriptive fitting. *Ear and Hearing, 11*(4), 299–305.

Lennenberg, E. H. (1967). *Biological foundations of language.* New York: John Wiley & Sons.

Leutje, D. M., Brackmann, D., Balkany, T. J., Maw, J., Baker, R. S., Kelsall, D., . . . Arts, A. (2002). Phase III clinical trial results with the Vibrant Soundbridge: A prospective controlled multicenter study. *Otolaryngology–Head and Neck Surgery, 126*(2), 97–107.

Lieu, J. E. C., Tye-Murray, N., Karzon, R. K., & Piccirillo, J. F. (2010). Unilateral hearing loss is associated with worse speech-language scores in children. *Pediatrics, 125*(6), e1348–e1355 10.1542/peds.2009-2448.

Ling, D. (2002). *Speech and the hearing-impaired child: Theory and practice* (2nd ed.). Washington, DC: Alexander Graham Bell Assoication for the Deaf.

Ling, D., & Ling, A. H. (1978). *Aural habilitation: The foundations of verbal learning in hearing-impaired children.* Washington, DC: Alexander Graham Bell Association of the Deaf, Inc.

Litovsky, R. Y. (2005). Speech intelligibility and spatial release from masking in young children. *Journal of the Acoustical Society of America, 117*(5), 3091–3099.

Lü, J., Huang, Z., Yang, T., Li, Y., Mei, L., Xiang, M., . . . Wu, H. (2011). Screening for delayed-onset hearing loss in preschool children who previously passed the newborn hearing screening. *International Journal of Pediatric Otorhinolaryngology, 75*(8), 1045–1049 10.1016/j.ijporl.2011.05.022.

Luckner, J. L. (2002). *Facilitating the transition of students who are deaf or hard of hearing.* Austin, TX. PRO-ED, Inc.

Luckner, J. L., Schauermann, D., & Allen, R. (1994). Learning to be a friend. *Perspectives in Education and Deafness, 12*(5), 2–7.

Luckner, J. L., Sebald, A. M., Cooney, J., Young, J., III, & Muir, S. G. (2006). An examination of the evidence-based literacy research in deaf education. *American Annals of the Deaf, 150*(5), 443–456.

Luterman, D. (2006). The emotional impact of hearing loss. In D. Luterman (Ed.), *Children with hearing loss: A family guide* (pp. 9–35). Sedona, AZ: Auricle Ink Publishers.

Luterman, D., & Kurtzer-White, E. (1999). Identifying hearing loss: Parent's needs. *American Journal of Audiology, 8,* 8–13.

Madden, C., Hilbert, L., Rutter, M., Greinwald, J., & Choo, D. (2002). Pediatric cochlear implantation in auditory neuropathy. *Otology & Neurotology, 23*(2), 163–168.

Madell, J. R. (1992). FM systems as primary amplification for children with profound hearing loss. *Ear and Hearing, 13*(2), 102–107.

Madell, J. R. (1996). FM systems: Beyond the classroom. *Hearing Journal, 30,* 44–46.

Madell, J. R. (2007). Using speech perception to maximize auditory function. *Volta Voices,* 16–20.

Madell, J. R. (2008a). Evaluation of speech perception in infants and children. In J. R. Madell & C. Flexer (Eds.), *Pediatric audiology: Diagnosis, technology, and management* (pp. 89–105). New York, NY: Thieme Medical Publishers.

Madell, J. R. (2008b). Selecting appropriate technology: Hearing aids, FM, and cochlear implants. *The Hearing Journal, 61*(11), 42–47.

Madell, J. R., & Flexer, C. (2008). *Pediatric audiology: Diagnosis, technology, and management.* New York: Thieme Medical Publishers.

Makdissi, H., & Boisclair, A. (2006). Modèle d'intervention pour l'émergence de la littératie. *Nouveaux cahiers de la recherche en éducation, 9*(2), 147–168.

Mancini, P., D'Elia, C., Bosco, E., De Seta, E., Panebianco, V., Vergari, V., & Filipo, R. (2008). Follow-up of cochlear implant use in patients who developed bacterial meningitis following cochlear implantation. *Laryngoscope, 118*(8), 1467–1471.

Marmot, M., & Wilkinson, R. (Eds.). (2006). *Social determinants of health* (2nd ed.). Oxford: Oxford University Press.

Marnane, V., & Ching, T. Y. C. (In preparation). How often do early- and late-identified children use their hearing devices: Findings from a longitudinal population study. *International Journal of Audiology.*

Marschark, M. (2007). *Raising and educating a deaf child* (2nd ed.). New York: Oxford University Press.

Marschark, M., Rhoten, C., & Fabich, M. (2007). Effects of cochlear implants on children's reading and academic achievement. *Journal of Deaf Studies and Deaf Education, 12*(3), 269–282 10.1093/deafed/enm013.

Maxwell, J., & Teplova, T. (2007). Social consequence of low language/literacy skills. *Encyclopedia of Language and Literacy Development.* Retrieved from http://literacyencyclopedia.ca/pdfs/Social_Consequence_of_Low_LanguageLiteracySkills.pdf.

Mayer, C. (2007). What really matters in the early literacy development of deaf children. *Journal of Deaf Studies and Deaf Education, 12*(4), 411–431.

McCauley, R. J. (2001). *Assessment of language disorders in children.* Mahwah, NJ: Lawrence Erlbaum Associates, Inc.

McCauley, R. J., & Swisher, L. (1984). Use and misuse of norm-referenced tests in clinical assessment: A hypothetical case. *Journal of* McCracken, W., Young, A., & Tattersall, H. (2008). Universal newborn hearing screening: Parental reflections on very early audiological management. *Ear and Hearing, 29*(1), 54–64.

McCracken, W., & Turner, O. (2012). Deaf children with complex needs: Parental experience of access to cochlear implants and ongoing support. *Deafness & Education International, 14*(1), 22–35.

McCracken, W., Young, A., & Tattersall, H. (2008). Universal newborn hearing screening: Parental reflections on very early audiological management. *Ear and Hearing, 29*(1), 54–64.

McDermott, H. (2011). Benefits of combined acoustic and electric hearing for music and pitch perception. *Seminars in Hearing, 32*(1), 103–114.

McGinnis, M. D. (2010). A support provider's goals. In E. A. Rhoades & J. Duncan (Eds.), *Auditory-verbal practice: Toward a family-centered approach* (pp. 349–377). Springfield, IL: Charles C Thomas Publisher, Ltd.

McKay, S., Gravel, J. S., & Tharpe, A. M. (2008). Amplification considerations for children with minimal or mild bilateral hearing loss and unilateral hearing loss. *Trends in Amplification, 12*(1), 43–54.

Meinzen-Derr, J., Lim, L. H. Y., Choo, D. I., Buyniski, S., & Wiley, S. (2008). Pediatric hearing impairment caregiver experience: Impact of duration of hearing loss on parental stress. *International Journal of Pediatric Otorhinolaryngology, 72*(11), 1693–1703.

Meinzen-Derr, J., Wiley, S., Grether, S., & Choo, D. I. (2011). Children with cochlear implants and developmental disabilities: A language skills study with developmentally matched hearing peers. *Research in Developmental Disabilities, 32*(2), 757–767.

Meinzen-Derr, J., Wiley, S., Grether, S., & Choo, D. I. (2010). Language performance in children with cochlear implants and additional disabilities. *Laryngoscope, 120*(2), 405–413.

Mildner, V., Sindija, B., & Zrinski, K. V. (2006). Speech perception of children with cochlear implants and children with traditional hearing aids. *Clinical Linguistics & Phonetics, 20*(2-3), 219–229.

Miller, J. F. (1981). *Assessing language production in children*. Boston, MA: Allyn & Bacon.

Miller, J. F., & Chapman, R. (2003). *Systematic Analysis of Language Transcripts (SALT)* [Computer porgram]. Madison, WI: University of Wisconsin–Madison.

Moeller, M. P., Donaghy, K. F., Beauchaine, K. L., Lewis, D. E., & Stelmachowicz, P. G. (1996). Longitudinal study of FM system use in nonacademic settings: Effects on language development. *Ear and Hearing, 17*(1), 28–41.

Moeller, M. P., Hoover, B., Peterson, B., & Stelmachowicz, P. G. (2009). Consistency of hearing aid use in infants with early-identified hearing loss. *American Journal of Audiology, 18*(1), 14–23.

Moeller, M. P., Tomblin, J. B., Yoshinaga-Itano, C., Connor, C. M., & Jerger, S. (2007). Current state of knowledge: Language and literacy of children with hearing impairment. *Ear and Hearing, 28*(6), 740–753.

Mohr, P. E., Feldman, J. J., Dunbar, J. L., McConkey-Robbins, A., Niparko, J. K., Rittenhouse, R. K., & Skinner, M. W. (2000). The societal costs of severe to profound hearing loss in the United States. *International Journal of Technology Assessment in Health Care, 16*(4), 1120–1135.

Moog, J. S., & Geers, A. E. (2003). Epilogue: Major findings, conclusions and implications for deaf education. *Ear and Hearing, 24*(Suppl. 1), 121S–125S.

Moog, J. S., Geers, A. E., Gustus, C. H., & Brenner, C. A. (2011). Psychosocial adjustment in adolescents who have used cochlear implants since preschool. *Ear and Hearing, 32*(1, Suppl), 75S–83S.

Moog, J. S., & Stein, K. K. (2008). Teaching deaf children to talk. *Contemporary Issues in Communication Science and Disorders, 35*, 133–142.

Most, T., & Zaidman-Zait, A. (2003). The needs of parents of children with cochlear implants. *Volta Review, 103*(2), 99–113.

Moodie, K. S., Sinclair, S. T., Fisk, T., & Seewald, R. (2000). Individualized hearing instrument fitting for infants. In R. Seewald (Ed.), *A Sound Foundation through Early Amplification: Proceedings of an international conference* (pp. 213–217). Stafa, Switzerland: Phonak.

Moore, B. C. (1995). *Perceptual consequences of cochlear damage*. New York: Oxford University Press Inc.

Moore, B. C., & Glasberg, B. R. (1986). A comparison of two-channel and single-channel compression hearing aids. *Audiology, 25*(4-5), 210–226.

Moucha, R., & Kilgard, M. P. (2006). Cortical plasticity and rehabilitation. *Progress in Brain Research, 157*, 111–122.

Mitchell, R., & Karchmer, M. (2004). Chasing the mythical ten percent: Parental hearing status of deaf and hard of hearing students in the United States. *Sign Language Studies, 4*, 138–163.

Morton, C. C., & Nance, W. E. (2006). Newborn hearing screening—a silent revolution. *New England Journal of Medicine, 354*(20), 2151–2164.

Most, T. (2007). Speech intelligibility, loneliness, and sense of coherence among deaf and hard-of-hearing children in individual inclusion and group inclusion. *Journal of Deaf Studies and Deaf Education, 12*(4), 495–503.

Murphy, J., & O'Donoghue, G. M. (2007). Bilateral cochlear implantation: An evidence-based medicine evaluation. *Laryngoscope, 117*(8), 1412–1418.

Nadol, J. B., Jr., Young, Y. S., & Glynn, R. J. (1989). Survival of spiral ganglion cells in profound sensorineural hearing loss: Implications for cochlear implantation. *Annals of Otology, Rhinology, and Laryngology, 98*(6), 411–416.

Nance, W. E., Lim, B. G., & Dodson, K. M. (2006). Importance of congenital cytomegalovirus infections as a cause for pre-lingual hearing loss. *Journal of Clinical Virology, 35*(2), 221–225.

National Institute for Health and Clinical Excellence. (2009). *Cochlear implants for children and adults with severe to profound deafness*. Retrieved from http://www.nice.org.uk/TA166 Nazzi, T., Berton-cini, J., & Mehler, J. (1998). Language discrimination by English-learning 5-month-olds: Effects of rhythm and familiarity. *Journal of Memory and Language, 43*, 1–19.

National Institute for Literacy. (2008). *Developing early literacy: Report of the National Early Literacy Panel.* Retrieved from http://www.pathsto literacy.org/sites/default/files/uploaded-files/NELPReport09.pdf

National Reading Panel. (2000). *Report on the National Reading Panel: Teaching children to read: An evidence-based assessment of the scientific research literature on reading and its implications for reading instruction.* Jessup, MD: National Institute for Literacy at ED Pubs.

National Workshop on Mild and Unilateral Hearing Loss. (2005). Workshop proceedings. Breckenridge, CO: Centers for Disease Control and Prevention.

Nelson, H. D., Bougatsos, C., & Nygren, P.; 2001 US Preventive Services Task Force. (2008). Universal newborn hearing screening: Systematic review to update the 2001 US Preventive Services Task Force Recommendation. *Pediatrics, 122*(1), e266–e276 10.1542/peds.2007-1422.

Nelson, P. B., & Blaeser, S. B. (2010). Classroom acoustics: What possibly could be new? *The ASHA Leader, 15*(11), 16–19.

Neuss, D., Fitzpatrick, E. M., Durieux-Smith, A., Olds, J., Moreau, K., Ufholz, L.-A., & Schramm, D. (In press.). A survey of assessment tools used by certified auditory-verbal therapists for children from birth to 3 years.

Neville, H. J., Schmidt, A., & Kutas, M. (1983). Altered visual-evoked potentials in congenitally deaf adults. *Brain Research, 266*(1), 127–132.

Nguyen, H., & Bentler, R. (2011). Optimizing FM systems: Verification of device function at fitting and follow-up preserves advantages of use. *The ASHA Leader, 16*(12), 5–6.

Nicholas, J., & Geers, A. E. (2007). Will they catch up? The role of age at cochlear implantation in the spoken language development of children with severe to profound hearing loss. *Journal of Speech, Language and Hearing Research, 50*, 1048–1062.

Nicholas, J. G., & Geers, A. E. (2006). Effects of early auditory experience on the spoken language of deaf children at 3 years of age. *Ear and Hearing, 27*(3), 286–298.

Nikolopoulos, T. P., Archbold, S. M., & Gregory, S. (2005). Young deaf children with hearing aids or cochlear implants: Early assessment package for monitoring progress. *International Journal of Pediatric Otorhinolaryngology, 69*(2), 175–186.

Nikolopoulos, T. P., Dyar, D., & Gibbin, K. P. (2004). Assessing candidate children for cochlear implantation with the Nottingham Children's Implant Profile (NChIP): The first 200 children. *Journal of Pediatric Otorhinolaryngology, 68*(2), 127–135.

Niparko, J. K., Tobey, E. A., Thal, D. J., Eisenberg, L. S., Wang, N. Y., Quittner, A. L., & Fink, N. E.; CDaCI Investigative Team. (2010). Spoken language development in children following cochlear implantation. *Journal of the American Medical Association, 303*(15), 1498–1506.

Nippold, M. (2007). *Later language development: School-age children, adolescents, and young adults* (3rd ed.). Austin, TX: Pro-Ed.

Nittrouer, S., & Chapman, C. (2009). The effects of bilateral electric and bimodal electric–acoustic stimulation on language development. *Trends in Amplification, 13*(3), 190–205.

Northern, J. L., & Downs, M. P. (2002). *Hearing in children.* Baltimore, MD: Lippincott Williams & Wilkins.

Nozza, R. J., Rossman, R. N. F., & Bond, L. C. (1991). Infant-adult differences in unmasked thresholds for the discrimination of consonant-vowel syllable pairs. *Audiology, 30*(2), 102–112.

Nyffeler, M., & Dechant, S. (2010). The impact of new technology on mobile phone use. *Hearing Review, 17*(3), 42–49.

Olds, J., Fitzpatrick, E., Schramm, D., & McLean, J. (2006). *Outcome of cochlear implantation in children with complex disabilities.* Paper presented at the 4th Widex Congress of Pediatric Audiology, Ottawa, Canada.

Olds, J., Fitzpatrick, E., Séguin, C., Moran, L., Whittingham, J., & Schramm, D. (2012). Facilitating the transition from the pediatric to adult cochlear implant setting: Perspectives of CI professionals *Cochlear Implants International, 13*, 5–15.

Olds, J., Fitzpatrick, E. M., Steacie, J., McLean, J., & Schramm, D. (2007). *Parental perspectives of outcome after cochlear implantation in children with complex disabilities.* Paper presented at the International Conference on Cochlear Implants in Children, Charlotte, NC.

Oller, D. K. (2000). *The emergence of the speech capacity.* Mahwah, NJ: Lawrence Erlbaum Associates Inc.

Oller, D. K., Eilers, R. E., Neal, A. R., & Schwartz, H. K. (1999). Precursors to speech in infancy: The prediction of speech and language disorders. *Journal of Communication Disorders, 32*(4), 223–245.

Olmstead, T., Mischook, M., & Doucet, S. P. (in press). Communication auditive-verbale en pratique à l'école. In E. M. Fitzpatrick & S. P. Doucet (Eds.). *Apprendre à écouter et à parler: La déficience auditive chez l'enfant.* Ottawa, ON: Les Presses de l'Université d'Ottawa.

Organization for Economic Co-operation and Development, Human Resources Development Canada, and Statistics Canada. (1997). Literacy skills for the knowledge society: Further results from the international adult literacy survey. Retrieved from http://abclifeliteracy.ca/adult-literacy.

Otto, S. R., Brackmann, D. E., & Hitselberger, W. E. (2004). Auditory brainstem implantation in 12- to 18-year-olds. *Archives of Otolaryngology and Head and Neck Surgery, 130*(5), 656–659.

Otto, S. R., Brackmann, D. E., Hitselberger, W. E., Shannon, R. V., & Kuchta, J. (2002). Multichannel auditory brainstem implant: Update on performance in 61 patients. *Journal of Neurosurgery, 96*(6), 1063–1071.

Ouelette-Kuntz, H. M. J., Coo, H., Lam, M., Yu, C. T., Bretenbach, M. M., Hennessey, P. E., . . . Crews, L. R. (2009). Age at diagnosis of autism spectrum disorders in four regions of Canada. *Canadian Journal of Public Health, 100*(4), 268–273.

Owens, R. E., Jr. (2012). *Language development: An introduction* (8th ed.). Upper Saddle River, NJ: Pearson.

Owens, R. O. (2008). *Language development: An introduction* (7th ed.). Boston: Allyn & Bacon Publishers.

Palmer, C., & Mormer, E. (1999). Goals and expectations of the hearing aid fitting. *Trends in Amplification, 4*(2), 61–71.

Papsin, B. C., & Gordon, K. A. (2008). Bilateral cochlear implants should be the standard for children with bilateral sensorineural deafness. *Current Opinion in Otolaryngology & Head & Neck Surgery, 16*(1), 69–74.

Paradis, J., Crago, M., Genesee, F., & Rice, M. (2003). French-English bilingual children with SLI: How do they compare with their monolingual peers? *Journal of Speech, Language, and Hearing Research, 46*(1), 113–127.

Paradise, J. L., & Bluestone, C. D. (2005). Consultation with the specialist: Tympanostomy tubes: A contemporary guide to judicious use. *Pediatrics Review, 26*(2), 61–66.

Paris, A. H., & Parish, G. S. G. (2003). Assessing narrative comprehension in young children. *Reading Research Quarterly, 38*(1), 36–76.

Paul, P. V. (1998). *Literacy and deafness: The development of reading, writing, and literate thought.* Needham Heights, MA: Allyn & Bacon.

Paul, R., & Norbury, C. F. (2012). *Language disorders from infancy through adolescence: Listening, speaking, reading, writing, and communicating* (4th ed.). St. Louis, MO: Elsevier, Inc.

Paul, P. V. (2009). *Language and deafness* (4th ed.). Sudbury, MA: Jones & Bartlett

Paul, P. V., & Whitelaw, G. M. (2011). *Hearing and deafness: An introduction for health and education professionals.* Sudbury, MA: Jones & Bartlett.

Pearce, W., Golding, M., & Dillon, H. (2007). Cortical auditory evoked potentials in the assessment of auditory neuropathy: Two case studies. *Journal of the American Academy of Audiology, 18*(5), 380–390.

Perfetti, C. A., & Sandak, R. (2000). Reading optimally builds on spoken language: Implications for deaf readers. *Journal of Deaf Studies and Deaf Education, 5*(1), 32–50.

Perkell, J. S. (2008). *Auditory feedback and speech production in cochlear implant users and speakers with typical hearing.* Paper presented at the 2008 Research Symposium of the Alexander Graham Bell Association International Convention, Milwaukee, WI.

Perreau, A. E., Tyler, R. S., Witt, S., & Dunn, C. (2007). Selection strategies for binaural and monaural cochlear implantation. *American Journal of Audiology, 16*(2), 85–93.

Peters, B. R., Litovsky, R., Parkinson, A., & Lake, J. (2007). Importance of age and postimplantation experience on speech perception measures in children with sequential bilateral cochlear implants. *Otology & Neurotology, 28*(5), 649–657.

Picard, M. (2004). Children with permanent hearing loss and associated disabilities: Revisiting current epidemiological data and causes of deafness. *The Volta Review, 104*(4), 221–236.

Pintner, R. (1918). The measurement of language ability and language progress of deaf children. *The Volta Review, 20,* 755–764.

Pipp-Siegel, S., Sedey, A. L., & Yoshinaga-Itano, C. (2002). Predictors of parental stress in mothers of young children with hearing loss. *Journal of Deaf Studies and Deaf Education, 7*(1), 1–17 10.1093/deafed/7.1.1.

Pittman, A. L., Stelmachowicz, P. G., Lewis, D. E., & Hoover, B. M. (2003). Spectral characteristics of speech at the ear: Implications for amplification in children. *Journal of Speech, Language, and Hearing Research, 46*(3), 649–657.

Pollack, D. (1977). *Educational audiology for the limited hearing infant* (4th ed.). Springfield, IL: Charles C Thomas Publisher.

Pollack, D., Goldberg, D., & Caleffe-Schenck, N. (1997). *Educational audiology for the limited-hearing infant and preschooler: An auditory-verbal program* (3rd ed.). Springfield, IL: Charles C Thomas.

Power, D., & Hyde, M. (2003). Itinerant teachers of the deaf and hard of hearing and their students in Australia: Some state comparisons. *International Journal of Disability Development and Education, 50*(4), 385–401.

Power, D., & Hyde, M. (2002). The characteristics and extent of participation of deaf and hard of hearing students in regular classes in Australian schools. *Journal of Deaf Studies and Deaf Education, 7*(4), 302–311.

Powers, S. (1996a). Inclusion is an attitude not a place: Part 1. *Journal of the British Association of the Teachers of the Deaf, 20*(2), 35–41.

Powers, S. (1996b). Inclusion is an attitude not a place: Part 2. *Journal of the British Association of the Teachers of the Deaf, 20*(3), 65–69.

Prieve, B. A., & Stevens, F. (2000). The New York State universal newborn hearing screening demonstration project: Introduction and overview. *Ear and Hearing, 21*(2), 85–91.

Punch, R., Hyde, M., & Creed, P. A. (2004). Issues in the school-to-work transition of hard of hearing adolescents. *American Annals of the Deaf, 149*(1), 28–38.

Ramsden, J. D., Papaioannou, V., Gordon, K. A., James, A. L., & Papsin, B. C. (2009). Parental and program's decision making in paediatric simultaneous bilateral cochlear implantation: Who says no and why? *International Journal of Pediatric Otorhinolaryngology, 73*(10), 1325–1328 10.1016/j.ijporl.2009.05.001.

Rance, G. (2005). Auditory neuropathy/dys-synchrony and its perceptual consequences. *Trends in Amplification, 9*(1), 1–43.

Rance, G., & Barker, E. J. (2008). Speech perception in children with auditory neuropathy/dyssynchrony managed with either hearing aids or cochlear implants. *Otology & Neurotology, 29*(2), 179–182.

Rance, G., Barker, E. J., Sarant, J. Z., & Ching, T. Y. C. (2007). Receptive language and speech production in children with auditory neuropathy/dyssynchrony type hearing loss. *Ear and Hearing, 28*(5), 694–702.

Rance, G., Beer, D. E., Cone-Wesson, B., Shepherd, R. K., Dowell, R. C., King, A. M., . . . Clark, G. M. (1999). Clinical findings for a group of infants and young children with auditory neuropathy. *Ear and Hearing, 20*(3), 238–252.

Rance, G., Cone-Wesson, B., Wunderlich, J., & Dowell, R. C. (2002). Speech perception and cortical event related potentials in children with auditory neuropathy. *Ear and Hearing, 23*(3), 239–253.

Rance, G., Roper, R., Symons, L., Moody, L. J., Poulis, C., Dourlay, M., & Kelly, T. (2005). Hearing threshold estimation in infants using auditory steady-state responses. *Journal of the American Academy of Audiology, 16*(5), 291–300.

Rance, G., & Starr, A. (2011). Auditory neuropathy/dys-synchrony type hearing loss. In R. Seewald & A.-M. Tharpe (Eds.), *Comprehensive handbook of pediatric audiology* (pp. 225–242). San Diego, CA: Plural Publishing, Inc.

Raveh, E., Buller, N., Badrana, O., & Attias, J. (2007). Auditory neuropathy: Clinical characteristics and therapeutic approach. *American Journal of Otolaryngology, 28*(5), 302–308.

Recanzone, G. H., Schreiner, C. E., & Merzenich, M. M. (1993). Plasticity in the frequency representation of primary auditory cortex following discrimination training in adult owl monkeys. *Journal of Neuroscience, 13*(1), 87–103.

Reese, E., & Cox, A. (1999). Quality of adult book reading affects children's emergent literacy. *Developmental Psychology, 35*(1), 20–28.

Rhoades, E. A. (2010). Core constructs of family therapy. In E. A. Rhoades & J. Duncan (Eds.), *Auditory-verbal practice: Toward a family-centered approach* (pp. 137–163). Springfield, IL: Charles C Thomas Publisher, Ltd.

Rhoades, E. A. (2010b). Enablement and environment. In E. A. Rhoades & J. Duncan (Eds.), *Auditory-verbal practice: Toward a family-centered approach* (pp. 81–96). Springfield, IL: Charles C Thomas.

Rhoades, E. A. (2008). Working with multicultural and multilingual families of young children with hearing loss. In J. R. Madell & C. Flexer (Eds.), *Pediatric audiology: Diagnosis, technology and management* (pp. 262–268). New York: Thieme Medical Publishers.

Rhoades, E. A., & Duncan, J. (Eds.). (2010). *Auditory-verbal practice: Toward a family-centered approach*. Springfield, IL: Charles C Thomas.

Rhoades, E. A., Price, F., & Perigoe, C. B. (2004). The changing American family & ethnically diverse children with hearing loss and multiple needs *Volta Review, 104*(4, monograph), 285–305.

Ricketts, T. A., & Galster, J. (2008). Head angle and elevation in classroom environments: Implications for amplification. *Speech, Language, and Hearing Research, 51*(2), 516–525.

Robbins, A. M., Renshaw, J. J., & Berry, S. W. (1991). Evaluating meaningful auditory integration in profoundly hearing-impaired children. *American Journal of Otology, 12*(Suppl.), 144–150.

Robbins, A. M., Svirsky, M. A., Osberger, M. J., & Pisoni, D. B. (1998). Beyond the audiogram: The role of functional assessments. In F. H. Bess (Ed.), *Children with hearing impairments: Contemporary trends* (pp. 105–124). Nashville, TN: Vanderbilt Bill Wilkerson Center Press.

Robertson, L. (Ed.). (2009). *Literacy and deafness: Literacy and spoken language*. San Diego, CA: Plural Publishing.

Rosenfeld, R. M., & Bluestone, C. D. (Eds.) (1999). *Evidence-based otitis media*. Hamilton, BC: Decker, Inc.

Ross, M. (1982). *Hard of hearing children in regular schools*. Englewood Cliffs, NJ: Prentice-Hall, Inc.

Rubinstein, J. T., Parkinson, W. S., Tyler, R. S., & Gantz, B. J. (1999). Residual speech recognition and cochlear implant performance: Effects of implantation criteria. *American Journal of Otology, 20*(4), 445–452.

Russ, S. A., Poulakis, Z., Barker, M., Wake, M., Rickards, F., Saunders, K., & Oberklaid, F. (2003). Epidemiology of congenital hearing loss in Victoria, Australia. *International Journal of Audiology, 42*(7), 385–390.

Sadato, N., Pascual-Leone, A., Grafman, J., Ibañez, V., Deiber, M. P., Dold, G., & Hallett, M. (1996). Activation of the primary visual cortex by Braille reading in blind subjects. *Nature, 380*(6574), 526–528.

Saffran, J. R., Werker, J. F., & Werner, L. A. (2006). The infant's auditory world: Hearing, speech and the beginnings of language. In R. Siegler & D. Kuhn (Eds.), *Handbook of child development* (Vol. 6, pp. 58–108). New York: Wiley.

Saint-Laurent, L., Giasson, J., Simard, C., Dionne, J. J., & Royer, É. (1995). *Programme d'intervention auprès d'élèves à risque: Une nouvelle option éducative*. Montréal: Gaetan Morin éditeur.

Sander, E. K. (1972). When are speech sounds learned? *Journal of Speech and Hearing Disorders, 37*(1), 55–63.

Schafer, E. C., Amlani, A. M., Seibold, A., & Shattuck, P. L. (2007). A meta-analytic comparison of binaural benefits between bilateral cochlear implants and bimodal stimulation. *Journal of the American Academy of Audiology, 18*(9), 760–776.

Schlessinger, H. (1992). The elusive X factor: Parental contributions to literacy. In M. Walworth, D. Moores, & T. O'Rourke (Eds.), *A free hand*. Silver Springs, MD: TJ Publishers.

Schramm, D., Fitzpatrick, E., & Séguin, C. (2002). Cochlear implantation for adolescents and adults with prelinguistic deafness. *Otology & Neurotology, 23*(5), 698–703.

Schramm, D., Fitzpatrick, E., Olds, J., & Sampson, M. (2007). *Systematic review of cochlear implants in children with multiple disabilities*. Paper presented at the 11th International Conference on Cochlear Implants in Children, Charlotte, NC.

Schum, D. J. (2010). Wireless connectivity for hearing aids. *Advance for Audiologists, 12*(2), 24–26.

Schwaber, M. K., Garraghty, P. E., & Kaas, J. H. (1993). Neuroplasticity of the adult primate auditory cortex following cochlear hearing loss. *American Journal of Otology, 14*(3), 252–258.

Scollie, S. D. (2008). Children's speech recognition scores: The Speech Intelligibility Index and proficiency factors for age and hearing level. *Ear and Hearing, 29*(4), 543–556.

Scollie, S. D., Ching, T. Y. C., Seewald, R. C., Dillon, H., Britton, L., Steinberg, J., & King, K. A. (2010a). Children's speech perception and loudness ratings when fitted with hearing aids using the DSL v.4.1 and the NAL-NL1 prescriptions. *International Journal of Audiology, 49*(Suppl. 1), S26–S34.

Scollie, S. D., Ching, T. Y. C., Seewald, R., Dillon, H., Britton, L., Steinberg, J., & Corcoran, J. (2010b). Evaluation of the NAL-NL1 and DSL v4.1 prescriptions for children: Preference in real world use. *International Journal of Audiology, 49*(Suppl. 1), S49–S63.

Scollie, S., Seewald, R., Cornelisse, L. E., Moodie, S., Bagatto, M., Laurnagaray, D., . . . Pumford, J. (2005). The Desired Sensation Level multistage input/output algorithm. *Trends in Amplification, 9*(4), 159–197.

Sedey, A. L., Carpenter, K., & Stredler-Brown, A. (2002). Unilateral hearing loss: What do we know, what should we do? Paper presented at the National Symposium on Hearing in Infants, Breckenridge, CO.

Seewald, R., Cornelisse, L. E., & Ramji, K. V. (1997). DSL v4.1 for Windows: A software implementation of the Desired Sensation Level (DSL [i/o]) method for fitting linear gain and wide-dynamic-range compression hearing instruments. Users' manual. London, Ontario: University of Western Ontario Hearing Health Care Research Unit.

Seewald, R. C., & Scollie, S. D. (2003). An approach for ensuring accuracy in pediatric hearing instrument fitting. *Trends in Amplification, 7*(1), 29–40.

Sexton, J. (2003). FM as a component of primary amplification. *Educational Audiology Review, 20*(4), 4–5.

Shanahan, T. (2006). Relations among oral language, reading, and writing development. In C. MacArthur, S. Graham & J. Fitzpgerald (Eds.), *Handbook of writing research* (pp. 171–183). New York: Guilford.

Sharma, A., Cardon, G., Henion, K., & Roland, P. (2011). Cortical maturation and behavioral outcomes in children with auditory neuropathy spectrum disorder. *International Journal of Audiology, 50*(2), 98–106.

Sharma, A., & Dorman, M. (2005). The clinical use of P1 latency as a biomarker for assessment of central auditory development in children with hearing impairment. *Audiology Today, 17*(3), 18–19.

Sharma, A., & Dorman, M. F. (2006). Central auditory development in children with cochlear implants: Clinical implications. *Advances in Oto-Rhino-Laryngology, 64,* 66–88.

Sharma, A., Dorman, M. F., & Kral, A. (2005). The influence of a sensitive period on central auditory development in children with unilateral and bilateral cochlear implants. *Hearing Research, 203*(1-2), 134–143.

Sharma, A., Dorman, M. F., & Spahr, A. J. (2002). A sensitive period for the development of the central auditory system in children with cochlear implants: Implications for age of implantation. *Ear and Hearing, 23*(6), 532–539.

Sharma, A., Dorman, M. F., Spahr, A. J., & Todd, N. W. (2002). Early cochlear implantation in children allows normal development of central auditory pathways. *The Annals of Otology, Rhinology, and Laryngology, 189*(Suppl.), 38–41.

Sharma, A. E., Martin, K., Roland, P., Bauer, P., Sweeney, M. H., Gilley, P., & Dorman, M. (2005). P1 latency as a biomarker for central auditory development in children with hearing impairment. *Journal of the American Academy of Audiology, 16*(8), 564–573.

Shaw, E. A., & Vaillancourt, M. M. (1985). Transformation of sound-pressure level from the free field to the eardrum presented in numerical form. *Journal of the Acoustical Society of America, 78*(3), 1120–1123.

Shriberg, L. D. (1993). Four new speech and prosody-voice measures for genetics research and other studies in developmental phonological disorders. *Journal of Speech and Hearing Research, 36*(1), 105–140.

Shulman, S., Besculides, M., Saltzman, A., Ireys, H., White, K. R., & Forsman, I. (2010). Evaluation of the universal newborn hearing screening and intervention program. *Pediatrics, 126*(Suppl. 1), S19–S27.

Silvern, S. (1985). Parent involvement and reading achievement: A review of reseach and implications for practice. *Childhood Education, 62*(1), 46–50.

Simser, J. (1993). Auditory-verbal intervention: Infants and toddlers. *Volta Review, 95*(3), 217–229.

Simser, J. (1999). Parents: The essential partners in the habilitation of children with hearing impairment. *Australian Journal of Education of the Deaf, 5,* 55–62.

Simser, J., & Steacie, P. (1993). A hospital clinic early intervention program. *Volta Review, 95*(5), 65–74.

Sindrey, D. (1998). *Cochlear implant auditory training guidebook.* Washington, DC: Alexander Graham Bell Association for the Deaf.

Sininger, Y. S., Grimes, A., & Christensen, E. (2010). Auditory development in early amplified children: Factors influencing auditory-based communication outcomes in children with hearing loss. *Ear and Hearing, 31*(2), 166–185.

Sininger, Y. S., & Oba, S. (2001). Patients with auditory neuropathy: Who are they and what can they hear? In Y. S. Sininger & A. Starr (Eds.), *Auditory neuropathy: New perspective on hearing disorders* (pp. 15–35). San Diego, CA: Singular, Thomson Learning.

Sjoblad, S., Harrison, M., Roush, J., & McWilliam, R. A. (2001). Parents' reactions and recommendations after diagnosis and hearing aid fitting. *American Journal of Audiology, 10*(1), 24–31.

Skarzynski, H., & Lorens, A. (2010). Electroacoustic stimulation in children. In P. Van de Heyning & A. Kleine Punte (Eds.), *Cochlear implants and hearing preservation: Advances in otorhinolaryngology* (Vol. 67, pp. 135–143). Basel: Karger. Clarion cochlear implants. *Advances in Oto-Rhino- Laryngology, 57,* 305–310.

Sloutsky, V. M., & Napolitano, A. C. (2003). Is a picture worth a thousand words? Preference for auditory modality in young children. *Child Development, 74*(3), 822–833.

Smaldino, J. J. (2011). New developments in classroom acoustics and amplification. *Audiology Today, 23*(1), 30–36.

Smaldino, J. J., & Flexer, C. (2012). *Handbook of acoustic accessibility: Best practices for listening, learning, and literacy in the classroom.* New York, NY: Thieme Medical Publishers.

Smoski, W. J., Brunt, M. A., & Tannahill, J. D. (1992). Listening characteristics of children with central auditory processing disorders. *Language, Speech, and Hearing Services in Schools, 23,* 145–152.

Snik, A. F. M., Leijendeckers, J., Hol, M., Mylanus, E. A. M., & Cremers, C. W. R. J. (2008). The bone-anchored hearing aid for children: Recent developments. *International Journal of Audiology, 47*(9), 554–559.

Snik, A. F. M., Mylanus, E. A. M., Proops, D. W., Wolfaardt, J. F., Hodgetts, W. E., Somers, T., . . . Tjellstrom, A. (2005). Consensus statements on the BAHA system: Where do we stand at present? *Annals of Otology, Rhinology, and Laryngology, 114*(12, Suppl. 195), 1–12.

Snow, C. E., Burns, M. S., & Griffin, P. (Eds.). (1998). *Preventing reading difficulties in young children.* Washington, DC: National Academy Press.

Spencer, L. J., Barker, B. A., & Tomblin, J. B. (2003). Exploring the language and literacy outcomes of pediatric cochlear implant users. *Ear and Hearing, 24*(3), 236–247.

Spencer, L. J., & Oleson, J. J. (2008). Early listening and speaking skills predict later reading proficiency in pediatric cochlear implant users. *Ear and Hearing, 29*(2), 270–280.

Spencer, P. E., & Marschark, M. (2010). *Evidence-based practice in educating deaf and hard-of-hearing students.* New York: Oxford University Press.

Spivak, L., Sokol, H., Auerbach, C., & Gershkovich, S. (2009). Newborn hearing screening follow-up: Factors affecting hearing aid fitting by 6 months of age. *American Journal of Audiology, 18*(1), 24–33.

Stacey, P. C., Fortnum, H. M., Barton, G. R., & Summerfield, A. Q. (2006). Hearing-impaired children in the United Kingdom, I: Auditory performance, communication skills, educational achievements, quality of life, and cochlear implantation. *Ear and Hearing, 27*(2), 161–186.

Stapells, D. R. (2000). Frequency-specific evoked potential audiometry in infants. In R.C. Seewald (Ed.), *A sound foundation through early amplification: Proceeedings of an international conference* (pp. 13–32). Stafa, Switzerland: Phonak AG.

Starr, A., Picton, T. W., Sininger, Y. S., Hood, L. J., & Berlin, C. I. (1996). Auditory neuropathy. *Brain, 119*(Pt. 3), 741–753.

Starr, A., Sininger, Y. S., & Pratt, H. (2000). The varieties of auditory neuropathy. *Journal of Basic and Clinical Physiology and Pharmacology, 11*(3), 215–230.

Steinberg, A. G. (2008). Understanding the need for language. *Odyssey: New Directions in Deaf Education, 9*(1), 6–9.

Stelmachowicz, P. G. (1999). Hearing aid outcome measures for children. *Journal of the American Academy of Audiology, 10*(1), 14–25, quiz 66.

Stender, T., Appleby, R., & Hallenbeck, S. (2011). V & V and its impact on user satisfaction. *Hearing Review, 18*(4), 12–21.

Stinson, M. S., & Antia, S. D. (1999). Considerations in educating deaf and hard-of-hearing students in inclusive settings. *Journal of Deaf Studies and Deaf Education, 4*(3), 163–175.

Stinson, M. S., & Liu, Y. (1999). Participation of deaf and hard-of-hearing students in classes with hearing students. *Journal of Deaf Studies and Deaf Education, 4*(3), 191–202.

Stinson, M. S., & Whitmire, K. A. (2000). Adolescents who are deaf or hard of hearing: A communication perspective on educational placement. *Topics in Language Disorders, 20*(2), 58–72.

Stoel-Gammon, C. (1987). Phonological skills of two year olds. *Language, Speech, and Hearing Services in Schools, 18,* 323–329.

Stoel-Gammon, C. (1991). Normal and disordered phonology in two year olds. *Topics in Language Disorders, 11*(4), 21–32.

Storch, S. A., & Whitehurst, G. J. (2002). Oral language and code-related precursors to reading: Evidence from a longitudinal structural model. *Developmental Psychology, 38*(6), 934–947.

Stredler-Brown, A. (2002). Developing a treatment program for children with auditory neuropathy. *Seminars in Hearing, 23*(3), 239–249.

Summerfield, A. Q., Lovett, R. E., Bellenger, H., & Batten, G. (2010). Estimates of the cost-effectiveness of pediatric bilateral cochlear implantation. *Ear and Hearing, 31*(5), 611–624 10.1097/AUD.0b013e3181de40cd.

Svirsky, M. A., Teoh, S. W., & Neuburger, H. (2004). Development of language and speech perception in congenitally, profoundly deaf children as a function of age at cochlear implantation. *Audiology & Neuro-Otology, 9*(4), 224–233.

Tait, M., De Raeve, L., & Nikolopoulos, T. P. (2007). Deaf children with cochlear implants before the age of 1 year: Comparison of preverbal communication with normally hearing children. *International Journal of Pediatric Otorhinolaryngology, 71*(10), 1605–1611.

Tait, M., Lutman, M. E., & Robinson, K. (2000). Preimplant measures of preverbal communicative behavior as predictors of cochlear implant outcomes in children. *Ear and Hearing, 21*(1), 18–24.

Tallal, P. (2004). Improving language and literacy is a matter of time. *Nature Reviews Neuroscience, 5*(9), 721–728.

Tattersall, H., & Young, A. (2006). Deaf children identified through newborn hearing screening: Parents' experiences of the diagnostic process. *Child: Care, Health and Development, 32*(1), 33–45.

Teagle, H. F. B., Roush, P. A., Woodard, J. S., Hatch, D. R., Zdanski, C. J., Buss, E., & Buchman, C. A. (2010). Cochlear implantation in children with auditory neuropathy spectrum disorder. *Ear and Hearing, 31*(3), 325–335 10.1097/AUD .0b013e3181ce693b.

Tharpe, A. M. (2008). Unilateral and mild bilateral hearing loss in children: Past and current perspectives. *Trends in Amplification, 12*(1), 7–15.

Thomas-Stonell, N. L., Oddson, B., Robertson, B., & Rosenbaum, P. L. (2010). Development of the FOCUS (Focus on the Outcomes of Communication Under Six), a communication outcome measure for preschool children. *Developmental Medicine and Child Neurology, 52*(1), 47–53.

Thompson, D. C., McPhillips, H., Davis, R. L., Lieu, T. L., Homer, C. J., & Helfand, M. (2001). Universal newborn hearing screening: Summary of evidence. *JAMA, 286*(16), 2000–2010.

Thoutenhoofd, E. D., Archbold, S. M., Gregory, S., Lutman, M. E., Nikolopoulos, T. P., & Sach, T. H. (2005). *Paediatric cochlear implantation: Evaluating outcomes.* London: Whurr Publishers Ltd.

Tieri, L., Masi, R., Ducci, M., & Marsella, P. (1988). Unilateral sensorineural hearing loss in children. *Scandinavian Audiology. Supplementum, 30,* 33–36.

Tierney, R. J., & Shanahan, T. (1991). Research on the reading-writing relationship: Interactions, transactions, and outcomes. In R. Barr, M. Kamil, P. Mosenthal & P. D. Pearson (Eds.), *Handbook of reading research 2* (pp. 246–280). New York: Longman.

Torgeson, J. K. (2000). Individual differences in response to early interventions in reading: The lingering problem of treatment resisters. *Learning Disabilities Research & Practice, 15*(1), 55–64.

Traxler, C. B. (2000). Measuring up to performance standards in reading and mathematics: Achievement of selected deaf and hard-of-hearing students in the national norming of the 9th edition Stanford Achievement Test. *Journal of Deaf Studies and Deaf Education, 5,* 337–348.

Trelease, J. (2006). *The read-aloud handbook* (6th ed.). New York: Penguin Group.

Trezek, B. J., Wang, Y., & Paul, P. V. (2010). *Reading and deafness: Theory, research, and practice.* Clifton Park, NY: Delmar Cengage Learning.

Truohy, J., Brown, J., Mercer-Moseley, C., & Walsh, L. (2005). *St. Gabriel's curriculum: A guide for professionals working with children who are hearing impaired (birth to six years).* St Gabriel's School for Hearing Impaired Children, Sydney, Australia.

Tsiakpini, L., Weichbold, V., Kuehn-Inacker, H., Coninx, F., D'Haese, P., & Almandin, S. (2004). *LittlEARS Auditory Questionnaire.* Innsbruck, Austria: MED-EL.

Tucci, D. L., & Pilkington, T. M. (2009). Medical and surgical aspects of cochlear implantation. In J. K. Niparko (Ed.), *Cochlear implants: Principles and practices* (2nd ed.) (pp. 161–186). Philidelphia, PA: Lippincott Williams & Wilkins.

Tyler, R. S., Kelsay, D. M., Teagle, H. F., Rubinstein, J. T., Gantz, B. J., & Christ, A. M. (2000). 7-year speech perception results and the effects of age, residual hearing and preimplant speech perception in prelingually deaf children using the Nucleus and Clarion cochlear implants. *Advances in Oto-Rhio-Laryngolgoy, 57,* 305–310.

Urbantschitsch, V. (1981). *Auditory training for deaf mutism and acquired deafness.* (S.R. Silverman, Trans.) Washington, DC: Alexander Graham Bell Association for the Deaf. (Original work published 1895).

Van Deun, L., van Wieringen, A., Scherf, F., Deggouj, N., Desloovere, C., Offeciers, F. E., . . . Wouters, J. (2010). Earlier intervention leads to better sound localization in children with bilateral cochlear implants. *Audiology & Neuro-Otology, 15*(1), 7–17.

Van Lierde, K. M., Vinck, B. M., Baudonck, N., De Vel, E., & Dhooge, I. (2005). Comparison of the overall intelligibility, articulation, resonance, and voice characteristics between children using cochlear implants and those using bilateral hearing aids: A pilot study. *International Journal of Audiology, 44*(8), 452–465.

Veneziano, E. (2010). Peut-on aider l'enfant à mieux raconter? Les effets de deux méthodes d'intervention: Conversation sur les causes et modèle de récit. In H. Makdissi, A. Boisclair, &

P. Sirois (Eds.), *La littératie au préscolaire: Une fenêtre ouverte vers la scolarisation* (pp. 107–144). Québec: Presses de l'Université du Québec.

Vlastarakos, P. V., Proikas, K., Papacharalampous, G., Exadaktylou, I., Mochloulis, G., & Nikolopoulos, T. P. (2010). Cochlear implantation under the first year of age—the outcomes: A critical systematic review and meta-analysis. *International Journal of Pediatric Otorhinolaryngology, 74*(2), 127–132.

von Ilberg, C. A., Baumann, U., Kiefer, J., Tillein, J., & Adunka, O. F. (2011). Electric-acoustic stimulation of the auditory system: A review of the first decade. *Audiology & Neuro-Otology, 16*(Suppl. 2), 1–30.

Voss, S. E., & Herrmann, B. S. (2005). How does the sound pressure generated by circumaural, supraaural, and insert earphones differ for adult and infant ears? *Ear and Hearing, 26*(6), 636–650.

Vouloumanos, A., Hauser, M. D., Werker, J. F., & Martin, A. (2010). The tuning of human neonates' preference for speech. *Child Development, 81*(2), 517–527.

Vouloumanos, A., & Werker, J. F. (2007). Listening to language at birth: Evidence for a bias for speech in neonates. *Developmental Science, 10*(2), 159–164.

Wagner, R. K., Torgesen, J. K., & Rashotte, C. A. (1994). Development of reading-related phonological processing abilities: New evidence of bidirectional causality from a latent variable longitudinal study. *Developmental Psychology, 30*(1), 73–87.

Wake, M., Hughes, E. K., Poulakis, Z., Collins, C., & Rickards, F. W. (2004). Outcomes of children with mild-profound congenital hearing loss at 7 to 8 years: A population study. *Ear and Hearing, 25*(1), 1–8.

Wake, M., Poulakis, Z., Hughes, E. K., Carey-Sargeant, C., & Rickards, F. W. (2005). Hearing impairment: A population study of age at diagnosis, severity, and language outcomes at 7-8 years. *Archives of Disease in Childhood, 90*(3), 238–244.

Wake, M., Tobin, S., Cone-Wesson, B., Dahl, H. H., Gillam, L., McCormick, L., . . . Williams, J. (2006). Slight/mild sensorineural hearing loss in children. *Pediatrics, 118*(5), 1842–1851.

Waltzman, S. B., Roland, J. T., Jr, & Cohen, N. L. (2002). Delayed implantation in congenitally deaf children and adults. *Otology & Neurotology, 23*(3), 333–340.

Warick, R. (1994). A profile of Canadian hard-of-hearing youth. *Canadian Journal of Speech-Language Pathology and Audiology, 18,* 253–259.

Watkin, P. M., & Baldwin, M. (2011). Identifying deafness in early childhood: Requirements after the newborn hearing screen. *Archives of Disease in Childhood, 96*(1), 62–66.

Weichbold, V., Tsiakpini, L., Coninx, F., & D'Haese, P. (2005). Development of a parent questionnaire for assessment of auditory behavior of infants up to two years of age. *Laryngo-Rhino-Otologie, 84*(5), 328–334 10.1055/s-2004-825232.

Werker, J. F., & McLeod, P. J. (1989). Infant preference for both male and female infant-directed talk: A developmental study of attentional and affective responsiveness. *Canadian Journal of Psychology, 43*(2), 230–246.

Werker, J. F., & Tees, R. C. (2005). Speech perception as a window for understanding plasticity and commitment in language systems of the brain. *Developmental Psychobiology, 46*(3), 233–251.

Werker, J. F., & Yeung, H. H. (2005). Speech perception bootstraps word learning in infancy. *Trends in Cognitive Sciences, 9*(11), 519–527.

Werner, L. A. (2002). Infant auditory capabilities. *Current Opinion in Otolaryngology & Head & Neck Surgery, 10*(5), 398–402.

Werner, L. A. (2007). What do children hear? How auditory maturation affects speech perception. *ASHA Leader, 12*(6–7), 32–33.

Whitehurst, G. J., Crone, D. A., Zevenbergen, A. A., Schultz, M. D., Velting, O. N., & Fishel, J. E. (1999). Outcomes of an emergent literacy intervention from Head Start through second grade. *Journal of Educational Psychology, 91,* 261–272.

Whitehurst, G. J., & Lonigan, C. J. (1998). Child development and emergent literacy. *Child Development, 69*(3), 848–872.

Wiley, S., Jahnke, M., Meinzen-Derr, J., & Choo, D. (2005). Perceived qualitative benefits of cochlear implants in children with multi-handicaps. *International Journal of Pediatric Otorhinolaryngology, 69*(6), 791–798.

Wiley, S., & Meinzen-Derr, J. (2009). Access to cochlear implant candidacy evaluations: Who is not making it to the team evaluations? *International Journal of Audiology, 48*(2), 74–79.

Wiley, S., Meinzen-Derr, J., & Choo, D. (2008). Auditory skills development among children with developmental delays and cochlear implants. *Annals of Otology, Rhinology, and Laryngology, 117*(10), 711–718.

Wilkes, E. (2003). *Cottage Acquisition Scales for Listening, Language and Speech (CASLLS)*. San Antonio: TX: Sunshine Cottage.

Williams, C. (2004). Emergent literacy of deaf children. *Journal of Deaf Studies and Deaf Education, 9*(4), 352–365.

Wilson, B. S., & Dorman, M. F. (2008). Cochlear implants: Current designs and future possibilities. *Journal of Rehabilitation Research and Development, 45*(5), 695–730.

Wilson, B. S., & Dorman, M. F. (2009). The design of cochlear implants. In J. K. Niparko (Ed.), *Cochlear implants: Principles and practices* (2nd ed.) (pp. 95–135). Philadelphia, PA: Lippincott Williams & Wilkins.

Wong, S. H. W., Gibson, W. P. R., & Sanli, H. (1997). Use of transtympanic round window electrocochleography for threshold estimations in children. *American Journal of Otolaryngology, 18*(5), 632–636.

World Health Organization. (2001). *International classification of functioning, disability and health: ICF.* Geneva: WHO.

Wright, B. A., & Zhang, Y. (2006). A review of learning with normal and altered sound-localization cues in human adults. *International Journal of Audiology, 45*(Suppl. 1), S92–S98.

Xu, Y. (2007). Empowering culturally diverse families of children with disabilities: The double ABCX model. *Early Childhood Education Journal, 34*(6), 431–437.

Yoshinaga-Itano, C. (2003). From screening to early identification and intervention: Discovering predictors to successful outcomes for children with significant hearing loss. *Journal of Deaf Studies and Deaf Education, 8*(1), 11–30.

Yoshinaga-Itano, C., Sedey, A. L., Coulter, D. K., & Mehl, A. L. (1998). Language of early- and later-identified children with hearing loss. *Pediatrics, 102*(5), 1161–1171.

Young, A., & Tattersall, H. (2005). Parents' of deaf children evaluative accounts of the process and practice of universal newborn hearing screening. *Journal of Deaf Studies and Deaf Education, 10*(2), 134–145.

Young, A., & Tattersall, H. (2007). Universal newborn hearing screening and early identification of deafness: Parents' responses to knowing early and their expectations of child communication development. *Journal of Deaf Studies and Deaf Education, 12*(2), 209–220.

Zeitler, D. M., Kessler, M. A., Terushkin, V., Roland, T. J., Jr, Svirsky, M. A., Lalwani, A. K., & Waltzman, S. B. (2008). Speech perception benefits of sequential bilateral cochlear implantation in children and adults: A retrospective analysis. *Otology & Neurotology, 29*(3), 314–325.

Zimmerman-Phillips, S., Robbins, A. M., & Osberger, M. J. (2000). Assessing cochlear implant benefit in very young children. *Annals of Otology, Rhinology, and Laryngology, 185*(Suppl.), 42–43.

Zimmerman-Phillipps, S., Osberger, M. J., & Robbins, J. M. (1998). Infant-Toddler: Meaningful Auditory Integration Scale (IT-MAIS). In W. Eastabrooks (Ed.), *Cochlear implants for kids* (pp. 379–386). Washington, DC: AG Bell Association for the Deaf.

Index

Note: Page numbers followed by *f* and *t* indicate figures and tables, respectively.